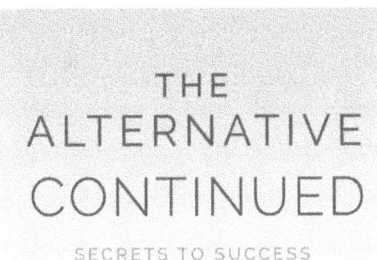

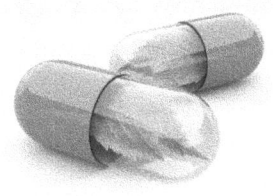

ELENA UPTON, D.Hom., Ph.D.

FREE DOWNLOAD…

To receive further information regarding remedies and protocols discussed throughout this book, download…

***THE ALTERNATIVE CONTINUED,* Secrets to Success** at the following link:

www.elenaupton.com/offer

You will receive FREE, over 150 pages of additional in-depth information that includes protocols not revealed in Volume I, as well as real cases to help to gain a better understanding of how remedies and protocols are utilized.

The combination of volumes is an invaluable resource for you and your loved ones to navigate through *first-aid* and *common conditions* quickly and easily.

THE ALTERNATIVE

YOUR FAMILY'S GUIDE TO WELLNESS

ELENA UPTON, Ph.D.

VOLUME 1

First-Aid & Common Conditions

Copyright © 2018 Elena Upton, Ph.D.

All rights reserved. No part of this book may be used or reproduced by any means, graphic, electronic, or mechanical, including photocopying, recording, taping or by any information storage retrieval system without the written permission of the author except in the case of brief quotations embodied in critical articles and reviews.

Edition: First Edition

Editor: A. Rosen

Because of the dynamic nature of the Internet, any web addresses or links contained in this book may have changed since publication and may no longer be valid.

The author of this book does not dispense medical advice or prescribe the use of any technique as a form of treatment for physical, emotional, or medical problems without the advice of a physician, either directly or indirectly. The intent of the author is to offer information of a general nature to introduce options available for your wellbeing.

If you choose to utilize information in this book for yourself, which is your constitutional right, the author assumes no responsibility for your actions.

Print ISBN: 978-0-9726417-7-7

eBook ISBN: 978-0-9726417-1-5

DEDICATION

For my sons Ryan and Jeremy who have been my greatest teachers. It has been a journey striving to find solutions for a healthy life. Now the journey continues with my grandchildren, Madelyn, Hailey, Brendan, Brady and Morgan.

CONTENTS

DISCLAIMER	xiii
ACKNOWLEDGMENTS	xv
FOREWORD	xvii
INTRODUCTION	xix

PART I
THE EVOLUTION OF HEALTH CARE

CHAPTER I

HOW DID WE GET HERE?	3
THE FLEXNER REPORT	5

CHAPTER II

EXPLORING NATURAL MEDICINE	8
HOMEOPATHY, TCM, CHIROPRACTIC MEDICINE, NATUROPATHC MEDICINE & OSTEOPATHIC MEDICINE AT A GLANCE	11
HOMEOPATHY	12
ACUPUNCTURE & CHINESE MEDICINE	19
NATUROPATHIC MEDICINE	21
CHIROPRACTIC MEDICINE	23
OSTEOPATHIC MEDICINE	26

CHAPTER III

ADVANCES UNDER THE RADAR	28
CELL SALT/TISSUE SALT CHART	31
GEMMOTHERAPY	33
PHENOLIC THERAPY	35
TRACE MINERAL THERAPY (OLIGOTHERAPY)	41
TRACE MINERAL THERAPY- 'OLIGOTHERAPY' REFERENCE CHART	42

CHAPTER IV

WHY WE GET SICK & HOW TO PREVENT IT	44

PART II
PUTTING IT ALL TOGETHER

CHAPTER V FIRST AID A-Z
CONVENTIONAL WISDOM & NATURAL RELIEF 51
  ALLERGIC REACTION (ANAPHYLACTIC SHOCK) 54
  ALTITUDE SICKNESS 56
  BITES 57
  BLEEDING 61
  BLISTERS 63
  BRUISE (CONTUSION) 64
  BURNS 65
  CARBON MONOXIDE POISONING 68
  CONCUSSION 69
  CUTS/ LACERATIONS/ WOUNDS 71
  DEHYDRATION 72
  DENTAL TRAUMA 74
  DISLOCATED JOINTS 76
  EYE INJURY 78
  FAINTING 79
  FOOD & WATER POISONING 82
  FRACTURES 84
  FRACTURES, SKULL 85
  FROSTBITE 87
  HEAD INJURIES (SEE CONCUSSION)
  HEAT EXHAUSTION (HEAT STROKE) 88
  HEAT RASH 90
  HYPERVENTILATION 91
  INSULIN SHOCK (HYPOGLYCEMIA) 94
  MARINE ANIMAL STINGS 96
  MOTION SICKNESS 98
  NOSEBLEED 99
  OPEN WOUND 101
  RIB FRACTURE 102
  SCRAPES (SEE CUTS)
  SHOCK 104

SPRAINS	106
SUNBURN	107
TEETH (SEE DENTAL TRAUMA)	
TICK BITES	108

CHAPTER VI COMMON CONDITIONS A-Z

CONVENTIONAL WISDOM & NATURAL RELIEF   110

ACID-REFLUX	114
ACNE	121
ACNE ROSACEA	125
ALLERGIES (SEASONAL)	126
ALLERGIES (FOOD)	127
ASTHMA & HOMEOPATHY	132
ATHLETE'S FOOT	134
BED-WETTING (ENURESIS)	135
BRONCHITIS	137
CANDIDA (CANDIDIASIS)	140
CANKER SORES	145
CARPAL TUNNEL SYNDROME (CTS)	147
CAVITIES, DENTAL CARIES (SEE TOOTH DECAY)	
CHOLESTEROL	149
COLDS AND FLU	151
COLIC	156
CONSTIPATION	161
COUGH	163
DEPRESSION	167
DERMATITIS	170
DIARRHEA	174
EAR INFECTION (OTITIS MEDIA)	176
ECZEMA (SEE DERMATITIS ALSO)	180
EDEMA	182
ENURISIS (SEE BEDWETTING)	
FEVER	185
FROZEN SHOULDER	188
FUNGAL INFECTIONS (SEE CANDIDA ALSO)	190
GERD/ACID REFLUX/ HEARTBURN	191

GINGIVITIS	*196*
HAY FEVER	*197*
HEADACHES	*199*
HEARTBURN (SEE ACID-REFLUX & GERD ALSO)	*202*
HEAVY METAL TOXICITY	*204*
HEMORRHOIDS	*208*
HIATAL HERNIA	*210*
HIVES (URTICARIA)	*212*
HYPERTENSION (HIGH BLOOD PRESSURE)	*214*
HYPOGLYCEMIA (ALSO SEE INSULIN SHOCK)	*216*
IMMUNE SUPPORT	*218*
INDIGESTION (DYSPEPSIA) (SEE ACID REFLUX ALSO)	*221*
INSOMNIA	*223*
JET LAG	*226*
LARYNGITIS	*228*
LEAKY GUT SYNDROME	*231*
MASTITIS (BREAST INFECTION)	*234*
MENOPAUSE	*237*
MENSTRUAL ISSUES	*244*
MEMORY ISSUES	*249*
MORNING SICKNESS	*251*
OTITIS MEDIA (SEE EAR INFECTION)	
PAIN	*253*
PARASITES	*257*
pH BALANCE (POTENTIAL OF HYDROGEN)	*262*
PRE-MENSTRUAL SYNDROME (PMS) (SEE MENSTRUAL ISSUES)	
RESTLESS LEG SYNDROME	*265*
RINGWORM	*267*
SCABIES	*269*
SCIATICA	*271*
SINUSITIS	*274*
SLEEP ISSUES (SEE INSOMNIA)	
SORE THROAT	*278*
TENDONITIS	*280*

TONSILLITIS	*282*
TOOTHACHE (TOOTH DECAY, CAVITY)	*285*
URTICARIA (SEE HIVES)	
VARICOSE VEINS	*286*
WEIGHT LOSS	*289*
WEIGHT LOSS AND MALNUTRITION	*292*

CHAPTER VII
WHAT'S IN YOUR HOME PHARMACY?   293

NOTES   299

INDEX   307

ABOUT THE AUTHOR   322
   CONTINUING YOUR JOURNEY TO VIBRANT HEALTH...   *323*

DISCLAIMER

The material presented in this volume is for educational purposes only. It is a culmination of health practices stretching over many generations and represents doctrines rooted in a natural approach to balancing the body.

The Federal Drug Administration (FDA) requires I tell you not to rely on the information in this volume as an alternative to medical advice from your doctor or other professional healthcare providers. If you have specific questions about any medical matter you should consult your doctor or other professional healthcare provider. If you think you may be suffering from a serious medical condition you should seek immediate medical attention. You should never delay seeking medical advice, disregard medical advice, or discontinue medical treatment based of information contained in this book. The author, editor and publisher cannot make any promise regarding individual effectiveness of treatments listed. It is hoped, however, that the information is of practical use to all who read this book.

Statements made in this book have not been evaluated by the FDA.

The Author receives NO remuneration from any manufacturer or distributor of products, or types of products mentioned in this book. Product references are based entirely on research, as well as personal and professional experience.

To locate a Holistic/Integrative/Alternative medical practitioner in your area, contact the American College For Advancement In Medicine (ACAM) at 800 532-3688, www.acam.org or the International College of Integrative Medicine (ICIM) at 866 464-5226, www.icimed.com

ACKNOWLEDGMENTS

I have been fortunate for the last three decades to have worked with many passionate educators and practitioners looking to improve the path to wellness. I will always hold dear the friendship and mentorship of Dr. Stuart Craig Wagstaff (3/15/1955-9/27/2012). Craig was a remarkable Naturopath who searched the globe for innovative therapies. As my business partner in our clinic "The Holistic Resource Center", he brought knowledge, compassion and a desire to always do better. He taught me more than I could begin to recount.

Dr. H.J. Carl is a scientist with extraordinary gifts who has helped me to pull together the knowledge I have acquired over the years. His guidance has been immeasurable and daily he continues to teach me the value of all life on this planet on many levels.

I extend sincere gratitude to my friend and editor Alan Rosen. Alan has not only had the patience to consistently review my words, but his long-time experience and knowledge of natural medicine helped to contribute an educated opinion for a clear delivery of the information.

Special thanks to Drs. Prasanta Banerji and Pratip Banerji of the PBHRF in Kolkata, India who so generously allowed me to include many of the Banerji's ground-breaking discoveries on modern uses of Homeopathic remedy protocols.

To all the dedicated Holistic/Integrative/Complimentary/Alternative doctors, scientists, researchers and educators who continue…in the face of controversy, to remain committed to the "Laws of Nature."

FOREWORD

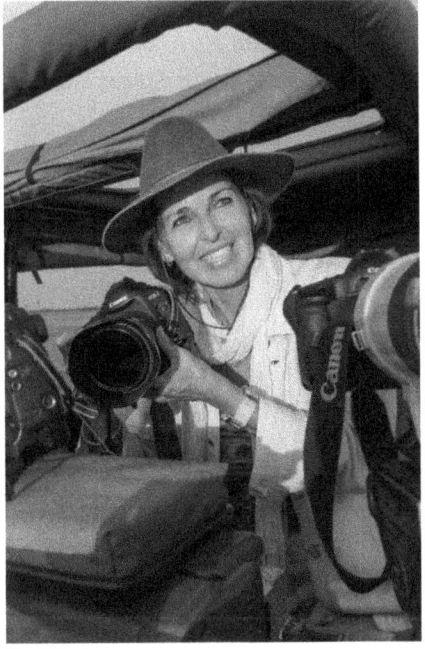

A view from the Bush…

After 32 years of bush living as filmmakers and National Geographic Explorers, my husband Dereck and I accumulated our fair share of parasites, diseases, bumps and scrapes. Our work makes our lives challenging and interesting and I would not change a thing.

When we arrived in Los Angeles to cut a film a number of years ago, I was really wrecked from life in the bush. At 41 I felt 65, largely because I was allergic to virtually everything. I was struggling to wade through the fatigue to discover exactly what it was all about.

Dereck and I gave a talk at the famous Matsuhisa restaurant in Los Angeles. Dereck was seated next to Elena who asked him what we did for our health in case of sickness and general prevention of illness in the bush. He said that I was in charge of that on our team, and that it was homeopathy. Elena's eyes lit up and said, "Well then I need to talk to Beverly."

She did and that day we started a journey together that saw my health steadily improve and my knowledge of the use of homeopathy vastly enhanced. I say it was a journey together because one of the things that Elena talks about is each person taking charge of their own situation, owning their own health. So while she was my guide, adding her knowledge and understanding from the perspective of a Homeopath, it was still my body and my investment in its future.

After some months of working with Elena I was feeling better and together we continued to chip away at the understanding of what I was reacting to and what could be done to improve my health.

Elena has a way with people, despite her knowledge she doesn't lord it over patients, but coaxes them into a better way of life. Leading to an understanding and partnership with their own bodies. She is a universal explorer in many ways since she goes into the unknown easily, exploring realms of natural medicines, not scared to make mistakes in her research to understand them. She will even reject those that she may have invested a lot of time in when the results of their teachings are not consistent.

It is an eternal quest for her to peel back layer after layer in this mission of hers. There are very few as committed to sharing the secrets to health and longevity with everyone as she is. Elena did this with me, secrets that I have lived by in Africa with lions and elephants in the untamed world. Dereck and I am now in far better health than ever before.

Beverly Joubert Johannesburg, S. Africa
February 2017

(Beverly Joubert is a National Geographic Explorer in Residence, a filmmaker and photographer with multiple awards of recognition, from Emmys to Peabodys and the World Ecology Award shared with the likes of Prince Charles, the Aga Khan, and Richard Leakey.)

INTRODUCTION

"A great deal of sickness is due to thoughtlessness, and the antidote is thoughtfulness."

-Manly P. Hall

The best person to heal you is you! That doesn't mean you need to become a doctor; it means you need to become aware. Become aware of your body, become aware of how to take care of your body, and become aware of choices when faced with a health issue needing attention.

Nearly thirty years ago I was developing health problems, as was some family members with no satisfaction from doctors. In fact, the suggestions and prescriptions usually exacerbated each situation. At about this time I was fortunate enough to be introduced to Homeopathy. I knew I needed to try something different, and the results were nothing less than spectacular.

Homeopathy cleared my son's chronic seasonal bronchitis (never to return), my husband's life-long allergies (now the cat he loved could sleep on his chest) and my health issues were much improved. From that time on I never looked back. I returned to school for a graduate degree in Homeopathy and went on to study with numerous medical doctors from around the world who had stepped outside the box of Western chemical based drug therapies and found a better way.

Tapping into this base of knowledge is easier than you might think. Whether it is a first-aid emergency, or a relatively common health condition **THE ALTERNATIVE, Your Family's Guide to Wellness**, helps you to quickly and easily find a solution, *naturally*.

Included within these pages is an opportunity to learn holistic options for your health care choices. The information is straightforward, and many conditions are presented as easy-to-read, illustrated 'cheat-sheets.'

You probably have some type of insurance, so it is logical to assume you only have one choice, your *primary care physician*, and his recommendations. If you already experienced that option with less than satisfactory results, it may be the very reason you picked up this book.

Recount the last time you or a family member needed medical care. The visit to a doctor's office probably went something like this…

- The doctor came in, listened for a couple of minutes to your complaints, then ordered testing.

- You went for the prescribed tests allowed by your insurance company, then waited for your next appointment.
- At the next appointment, the doctor looked at test results, spoke to you for a couple of minutes, then wrote a prescription. (For a more serious issue, surgery or a treatment procedure allowed by your insurance provider, may have been prescribed.)

During the entire process, you probably spent less time with the doctor making serious health decisions than you spend with your hairdresser or barber. In fact, your hair cutter probably knows more about you than your doctor.

Welcome to conventional Western medicine in the 21st Century. We seem to have arrived at a place where doctors depend on test results, rather than direct investigation of the patients themselves. The prognosis is followed by solutions that are either chemically induced or surgical in nature.

This brings me to the second reason you may be interested in this book. Are you tired of the pharmaceutical drug treadmill? The one you stepped onto and now can't get off. It started with one prescription (that did not cure your complaint), to another, then another. Soon you have far more symptoms than when you started. This may be because you've added even more chemicals to your body in this day and age of pollution and contamination at every turn.

If any of these scenarios represent your philosophy and desires, answers to your situation, or that of a loved one, lay within these pages.

If I were in an accident, I would want to be rushed to the finest medical facility to be patched up. But then I would check out as soon as possible, go home and take the natural remedies I know, through decades of experience, that will hasten my recovery.

If I needed lab testing for an acute digestive disorder after returning from a foreign land I would not hesitate; but then I would opt to take the most effective natural remedy to treat the parasitic infestation discovered.

If I fell ill after the removal of dental amalgam fillings, I would not hesitate to use modern testing methods for heavy metal poisoning; if shown to be positive I would then use a proven natural protocol for detoxification of the mercury poisoning.

These are just a few examples of ways in which alternative medicine can be easily integrated into your life. The biggest news flash about using natural based substances is that there are no known side effects (especially with the use of Homeopathic medicines). Best of all, the cost of the FDA approved remedies is far lower than that of pharmaceutical drugs and treatments.

'Modern' medicine has created a science with its own language. This science explains only what they know; it cannot explain what they don't know. Medical education entails the training of anatomy, physiology, and biochemistry. Knowing the position of internal organs, bone structure and muscles and tissues does not, however, translate to a complete understanding of how the human body works.

There is a reason plants and other living organisms have the ability to heal us. They carry an energetic signature key to all life. Our dense physical bodies that we see, feel and touch is driven by a much greater factor than blood flow and cell division. In fact, there would be no cell division without the energy to drive reproduction at every level. Also, the body innately recognizes medicines from nature. They are a match, which is why they do not produce side-effects. This in contrast to chemical compound structures that suppress, as well as confuse and complicate an already compromised body.

As you continue to read you will follow a path of connectedness of energetic-based modalities and medicines that distinguish *Alternative Medicine, Holistic Medicine, Natural Medicine* from drug based therapies and philosophies.

THE ALTERNATIVE takes you on a journey into understanding the five most well-known and accepted methods of natural/ holistic/alternative medicine available today. Beyond that, it is a manual for you to readily find holistic methods of treating hundreds of First-Aid situations, as well as many Common Conditions.

You can be in your own authority by taking control of your health and peering over the fence to a more natural way of life. If you already embrace a holistic lifestyle, you will be pleasantly surprised with the tools revealed in this book that can easily be added to your toolbox.

This resource is a litany of information gathered over nearly three decades of research into health solutions that work. Many are not freely written about since the modalities and products are reserved for practitioners. However, in this day and age of the world-wide-web, information and products not previously sold to the masses are more easily obtainable.

Absorb the information and investigate appropriate products and protocols before you dive in and self-treat, or attempt to treat others. Above all, it is important to know when to take control of your health choices and when to defer to professionals.

What brings health to the body brings peace to mind and soul. All the values of life are clarified when we decide to put ourselves in order.

To your health…**the Author**

PART I

THE EVOLUTION OF HEALTH CARE

"The natural healing force within each of us, is the greatest force in getting well."

-Hippocrates

CHAPTER I
HOW DID WE GET HERE?

To understand the scope of medical choices offered today (or lack thereof) it is important to know how we got here. Holistic medicine did not lose ground within the conventional medical community because of the advent of aspirin, penicillin and vaccines. Great advances in the world of natural medicine continues concurrently. We see this as Homeopathy continues to be the second largest system of medicine world-wide, the advent of Osteopathic medicine and Naturopathic medicine, as well as Chinese Medicine and Acupuncture spreading across continents. Alternative medicine is a multi-billion-dollar industry in America alone.

What we now refer to as 'Modern Medicine' emerged during the twentieth century. In 1901, the average life expectancy in the civilized world was 47 years. During the 20th century access to clean running water, improved nutrition and an understanding of proper hygiene by doctors who began to regularly wash their hands, contributed to the steady increase of 64% in life expectancy. This brought us to an average life expectancy of 77.

As far as health care, a new science evolved and with it an era of chemical compounds and medical testing procedures. The new science looks at the body in a different way, quantifying symptom pictures for individual organs and diseases.

The body began to be looked at less as an integrated hologram of life and more as individual unconnected parts.

During this era natural medicine struggled to survive, since attention and funding was directed to the new science. This however, has not stopped the evolution of natural methods of healing as it advances consistently around the world with new discoveries and therapies.

Researchers are beginning to predict however that life expectancy rates will begin to reverse themselves in the 21st century. Lifestyle factors leading to obesity is named as the number one cause, but there is also evidence emerging of a growing number of premature pharmaceutical drug related illnesses and deaths. There is controversy surrounding vaccines, statin drugs and the over-prescribing of opiates.

We have gone from a long history of relying on natural medicines to government-mandated health care that subscribes exclusively to chemical drugs and surgery. How did this happen? It is a curious evolution, but was it evolution or did something else occur to create the present lack of choice? It appears to be an unnatural imbalance in America, since in many countries of the world holistic medicines are readily used alongside pharmaceuticals and surgical intervention.

At the turn of the 20th century a battle was brewing in America within the medical community. A new medical science based on blood tests and the preparation of chemical compounds was gaining ground. This, along with anesthetics, made possible a new intensity for surgical procedures.

Some sixty years before, in 1844, *Homeopathic* Physicians founded the *American Institute of Homeopathy*. It was the first national medical organization in the United States and predated the American Medical Association (AMA) which was not established until 1847. Immediately on its inception the AMA began mandating rules and parameters by which *all* types of physicians should be trained.

In other words, this was the pivotal moment when the establishments' definition of "science" based empirical medicine took over as the voice of *all* health practices.

A new rating system was imposed that had many schools complaining, especially the holistic based systems like Homeopathy. Their practices did not fit the model proposed by the AMA. Further, all the eclectic groups questioned the right of this association to assert their evaluation on them. This is when the Council on Medical Education called on the *Carnegie Endowment for the Advancement of Teaching* as a presumably "objective" outside authority to lend its support and prestige to settle the matter once and for all.

THE FLEXNER REPORT

How the Face of Medicine in America Changed Forever

It was 1908 when the Carnegie Foundation commissioned Abraham Flexner (1866-1959) to study and report on the efficacy of medical schools in America. Abraham Flexner was a secondary school teacher and principal for 19 years in Louisville, Kentucky. Flexner also did some graduate work at Harvard and the University of Berlin before joining the research staff at the Carnegie Foundation for the Advancement of Teaching. He did not, however, have any education or experience in medicine.

The AMA had already completed a study in 1906 of the existing medical schools in America and had found much of the training *different* and therefore unacceptable to them. These findings had never been published. Instead, Dr. Arthur Bevan (1861-1943), head of the AMA Council on Medical Education, decided, "If we could obtain the publication and approval of our work by the Carnegie Foundation for the Advancement for Teaching, it would assist materially in securing the results we are attempting to bring out."

'The Flexner Report', as it is referred to, may have triggered much needed reforms in the standards, organization and curriculum of American medical schools, but at what cost and did it go too far? It is curious that Flexner and the AMA delivered an opinion on doctrines of medical practices of which they had no knowledge (such as Homeopathy and Chinese medicine).

The Flexner Report provided very specific recommendations for state education, medical education, licensure, public health, scientific research, public hospitals and last but not least, the *elimination of several competitors of allopathic medicine*. In other words, he described what the proper basis for medicine should be according to his views, which he established as a student at Johns Hopkins. It was clear that Flexner had a prejudice toward the medicine of his alma mater.

Flexner asserted that any discipline that did not employ drugs to help cure the patient was tantamount to 'quackery and charlatanism.' Any medical schools offering courses in bioelectric medicine, homeopathy, chiropractic, or eastern medicine were told to either drop the courses from the curriculum or loose accreditation and underwriting support.

Fast-forward a few years and it is easy to measure the repercussions Flexner's recommendations brought forth. Within a few years of the report a majority of the M.D. and D.O. (Osteopathic) granting institutions closed. Previously there were over 160 M.D. granting institutions, and by 1935 there were only 66 with 57 of these being part of a University. It is well documented that the decline in the number of medical schools was largely due to the implementation of Flexner's recommendation that all "proprietary" schools (small trade schools unaffiliated with universities) be closed and that medical schools should all be connected to Universities.

Minority medical schools felt the biggest blow. By 1914 four of the seven medical schools for "negroes" disappeared. Flexner suggested that two remain open, since there would always be a need for black physicians. He outrageously stated, "'negroes' being a potential source of infection and contagion, need their own physicians." Flexner also recommended the closing of all 3 women's medical schools, saying, "it is clear that women show a decreasing inclination to enter the profession because any strong demand for women physicians or any strong ungratified desire on the part of women to enter the profession is lacking." The three female institutions did in fact close.

The twenty-two Homeopathic colleges in 1900 became seven by 1918. This led to the decline of the 100 Homeopathic hospitals, 60 Homeopathic based orphanages and homes for the elderly and the 1,000+ Homeopathic pharmacies. By the 1930s Homeopathic education had all but ceased in America. This was at a time when the popularity of Homeopathy was quickly expanding across Europe. (Homeopathy is favored by the Royal Family of England to this day.)

Osteopathic institutions were hit particularly hard. Flexner's report concluded that their standards were in fact substantially lower. He showed outward contempt for Homeopathy, which at that time was already 100 years older than the new "science" based medicine he was proposing exclusively. He referred to Chiropractors as "unconscionable quacks!"

The findings of the Flexner Report and the ongoing evaluation of medical schools by the AMA were soon accepted by state examining boards. The benefactors of medical education such as Rockefeller, Carnegie and the US government, followed AMA recommendations and pulled funding accordingly. (It is curious that Rockefeller, who lived to age 99, traveled with a Homeopathic physician and favored the use of Homeopathic remedies.)

The other question regarding the AMA's motivation is in regards to supply and demand. Flexner's intent was also to reduce the physician supply, since he believed that far too many physicians were practicing, due to an over production of doctors.

Worldwide we see Homeopathy and other natural modalities freely practiced by medical doctors. It is unfortunate that so few Americans are aware of and continue to have difficulty accessing other forms of health care.

The turning point in medical choices in America created by the Flexner report was repeated internationally in 1948 with the creation of the World Health Organization (WHO) by the United Nations. It was created with the goal of standardizing international health policies and practices. The WHO has been responsible for any number of wonderful health achievements around the world, but again, if you review their doctrines they come up exclusively on the side of expensive pharmaceutical-based drugs and western medical practices. With this comes the continual rise in the cost of health care worldwide, since natural medical practices can be administered at a far lower cost. As a result, their budget does not stretch around the globe as easily as it could if some aspects of medical care were garnered through the use of natural medicines.

When we look at the series of events that took place a little over 100 years ago it is clear why natural medicine in America is not accessible to the masses and limited to those who can afford to pay health care costs out of their own pockets. Also, the prejudice that exists between AMA doctors and those trained within any of the natural modalities continues. This lack of cooperation makes for a prickly situation for many patients seeking to use traditional natural medicines along with conventional medicines and therapies.

If it hadn't been for the Flexner Report would natural medicine be commonly practiced in America as it is in so many parts of the world? Would it have become an integrated common practice and even part of our national health care system? We'll never know because we were not given the opportunity of choice. At this time the only choice available is your insurance mandated drug-based system, or dipping into your pocket and paying directly for natural health care, or what is now referred to as alternative medicine.

There is however, an even larger travesty heaped onto the American public robbing us of affordable, choice driven, health options. The person to blame is President Richard M. Nixon.

In 1973, Nixon met with his friend and campaign financier, Edgar Kaiser, then president and chairman of Kaiser-Permanente. Subsequent to this meeting Nixon signed into law, the <u>Health Maintenance Organization Act of 1973,</u> *in which medical insurance agencies, hospitals, clinics and even doctors, could begin functioning as* **for-profit** *business entities instead of the service organizations they were intended to be. The insurance company that received the first Federal subsidies from the implementation of HMOA73 was Kaiser-Permanente.*

Unfortunately, so many years have passed since this horrible turn of events that American society is completely unaware their medicine is not based on healing, but instead on **profit**!

As you continue to read you will ascertain the aspects of natural health care you can confidently manage for yourself and your family. *It can be liberating to transition from a system of medical management to self-directed health and wellness.*

CHAPTER II
EXPLORING NATURAL MEDICINE

The five most popular natural therapies thriving in America today are:
- Homeopathy
- Acupuncture & Traditional Chinese Medicine (TCM)
- Naturopathic Medicine
- Chiropractic Medicine
- Osteopathic Medicine

These popular therapies are based on natural laws of healing and continue to thrive today world-wide more than ever. I have experienced each of them for myself, for my family and recommended them for clients.

Alternative (Traditional) Medicine modalities all have one factor in common.

A respect for the innate nature of the body to heal itself through its own intelligence.

That intelligence is driven by its own *energy*. Health is only possible when there is complete harmony of the energies that drive the functions of the body. If those energies are ignored, distorted, corrupted or violated, then there can be no health.

Each form of holistic medicine is an approach to healing through an inborn intelligence and incorporate the natural forces that abide by the power of its *vital force*.

- Homeopathy is the use on minimal doses of plant, animal or mineral elements diluted and 'succussed' (shaken) to expand their energetic signatures, repeating the process to create additional potencies.
- Acupuncture is the use of needles inserted into specific energy points on the body to release the free-flow of natural energy patterns.
- Naturopathic Medicine uses supplements and treatments to support the bodies' natural flow of energy.

- Chiropractic Medicine adjusts the body to enable free-flow of energy.
- Some forms of Osteopathic medicine apply gentle touch to help guide the movement of energy into its proper patterns.

The major thrust of Natural Medicine is to treat the *whole person*, including their emotional state.

When a Homeopath "takes your case" he or she is listening to a description of your physical symptoms and sensations, as well as clues to your emotional state.

When the Osteopathic doctor brings his or her hands to the body to determine the sensations of energy movements there is a connection with your *emotional* patterns.

When a doctor of Chinese medicine is 'reading' your pulse he is interpreting information transmitted by your organ systems, as well as nuances from your *mental/emotional* state.

Each of the modalities is an approach…a very different approach from what we have come to know as the western medical model. Many individuals have been helped by western medicine. Emergency medical care can set bones perfectly, arrest heart failure and efficiently sew up mangled limbs. This is part of an advancement we are all fortunate to benefit from in the 21st century. However, there are methods of healing that exist within holistic medicine practices that can further assist in conventional settings to gently guide the body back to a balanced state.

In the April/May 2015 issue, *National Geographic Magazine* featured an article titled "Aztec Healing: Medicine, Magic and Prayer." The story outlines the advanced natural medicine practices of the Aztec Empire and how their good health and longevity impressed their Spanish conquerors. So much so that Fray Bernardino deSahagun, who compiled the 16th century study of Aztec life known as the "Florentine Codex" wrote, "Some (physicians) have experience of grave illnesses that Spaniards have long endured without hope, and which these doctors are able to cure."

The same still holds true today. There are many illnesses that meet with superior results with the use of holistic medicine.

Before we move on to a more in-depth description of the five modalities I want to give a shout out to **Ayurvedic Medicine**. *Ayurvedic medicine* (also called *Ayurveda*) is one of the world's oldest medical systems. It originated in India more than 3,000 years ago and widely remains the country's traditional system of health care.

Its concepts about health and disease promote the use of herbal compounds, special diets, and other unique health practices. India's government and other institutes throughout the world support clinical and laboratory research on Ayurvedic medicine, within the context of the Eastern belief system.

Key concepts of Ayurvedic medicine include:
- Universal interconnectedness (among people, their health, and the universe)
- The body's constitution *(prakriti)*
- Life forces *(dosha)*

Using these concepts, Ayurvedic physicians prescribe individualized treatments, including compounds of herbs or proprietary ingredients, as well as diet, exercise and lifestyle recommendations.

Ayurvedic medicine is not covered in this text because there are few Ayurvedic doctors in the west. However, if you live or travel abroad, do not hesitate to look into this complete ancient system of wellbeing.

The following holistic modalities survive the scrutiny of the AMA today because they are safe, efficient and ultimately cost effective.

You may be familiar with most, if not all of the following therapies. Maybe you've even experienced one or more of them. However, for those who think Homeopathy is herbs and an Osteopath is a medical doctor who specializes in bones, the following explanations into the more widely used and accepted holistic modalities will help to clear any confusion.

Each modality requires a high level of training and most requires licensure. Education, training and licensing varies from state to state.

HOMEOPATHY, TCM, CHIROPRACTIC MEDICINE, NATUROPATHC MEDICINE & OSTEOPATHIC MEDICINE AT A GLANCE

HOMEOPATHY
- Treats the whole person
- Energy Medicine derived from animal sources, plants & minerals
- In-depth case taking and observation
- Addresses mental, emotional & physical issues
- Treats the cause, does not suppress symptoms

TRADITIONAL CHINESE MEDICINE
- Treats the whole person
- Acupuncture moves energy with needles placed in meridians
- Pulse reading diagnoses the health of organs
- Addresses mental, emotional & physical issues
- Utilizes Chinese Herbs to treat cause, does not suppress symptoms

CHIROPRACTOR
- Adjusts spine in relation to imbalances
- Various techniques of gentle body manipulation
- Treats symptoms that address cause

NATUROPATHIC DOCTOR
- Treats the person as a whole
- Utilizes western medical testing as well as energetic
- Can use meds, herbs, supplements & remedies
- Treats cause, not symptoms

OSTEOPATHIC DOCTOR
Two different styles
- Uses traditional Western testing and pharmaceuticals in America

    OR:

- Treats the whole person
- Uses natural medicines
- Hands on therapy to stimulate energy balancing

HOMEOPATHY

German Wisdom Brings Forth Energetic Medicine

When I was first introduced to Homeopathy I thought I'd stepped into a land of make believe. I was visiting friends in Colorado during a ski trip with my husband and two sons. My friend Colleen was at the beginning stages of a cold. I watched her open a small case with vials that contained little white pellets. She referenced a booklet, chose one of the remedies and placed a few pellets under her tongue. She repeated the process two more times every fifteen to thirty minutes. Within a couple of hours, she was free of symptoms and the cold never materialized.

I was shocked and wanted to know everything about the little miracle she had just performed. She gave me a short explanation of Homeopathy and I never looked back. As soon as I went home to Massachusetts I started to search for any means available to learn about this amazing system of medicine that I later discovered was over two hundred years old.

I couldn't imagine why I'd never heard of Homeopathy and why no one I knew hadn't either. As I searched further I continued to be amazed that in 1987 it was the best-kept secret in America. There was no Internet to consult back then, but fortunately for me, in the 1980s Homeopathy was experiencing a resurgence in North America.

Homeopathy, from the Greek *homoeo* (meaning similar) and *pathos* (meaning suffering) is a system of medicine based on treating symptoms and conditions with substances from nature that exhibits the same symptom picture. In other words, if you have an itchy rash, a remedy for cure is a plant that creates an itchy rash on exposure. It is the introduction of an artificial disease that neutralizes the natural disease. The same principle is used with some conventional medicine, the most notable examples being the use of vaccines and anti-biotics. Homeopathy however, utilizes much smaller doses of the original substance kept pure in manufacture and not mixed with other chemical components. As a result, there are no side effects.

Homeopathy also treats the whole person based on their specific symptoms, rather than a "disease."

The manner in which a remedy is chosen is unique to Homeopathy. There are very specific dictates that sets Homeopathy apart from other systems of medicine:

- The manufacturing process is unique including numerous dilutions (creating the different potencies or strengths) and succussing (shaking) of the remedy to expand the energy of the base material.
- A very small amount of the original material remains in the end product.
- A case taking method that embraces specific observation of the patient to determine which remedy best suits the individual mentally, emotionally and physically.
- The dispensing of one remedy at a time and observing the action of the remedy before changing potency or moving on to a different remedy (this method is referred to as 'Classical' Homeopathy, and has evolved to more complex prescribing in recent years.)

An example would be the onset of a cold. There is no one specific Homeopathic "cold" remedy. The proper remedy choice would instead suit the particular symptoms exhibited by the patient, including their mental and emotional state. It would be observed whether or not there is cough that is wet or dry; is there a stuffy nose or drippy, or a combination; sore throat or respiratory issues; is the patient irritable, wanting of fresh air or are they easily chilled; are they thirsty or thirstless? It is important to note all the symptoms of the person. This observation is crucial, since the proper remedy reveals itself based on the collective of symptoms. The remedy that best fits the symptoms will also bring about a resolve to the root cause of the illness.

Example: A mom called me saying her four-year-old was complaining of an earache. She was attempting to describe his symptoms when I heard a shout out from the background, "Mommy it hurts to hear." That statement told me the correct remedy was *Pulsatilla*. She later reported that within an hour of dispensing the remedy the earache resolved, never to return.

If instead the child had said he was having sharp, splinter-like pain and on investigation there was discharge with an odor, the remedy would have been *Hepar Sulph Calcarea*.

The theory of Homeopathy was developed by Samuel Hahnemann (1755-1843) into a systematic medical science. Dr. Hahnemann was a German physician who stumbled upon the concept of substances from nature matching symptoms of illness when he was working to translate the writings of Dr. William Cullen in 1789. Dr. Cullen, one of the leading physicians of the era had written about the use of Peruvian bark (Cinchona) in treating Malaria. He reasoned that its efficacy was due to its bitter and astringent properties.

Hahnemann disputed Cullen's deduction, since there were many other plants that were bitter and astringent that did not affect the symptoms of malaria.

Hahnemann decided to take the Peruvian bark himself, repeatedly, until he came down with fever, chills and other symptoms that mimicked malaria. Hahnemann concluded that the reason Peruvian bark cured malaria was not because it was a bitter astringent, but because it caused similar symptoms (like cures like) of the disease itself. This experiment proved to be the beginning of the development of Homeopathy as a science and system of medicine.

Hahnemann tested remedies (called provings) by giving doses of various substances to both himself and healthy individuals in small quantities for days or weeks until they would manifest the set of symptoms peculiar, or specific to that substance.

Hahnemann chanced upon one of the more puzzling aspects of Homeopathy when he experienced that the more dilute a substance was, the more effective it became in treating illness. At that time in our history, the science of water molecules inherently possessing memory had not yet been proven, along with little to no understanding of the body's energetic *vital force*.

Hahnemann found over and over that the healthy subjects' proving symptoms were a milder version of the well-known poisonous symptoms of diseases, leading to the realization that "poisons" when suitably prepared and administered in sufficiently small doses, possess powerful medicinal properties.

The *proving* process, besides the concept of tiny doses, is the major difference between this system of medicine and the methods of conventional pharmaceutical medicine. The substances are not given to animals in the laboratory to produce pathological changes, nor is it first given to sick individuals to see how they react. The method of seeing the efficacy of a homeopathic medicine does not go from test tube to laboratory animals to the sick, but instead is observed by meticulously recording the changes that occur to healthy individuals when they are given the medicine. *Those changes, mental, emotional and physical, mimic the symptoms of the illness the medicine will affect.*

Whenever there is controversy in regards to Homeopathy it is in relation to the fraction of original substance left in the end product. Pharmaceutical medicines are the opposite and contain large doses of chemical substances. As a result, the benefits of feeding the body information to heal itself goes unrecognized and ignored by western science.

Sixty Minutes aired a story in March of 2015 about doctors at the Duke University Medical Center working on a cure for brain cancer using the polio virus. They were having great success injecting small doses of the virus directly into the tumors, but decided to increase the dosage. The next eleven patients died as a result of the higher dosing, at which time the researchers returned to the original lower dose treatment. An understanding of the long history of Homeopathy successfully using infinitely small doses of poisonous substances to cure may have helped to avoid the tragedy of losing the eleven lives.

Hahnemann went on to prove over one hundred Homeopathic remedies carefully documenting the complete action of each substance in his **Materia Medica Pura**, as well as producing the **Organon of the Healing Art**. This important work is a detailed account of what he saw as the rationale of Homeopathic medicine and included many aspects of how true medical care should be practiced with specific guidelines presenting a revolutionary system of medicine.

Hahnemann's mantra was, *"Restore health and annihilate the whole, the entire disease, not SUPPRESS certain symptoms."*

An important part of Hahnemann's writings referred to the *'vital force'* that he claimed exhibited itself in the method of preparing the remedies through dilution and succussion. Einstein, through his renowned equation $E=mc^2$, determined that energy and matter are dual expressions of the same universal substance. A slowly vibrating substance is referred to as physical matter, whereas the subatomic (which vibrates at or above the speed of light) is subtle matter or pure *light* energy. The life principal does not depend on matter and its compounds for existence, but only for its *manifestation*.

The *vital force* that exists within Homeopathy is a form of energy, like heat, light, electricity and magnetism. As with these forces, it can only manifest under certain well-defined conditions. They are simply *alive*, expressing the four basic fundamental principles of physical life:

- Attraction
- Repulsion
- Sensation
- Volition

They are dominated by these powers. They need no other qualities, other than chemical *composition* for them to be alive. This power of becoming alive, therefore does not reside inherently in matter, but in the vital force that dominates it. This is the basis of the principal of the energies within the remedies we know as a Homeopathic preparation.

Homeopathy works. It is the understanding of *how* it works that has alluded many, even within the realm of science. We have grown accustomed to large material doses of medicines to 'get the job done'. However, this is not without a myriad of resulting side-effects. Homeopathy, on the other hand, is very tiny doses of natural substances that are 'shaken' each time they are diluted to expand their energetic field. These diluted substances, when dispensed, deliver *information* to the body at the energetic level. This then translates to physical change.

CONSTITUTIONAL PRESCRIBING

Dr. Hahnemann developed his system of medicine by dispensing one medicine at a time. He observed changes (or lack thereof) and moved on to the next appropriate prescription. This method takes into account the person's mental, emotional and physical state. This method of dispensing remedies is referred to as 'Constitutional' or 'Classical' Homeopathy.

In other words, constitutional prescribing is based on presenting symptoms, as well as personal characteristics. Meaning, in regards to a person's temperament. An example would be a case of a person with a chronic skin condition. Two remedies that fit his symptoms are *Sulphur* and *Arsenicum album*. If his unhealthy skin symptoms coincide with a condition of excess body-heat, we know the correct choice is *Sulphur*. If on the other hand, he is a chilly person, the remedy choice would be *Arsenicum album*.

In the 230+ years since the inception of Homeopathy many medical doctors have traveled down its path, along with societal changes. As a result, Homeopathy has evolved to other methods of prescribing.

ACUTE PRESCRIBING

Acute illness such as a cold, headache or indigestion can be treated quickly and efficiently with remedies known to work for those particular issues. Much of what is written in this book is for the purpose of acute prescribing. Practitioners who follow classical prescribing may repeat the 'constitutional' remedy instead to restore balance. When searching *First Aid* or *Common Conditions* you will read a list of symptoms and when pertinent, temperament differentials are listed.

COMPLEX HOMEOPATHY

Complex Homeopathy is a description usually reserved for combination remedies. This means a number of complimentary, or similar remedies have been combined for a specific issue. Common combination remedies include teething formulas, sinus formulas, headache, or cold/flu remedies.

THE BANERJI PROTOCOLS™

The Banerji Protocols™ have been developed over the last 80 years in a clinical setting in Kolkata, India. Based on the thousands of patients that have graced their medical clinic numerous protocols have been developed for specific conditions. You will find some of them listed under Common Conditions.

DISCLAIMER

Some of the potencies included in The Banerji Protocols™ are unavailable in countries outside of India, including the US. As a result, I suggest sourcing a potency as close to the original protocol as possible. An example would be sourcing **Belladonna 6C** or **Arsenicum album 6C** if **3C** is unavailable. Dr. Pratip Banerji has stated however, that the desired effect when making a change may diminish the desired result.

POTENCY

Potency in Homeopathy is unlike milligrams in chemical drugs. Each potency represents a system of dilution. X potencies represent the Roman numeral for 10. This designates a strength of 1:10 dilution. C dilutions represent the Roman numeral for 100. This designates a strength of 1:100 for each dilution. M designates 1:1,000 and so on. This is where Homeopathy becomes very confusing, since the infinite number of dilutions at first thought can be mind-boggling. However, there is an entire body of science describing the energy of molecules that survive the dilutions that can be sourced in other texts.

Potency choice can depend on both the sensitivity of the person and the depth of illness. A general rule followed by many Homeopaths is when prescribing for chronic illnesses (i.e. those that you've had for a long time) treat with high dilution numbers and for acute prescribing (i.e. issues relatively new or first-aid), with low dilutions.

However, there are exceptions, particularly when symptoms are triggered by an accident or trauma. You might in this case dispense a higher, more powerful potency, such as *Aconitum* 200c or 1M for shock or trauma, or *Arnica* 200C for severe bruising.

Another general rule is that high potency Homeopathic medicine should be taken when there is certainty about the prescription. If not, begin with a lower potency and increase the potency if there is improvement, though incomplete or unsustained. In any given situation dispense the potency you have on hand at the time. *Choosing the correct remedy is much more critical than the dispensing of an exact potency.* For this reason I have not specified potency for most remedies. Where they are mentioned is mostly under the Banerji Protocols, since their success is largely due to specific guidelines.

Most commonly, health food stores and pharmacies carry 6x, 6c and 30c potencies. In metropolitan areas you may also find 200c potencies. Most potencies can be accessed online. (Refer to Chapter VII, "What's in Your Home Pharmacy?" for options.)

DOSAGE

In acute situations remedies can be repeated as often as every 10-15 minutes. This would include situations such as shock and trauma, excessive bleeding, severe bruising, etc.

For less dramatic issues like cough or fever repeat as often as every thirty minutes. As soon as there is a response repeat less often.

For chronic issues such as sinusitis, acne, or heartburn, remedies are usually repeated twice daily. Many chronic issues listed throughout the book call for protocols to be followed for as long as 12-13 weeks.

When in doubt seek the guidance of a professional.

LEARNING HOMEOPATHY

Since remedies are made from natural substances and dispensed in tiny doses, they have shown to be safe and effective. As a result, the practice of Homeopathy has spread to many avenues of treatment. Chiropractors commonly study Homeopathy, as well as Acupuncturists, Naturopaths and other natural health practitioners. Acute prescribing of Homeopathy has also been taught to nurse practitioners, yoga instructors, therapists and those with no prior medical training. A mom armed with Homeopathic books and remedies, having had some Homeopathic instruction can efficiently choose remedies for herself and her family.

There is nothing more rewarding than successfully dispensing a remedy in the middle of the night to a child awakened by a fever, cough or a tummy ache. Anyone with intention and determination can learn basic Homeopathic prescribing. It is what our Great Grandmothers did before we gave over our power to a complicated system of 'modern' medicine.

KNOWING WHEN TO CHOOSE HOMEOPATHY

Homeopathy provides a safe, effective, natural, nontoxic treatment for many acute and chronic illnesses. Homeopathy is safe for newborns, pregnant women, the elderly, and animals. There is also a growing base of knowledge in the use of homeopathy on plants and in agriculture. Since remedies are made from very small amounts of natural substances they are gentle, yet extremely effective when used properly.

To prescribe a homeopathic medicine specific symptoms are observed, as well as changes in mood which will lead to the correct remedy. This process may be simple or complicated, depending on the disease and/or the cooperation of the patient. A minor illness with a few well-defined symptoms can be simplistic or a complicated, chronic illness with many factors can be much more difficult. It is helpful to divide medical conditions into three different categories: first aid, acute, and chronic conditions.

The easiest way to get started is to find a qualified Homeopath in your area and make an appointment. If none exists, go to the world-wide-web and start searching. There are a number of legendary Homeopaths who do phone or Skype consultations. There are also many opportunities for Homeopathic training online.

Once you have experienced Homeopathy in this way keep going…you will know pretty quickly if this is your ticket to health. Start reading as much as you can for free online or in the library, go to health food stores and start sharing your knowledge with friends and family.

The following is a small sampling of some of the top FDA approved Homeopathic remedies. Safe for all ages, including animals, and free from side-effects.

- **ACONITUM-** shock & trauma
- **APIS-** bee stings, bug bites, rashes
- **ARSENICUM ALBUM-** food poisoning, diarrhea, vomiting
- **ARNICA-** wounds, contusions, bleeding
- **BELLADONNA-** fever, rash, irritability
- **BRYONIA-** cold/flu
- **CALC CARB-** allergies, frequent colds
- **EUPHRASIA-** eye infections
- **FERRUM PHOS-** fever, anemia
- **GELSEMIUM-** anxiety, flu
- **HEPAR SULPH-** abscesses, infection
- **HYPERICUM-** nerve damage
- **LEDUM-** puncture wounds
- **MERCURIUS-** glandular infections
- **NUX VOMICA-** overindulgence in food or drink
- **PHOSPHORUS-** fever, cough, bleeding
- **SULPHUR-** skin issues, hot flashes

ACUPUNCTURE & CHINESE MEDICINE

Traditional Medicine of the Far East

I have long been familiar with Acupuncture and Chinese Medicine and have experienced it for the successful treatment of back pain and sciatica. I became much more intimately exposed to it when my oldest son decided to study Acupuncture. A number of years later he is a skilled practitioner at the hands of this ancient art of healing. We have since found that Acupuncture and Homeopathy can be a wonderful compliment to each other.

TCM nurtures health, rather than the treating of disease. TCM, using the principles described above, is a system of diagnosis and health care that has reportedly evolved over the last 5,000 years. Chinese practices include acupuncture, herbal remedies, diet, Tui na, massage, meditation and both static and moving exercises called Qi Gong and Tai Chi. Although all these practices appear different in approach, they all share the same underlying sets of assumptions about the nature of the human body and *the importance of moving energy throughout the body.*

The first Basic Principal of Traditional Chinese Medicine (TCM) is that all dis-harmony begins with the emotions, except for the extraordinary others. These would be those things out of our control, such as being hit by a car or breaking a leg skiing, but ultimately they may still relate to our emotional state.

The second Basic Principal is Qi and blood. Blood is the Mother of Qi and Qi is the mover of blood. Qi is an *energetic response*. If there is no circulation, then there is no synapse (place where a signal passes from one nerve cell to another). The movement in the body is Qi and blood creates the Qi.

The third Basic Principal is the repolarization (restoration of the difference in charge between the inside and outside of the cell) to cells either being turned on or turned off. It is the same principal as the 0 or 1 of the binary numbers system. There is feedback created to the brain that moves the blood increasing circulation and conductivity.

These principles relate to the tracking of patterns. *TCM treats the patterns*

Meridians, or energy pathways of the body, have been mapped out and acu- points determined along them. These points and meridians are stimulated by acupuncture, the insertion of fine needles into the skin, or acupressure (massaging and pressing on these acu-points).

The needles help to unblocked energy that has become trapped, causing disturbances to the natural flow within the bodily functions.

The term 'meridian' describes the overall energy distribution system of TCM and helps with the understanding of how basic substances of the body (Qi, blood and body fluids) permeate the whole body. The individual meridians themselves are often described as 'channels' or 'vessels' that reflects the notion of carrying, holding, or transporting Qi, blood and body fluids around the body.

Practitioners of Chinese Medicine must be as knowledgeable about these meridian channels as the western doctor is about anatomy and physiology of the physical body.

Without this thorough understanding, successful acupuncture treatments would be difficult. A doctor of Chinese Medicine must know how and where to access the Qi energy of the body to facilitate the healing process.

Traditional Chinese medicine is highly respected worldwide for effectively treating both common ailments and difficult health conditions. Millions of people throughout China's long history have maintained their wellness with Chinese medicine, used either as primary or complementary care.

Traditional Chinese Medicine also uses herbal medicines. For thousands of years the Asians have utilized a very wide variety of botanicals, animal products and minerals and have developed an herbal system that is a sophisticated form of natural health maintenance.

Asian herbalism is founded on the principle that health *promotion* is fundamental to any health care program.

Chinese tonic herbs have yin and yang properties, which are thought to influence certain organs and functions in the body. Yin tonics *replenish* the body's resources, blood and essence; yang tonics *build* the body's capacity to use its resources and convert them into energy (Qi) and warmth.

There is a 'Superior Class' consisting of 120 herbs. They are the rulers. They control the maintenance of life. These herbs are not considered as medicines and can be taken in larger amounts or over a long period of time. They can be compared to the use of supplements in the western world. If one wishes to supplement the energies and nutrients circulating in the body, and to prolong the years of life without aging, they can concentrate their efforts on the herbs within the Superior Class.

NATUROPATHIC MEDICINE

A Culmination of Natural Modalities

I was fortunate to meet a wonderful Naturopath when I was completing Homeopathic graduate school. He was unique in that he had been to Germany to learn many medicines and techniques little known in the west. Dr. Craig Wagstaff (1955-2012) was from Kelowna, B.C. Canada and traveled regularly to wherever he heard there was something innovative to learn. He honed his craft into becoming a much sought after allergy specialist.

Dr. Wagstaff agreed to come and work with me in my new clinic. For the first two years I followed him around like a puppy dog absorbing as much as I could about many different aspects of Naturopathic Medicine. Chapter III talks about many of the therapies we integrated including *Phenolic Therapy*. Although I had been trained as a Classical Homeopath, using one remedy at a time, I quickly saw the value of adding other natural therapies to develop cohesive protocols. Within a short period of time the clinic gained a glowing reputation for treating patients with complicated issues.

Naturopathic medicine, sometimes referred to as *Naturopathy, is a system of primary health care focused on prevention and self-healing through the use of natural medicines and therapies.* Naturopathic doctors are referred to as NDs and are trained in a similar manner to conventional medical doctors. The difference lies in the use of natural medicines, rather than pharmaceutical drugs.

Naturopathic medicine is a collective of other holistic modalities and is derived from an outgrowth of what was called "botanical medicine" or "Eclecticism" in the nineteenth century. The preferred method of diagnosis is focused on identifying the underlying cause of disease. Many Naturopaths use specific testing devices, as well as kinesiology (muscle testing) to accomplish this.

Naturopathic medicine combines the use of clinical nutrition, Homeopathy, botanical medicine, Acupuncture and Chinese medicine, midwifery, herbalism, psychology, and even spirituality. Their scientific and empirical methodology is based on six principles as stated by Bastyr University, a Washington state Naturopathic college.

- First do no harm
- The healing power of nature
- Discover and treat the cause
- Treat the whole person
- The physician is the teacher
- Prevention is the best "cure"

Educated in all of the same basic sciences as a medical doctor (MD), a Naturopathic doctor uses the Western medical sciences as a foundation for diagnosis and treatment. Just like MDs, Naturopathic physicians must pass rigorous professional board exams before they can be licensed by a state or jurisdiction. And, for at least the final two years of the medical program, Naturopathic medical students intern in clinical settings under the close supervision of licensed professionals.

The term "naturopathy" was first coined around the turn of the 20th century to describe a rapidly growing system of natural therapeutics, originally organized in response to the increasing disillusionment of physicians and patients with toxic and ineffective methods. It was in the late 1800s, that practitioners from several medical disciplines, Homeopathy, Osteopathy, Herbal medicine, Chiropractic and Nutritional medicine were coming together to form the first Naturopathic professional societies.

Naturopathic medicine was born out of the never-ending different points of view over medicine. *The Naturopath holds true to the belief that health is the natural order of things, a positive attribute to which all are entitled if we lead a healthy lifestyle.*

Most NDs provide primary care through office-based private practice. Because NDs view natural remedies as complementary, as well as primary, many cooperate with other medical professionals, referring patients to (and receiving patients from) conventional medical doctors, surgeons and other specialists when appropriate. Some cancer clinics employ NDs as doctors on their staff.

As stated by the North Carolina Association of Naturopathic Physicians (NCANP) "Today's naturopathic physician easily blends modern, state-of- the-art diagnostic and therapeutic procedures and research with ancient and traditional methods. They represent a thoroughly rational, evenhanded balance of tradition, science and respect for nature, mind, body and spirit."

Dr. Wagstaff spent five years in my clinic and over that period we saw hundreds of patients. His skills using German medicines and allergy desensitization combined with my skills in Homeopathy were a winning combination. It was most gratifying to offer treatments that resolved health issues, while supporting the immune system.

CHIROPRACTIC MEDICINE

An American Innovation

"Life is the expression of Tone"

-David Palmer

Chiropractic work is based on the theory that the *brain and nervous system connects to every cell in the body*. When there is misalignment in the spine it can put pressure on the nerves and reduce communication to their target tissues. This can adversely affect organs, muscles, joints, etc. leading to pain and/or reduction of function. The chiropractic philosophy is to treat the cause not the symptom, and chiropractic treatment reflects the disturbance in the nervous system as the cause.

Chiropractic focuses attention on the correct alignment of the vertebrae as they affect the propagation of impulses and thereby the overall state of the nervous system.

Back pain ranks among the most common problem that brings people to chiropractors. In fact, it is said that one out of every three people who suffers from low back pain seeks chiropractic care, making it the most utilized healthcare practice outside of conventional medicine.

Doctors of chiropractic have a deep respect for the human body's ability to heal itself without the use of surgery or medication. Chiropractors devote careful attention to the biomechanics, structure and function of the spine, its effects on the musculoskeletal and neurological systems, and the role played by the proper function of these systems in the preservation and restoration of health. A Doctor of Chiropractic is one who is involved in the treatment and prevention of disease, as well as the promotion of public health, and a wellness approach to patient healthcare.

Doctors of chiropractic frequently treat individuals with:

- Joint pain
- Neck pain
- Low back pain
- Sciatica
- Osteoarthritis
- Spinal disk conditions
- Carpal tunnel syndrome
- Tendonitis
- Sprains and strains
- Neuro-musculoskeletal complaints

Chiropractors also treat patients with osteoarthritis, spinal disk conditions, carpal tunnel syndrome, tendonitis, sprains, and strains. However, the scope of conditions that Doctors of Chiropractic manage or provide care for is not limited to neuro-musculoskeletal disorders. Chiropractors have the training to treat a variety of non-neuro-musculoskeletal conditions such as: allergies, asthma, digestive disorders, otitis media (non-suppurated) and other disorders as new research is developed.

Chiropractors who choose to extend their training treat a variety of health issues with the use of Homeopathy, nutritional training and other holistic therapies. The parameters for treatment guidelines vary from state to state.

The roots of chiropractic care can be traced all the way back to the beginning of recorded time. Writings from China and Greece written in 2700 B.C. and 1500 B.C. mention spinal manipulation and the maneuvering of the lower extremities to ease low back pain. Hippocrates, the Greek physician, who lived from 460 to 357 B.C., also published texts detailing the importance of chiropractic care. In one of his writings he declares, "Get knowledge of the spine, for this is the requisite for many diseases."

The American Chiropractic Association (ACA) writes that in the United States, the practice of spinal manipulation began in the late 19th century. In 1895, Daniel David Palmer founded the Chiropractic profession in Davenport, Iowa. Palmer was well read in medical journals of his time and had great knowledge of the developments that were occurring throughout the world regarding anatomy and physiology.

Palmer conceived chiropractic theory in terms of "intelligence." He believed the entire universe permeated by the "universal intelligence of God" bestows on every human the innate intelligence governing bodily activities. In other words, he believed man has a natural healing power bestowed by God; the body's *vital force* or vitality.

He believed that the vitality regulates "tone" through "nervous" or "mental" impulses traveling as vibrational waves to all parts of the body.

In 1897, Daniel David Palmer went on to begin the Palmer School of Chiropractic, which has continued to be one of the most prominent chiropractic colleges in the nation.

Palmer said in 1910, "Life is the expression of Tone. Tone is the normal degree of nerve tension. Tone is expressed in functions by normal elasticity, activity, strength, and excitability of the various organs, as observed in a state of health."

A variety of techniques, treatments and procedures are used to restore healing within the scope of Chiropractic. Since the original basic chiropractic method, referred to as "Diversified Technique" a number of advanced treatments have been developed. All continue to respect the original concept of a natural approach to health care without the use of surgery or drugs.

APPLIED KINESIOLOGY- A POPULAR TESTING METHOD

Applied Kinesiology (AK) as explained by the International College of Applied Kinesiology is a system that evaluates structural, chemical and mental aspects of health using *manual muscle testing* with other standard methods of diagnosis.

The Chiropractor using AK finds a muscle that is unbalanced and then attempts to determine why that muscle is not functioning properly. The doctor works out the treatment that will best balance the patient's muscles.

Simply stated, Applied Kinesiology (AK) is a form of diagnosis using muscle testing as a primary feedback mechanism to examine how a person's body is functioning. When properly applied, the outcome of an AK diagnosis will determine the best form of therapy for the patient.

Treatments may involve specific joint manipulation or mobilization, various myofascial therapies, cranial techniques, clinical nutrition, dietary management, counselling skills, evaluating environmental irritants and various reflex procedures.

Many Chiropractors utilize Applied Kinesiology as a means for the body to "talk." It can help to reveal what needs adjusting and when adjusting is complete, as well as other important factors.

Doctors of Chiropractic have become pioneers in the field of non-invasive care promoting science-based approaches to a variety of ailments. A continuing dedication to chiropractic research could lead to even more discoveries in preventing and combating maladies in future years.

Chiropractic spinal manipulation has now witnessed about three decades of very active research, and hundreds of studies have been published in peer- reviewed medical journals examining its clinical usefulness.

Chiropractic doctors have become pioneers in the field of non-invasive care promoting science-based approaches to a variety of ailments. Chiropractic research continues and looks to lead to even more discoveries in preventing and combating health maladies in the future.

OSTEOPATHIC MEDICINE

"Life is matter in motion."

-Andrew T. Still

I was fortunate to have access to an amazing Osteopath shortly after the birth of my third grandchild. Brendan was about eight or nine months old when I noticed he was dragging his right leg when he crawled. I brought my observation to the attention of his parents and we discussed his difficult birth. I told them I felt there was a connection and suggested a visit to the Osteopath for a diagnosis. As it turned out, without giving the doctor much detail, he was able to immediately track an energy blockage in the cranium. He worked on our little guy for over an hour that day to assist his body in releasing the trauma. Within seventy-two hours the baby was crawling normally.

I chose this type of hands-on Osteopathic treatment for my grandson because I previously had had the good fortune of experiencing this therapy for a health issue of my own. I had been pleasantly surprised at the efficiency with which opening up blocked energy in this way hastened recovery.

This type of Osteopathy treats by restoring the body's musculoskeletal system to "normality." Osteopathy, in its inception, held similarities to Chiropractic practices. What is referred to as "sublexation" (displaced, pinched off, or blocked nerve impulses in the spine) in chiropractic practices, is referred to as "osteopathic lesion" in Osteopathic practice. It is believed that the disturbance of "structure-function" leads to changes in the tissues resulting in subjective or objective signs and symptoms.

In and of itself this may sound like the description of what is commonly referred to as "spinal adjustment." Most envision this experience as crudely manipulating the spinal structure by popping a rib into place, adjusting neck vertebrae, or manipulating the pelvis. However, there is much more involved in restoring the body's musculoskeletal system than manually manipulating bones. There are muscles, tendons, nerves, but most importantly, an *energy flow* that innately assists in keeping the body functioning properly. It is the energetic release that can help to restore normality.

As Bonnie Gintis, DO, states in her book **Engaging the Movement of Life**, "Alignment is a static quality and the body is a dynamic unit of function. It is not a useful concept to isolate individual parts and look at how they line up. *If every part of the body were free to move the way it was designed to, the alignment would take care of itself.*"

Near the turn of the 19th century, the son of a pioneer physician viewed the methods of medical practices of the day and saw a better way. Andrew Taylor Still (1828-1917) theorized there is a presence of a natural healing power in the body operating through a homeostatic mechanism to counteract disturbances that lead to illness.

Still believed the body had much in common with a machine, one that should function well if it is mechanically sound. This was a departure from the medical thinking of the time. He believed that the human body should be studied as a whole, and that all elements of a person's body, mind and spirit had to be incorporated into the total care of that person. He also believed that the body had self-regulatory and self-healing powers, that the body contained within it all the substances necessary for maintaining health. When the body was properly stimulated, these substances would also assist in recovering from illness. He did not view disease as an outside agent somehow inflicting itself on the body. Rather, disease was the result of alterations in the structural relationships of the body parts that led to an inability of the body to resist or recover from illness.

He said that by correcting problems in the body's structure, through the use of manual techniques, now known as "osteopathic manipulative treatment," the body's ability to function and to heal itself could be greatly improved. Still further stated, "Osteopathy is based on the perfection of Nature's work. When all parts of the human body are in line we have health. When they are not the effect is disease. When the parts are readjusted disease gives place to health.

The work of the osteopath is to adjust the body from the abnormal to the normal; then the abnormal condition gives place to the normal and health is the result of the normal condition."

A Chiropractor is trained to focus on alignment, range of motion, pain and physical release to relax physical patterns of strain. Osteopathic treatment works with movement of the fluids of the body. When there is movement of fluid at the cellular level nutrients and other information-containing substances can be delivered throughout the body. This process of exchange of fluids can accomplish stimulation of blood flow, lymphatic drainage, fluctuation of cerebral spinal fluid and visceral mobility and motility, to name a few. When there is flow and movement within the functional fluid system, alignment, relief of pain and physical release will follow. Emotional shifts also occur when energy is released in this way.

Still, in his rudimentary understanding of the fluids in the body at that time described it by saying, *"I suspended the action of the great occipital nerves, and given harmony to the flow of the arterial blood to and through the veins."*

There are two very different types of Osteopaths in practice today. There are those who use their medical training as other conventional physicians and incorporate the prescribing of both natural medicines and pharmaceutical drugs. Then there are those who subscribe to the above description of working directly on the body to create stimulation of both energy and fluids to restore health.

CHAPTER III
ADVANCES UNDER THE RADAR

I refer to this chapter as "Advances Under the Radar" for two reasons. Firstly, they are therapies not taught to western medical doctors, so most are unaware of the possibilities these methods hold for the health of their patients. Secondly, doctors trained in holistic medicine may not be aware of all the therapies available either. It can become comfortable to stick to what we know, especially if we are happy with the results and therefore don't look outside the box.

Conventional medical schools follow standard guidelines of education for the diagnosis of disease, drug therapy and surgery. Holistic schools of medicine have standard guidelines within their own defined modality. Therapies from outside the US or recent discoveries are taught at the discretion of each individual school.

There are a number of philosophies, modalities and natural medicine protocols that follow a specific doctrine and are successfully practiced by holistic doctors around the world. Many of them have been in existence for decades, some even centuries and have helped countless people with numerous illnesses and conditions.

I have found that a Naturopath might specialize in functional medicine and nutrition, but may not have been exposed to more modern uses of remedies. Or a Homeopath may be well trained in the use of classical remedies and not *Phenolic Therapy* or *Organ Drainage*.

I have been fortunate to study with doctors from varying backgrounds who utilize numerous techniques to reach their goals. Included in this chapter are therapies I have had success with through the years.

The following therapies are listed in alphabetical order and not in order of preference or efficacy.

CELL SALT THERAPY

In the human body mineral salts form the life core of its functions. They shift fluids, raise and lower blood pressure, cause the stability of bones, fire nerve endings, make muscles contract and keep order in the brain. Without salts, (also referred to as tissue salts), there would be no life.

When the body is kept in balance with the necessary nutrients, harmony can be restored much more readily when a stressful or abnormal condition arises. In actuality, the body is like a storage battery and must be supplied with the necessary cell salts to run efficiently.

Dr. Wilhelm Heinrich Schuessler (1821–1898) was a medical doctor and Homeopath from Oldenburg, Germany. In 1873 Schuessler published an article in the General Homeopathic Journal titled, "An Abbreviated Therapy" (English translation.) Schuessler said he did not like the Homeopathic practice of having to use hundreds of remedies, and was searching for a simpler method of healing.

While studying the ash of cremated corpses he discovered that the human body is made up of only a dozen inorganic compounds, or mineral salts.

- Calcium Phosphate
- Calcium Fluoride
- Calcium Sulphate
- Sodium Chloride
- Silicic Acid
- Potassium Chloride
- Potassium Sulphate
- Potassium Phosphate
- Magnesium Phosphate
- Iron Phosphate
- Sodium Sulphate
- Sodium Phosphate

The minerals that make up the ash after burning a human body and all of its tissues are the immortal part of the physical body that remains.

Schuesslers' work brought him to the determination that it was the missing inorganic mineral salts that cause disruption to the processes of the body and therefore create illness. He believed where there was illness there was a missing mineral, or minerals. If the missing mineral was supplied the disrupted cell metabolism began working properly.

When the inorganic substances present in the blood and tissues are balanced, then they are capable of carrying out the major regulatory functions of the body, including removal of toxins and disease causing agents.

The body's defense mechanisms usually keep the body cells naturally in balance; however, improper diet and processed food, lack of exercise and modern-day stress can create a tissue salt imbalance or deficiency. Through use of the appropriate tissue remedies the cells are brought back into proper balance. This results in normal body functions. There are twelve Cell Salts that, when used accordingly as nutritional supplements, can ensure optimal health maintenance.

Schuesslers' principal objective was not to supply the body with the deficient minerals, but to stimulate the body to rebalance itself where mal-absorption of minerals was taking place. In other words, the cell salts, (or tissue salts) helped to activate healing by allowing regeneration and stabilization. This is why he recommended taking the indicated salt only until symptoms subside.

SCHUESSLER THEORIZED:

- Disease does not occur if cell metabolism is normal
- Cell metabolism is in turn normal if cell nutrition is adequate
- The body can determine whether nutritional substances are either of organic or inorganic nature
- The ability of the body's cells to assimilate and to excrete and utilize nutritional material if there is a deficiency in the inorganic (mineral or cell salt) constituent of tissue

EXAMPLES OF CELL SALT USE:

- **Calcium Sulphate** for skin conditions such as wounds, acne and eczema.
- **Ferrum Phosphate** is an oxygen carrier and anti-inflammatory useful in fevers, colds, congestion, anemia and fatigue.

(Recently I suggested a dose of **Ferrum Phosphate** to the mom of an 18-month old who had a fever. Within 30 minutes it subsided. The fever was not suppressed as with chemical drugs, but instead the body was able to bring itself back into balance.)

- **Magnesium Phosphate** is essential to nerve and muscle communication. Helps with leg cramps, menstrual cramps, spasms and sciatic nerve pain.
- **Calcium Phosphate** works well to regulate calcium to build strong bones and is especially helpful to children with growing pains.

CELL SALT/TISSUE SALT CHART

The following serves as a brief description for the many uses of the twelve cell salts.

DOSAGE: Adults (12 years +) 4 tablets; children (6-11 years) 2 tablets; children (1-5 years) 1 tablet, all ages take 3 times daily, or as directed by a health care practitioner. The most common potencies are 3X and 6X.

1. **CALCIUM FLUORIDE** (Calc. Fluor.)
   TISSUE ELASTICITY; RESTORES FLEXIBILITY, DISPURSES BONY GROWTHS, TOOTH ENAMEL

2. **CALCIUM PHOSPHATE** (Calc. Phos.)
   GROWTH & NUTRITION OF BONES; GROWING PAINS, TEETHING, STIFFNESS

3. **CALCIUM SULPHATE** (Calc. Sulph.)
   SKIN CONDITIONS; ACNE, BOILS, MINOR WOUNDS, GLANDS, YELLOW DISCHARGES

4. **FERRUM PHOSPHATE** (Ferr. Phos.)
   ENERGIZER; OXYGEN CARRIER, ANEMIA, FEVER, COUGH, MINOR INFLAMMATION

5. **KALI MURIATICUM** (Kali Mur.)
   CONGESTION; COLDS WITH WHITE DISCHARGES, CONGESTED EARS, SORE THROAT

6. **KALI PHOSPHATE** (Kali Phos.)
   MENTAL EXHAUSTION; HEADACHES, NEURALGIA PAIN, IRRITABILITY, SADNESS, ANXIETY, SPASMODIC PAIN, WEAKNESS

7. **KALI SULPHURICUM** (Kali Sulph.)
   OXYGEN CARRIER, SKIN ISSUES, DEEP YELLOW DISCHARGES, DANDRUFF

8. **MAGNESIUM PHOSPHORICA** (Mag. Phos.)
   ANTI-SPASMODIC; CRAMPS, RADIATING PAINS, SPASMS

9. **NATRUM MURIATICUM** (Nat. Mur.)
   WATER DISTRIBUTION; CHILLINESS, MOUTH BLISTERS, CRACKED LIPS, NUMBNESS, TINGLING

10. **NATRUM PHOSPHORICUM** (Nat. Phos.)
    ACID NEUTRALIZER; INDIGESTION, FLATULENCE, SOUR BELCHING

11. **NATRUM SULPHURICUM** (Nat. Sulph.)
    STOMACH CONDITIONS; BELCHING, DIARRHEA, FLATULENCE, NAUSEA

12. **SILICEA** (Silica)
    CLEANSER; BRITTLE NAILS, BOILS, ACNE, PUS FORMATION

GEMMOTHERAPY

Gemmotherapy, also known as *Plant Stem Cell Therapy*, are European tinctures made from baby buds of wild harvested plants. The materials are gathered from the plants mostly in the spring at a key stage of their natural growth cycle. The buds and young shoots are then freshly prepared by maceration and put into a solution of water, alcohol and glycerin to extract their active ingredients.

They are most often used for *drainage* and *detoxification* since they are gentle and efficient.

We know that within a tiny acorn lives a giant oak tree. It is also true that within the bud of a plant is the genetic material for the entire plant. It is the plant's form of stem cells contained in their fresh buds, sprouts, seeds, sap and barks that can be harvested from the growing plant. It is these elements of the plant that contain the highest concentrations of the active ingredients necessary for tissue regeneration, growth development and essential drainage properties. Each contains a large amount of genetic information and also contains what is referred to as phytonutrients that consist of minerals, trace elements, vitamins, and enzymes.

From these pure living plant sources springs Gemmotherapy. Gemmotherapy is a method of creating concentrated tinctures and captures the essential life essence of the strongest and most active elements of the naturally harvested plants. *Through scientific investigation the pharmacological superiority of the bud versus the fully developed plant has been discovered*, along with their specific clinical indications.

Plants naturally produce more than eight thousand different compounds called *phenols* for functions as varied as cell wall chemical compounding, flower pigmentation, and host defense.

A few of the many uses for Gemmotherapy tinctures are:
- Adrenal insufficiency
- Inflammation
- Blood thinner
- Circulation
- Hormone balancing
- Immune modulators
- Organ drainage and detoxification
- Sugar Regulation
- Skin Issues
- Viral, bacterial and fungal infections

The following are a few examples of plant stem cell uses:

Black Currant (Ribes Nigrum) is very high in Vitamin C and is an excellent anti-inflammatory by directly stimulating the adrenals.

The bud of the **Fig Tree** (Ficus Carica) is useful for nervous conditions such as anxiety, anguish, anger, excessive thinking while trying to fall asleep, and depression.

Linden Tree (Tilia Tomentosa) buds have shown to have great tranquilizing properties, can detoxify the nerve cells, and help with nervous headaches.

Hazel (Corylus Avellana) is a liver and lung remedy and can reduce cholesterol.

Ask your holistic practitioner if they are trained in the use of Gemmotherapy tinctures. Most brands are imported from Europe and should be used under the guidance of a health care practitioner.

PHENOLIC THERAPY

Runny noses and persistent post-nasal drip are often the result of the body's reaction to simple components of food or pollen molecules called *phenolics*. Intolerance to phenolic substances causes a wide variety of complaints. Allergic reaction to nuts, a headache and bloating from gluten intolerance, or joint pain after eating tomatoes are a few reactions to natural substances. Phenolics are one of the causes of these maladies. Scientific studies and numerous clinical experiences demonstrate that phenolics play a large part in many illnesses, especially allergies.

Phenolics are six-sided chemical rings that are part of basic food and pollen molecules. They include amino acids, hormones and neuro-chemicals. Conventional medicine describes allergies as "reactions caused by the production of IgE antibodies to inhaled foreign proteins," according to Martin D. Chapman, Ph.D. Dr. Chapman's statement is true, to an extent, but looking deeper into chemistry it has been discovered that the *phenolics* attached to protein molecules are the real culprits.

The chart below shows the specific six-sided phenol rings that comprise the makeup of all foods. In some cases, they are valuable nutrients and in others create havoc as allergens.

Phenolic therapy is the compounding of the specific chemical ring within the protein that causes the allergic reaction. As an example, gallic acid is found in approximately 22 foods, especially fruits, cheeses, lettuce and tomatoes. If a patient has allergic symptoms after eating strawberries and their allergy shot therapy focuses on the strawberry, many other foods that include the real culprit, the gallic acid phenolic ring, will be missed. Perhaps this is why allergy shots are usually an incomplete therapy that offers some relief, but usually not a cure.

People who react negatively to drinking red wine may believe it is the sulfites in the wine causing the reaction when in reality it may be the phenolic ring responsible for the red color of the skin. Phenolics are important to nature in many ways. The chart below demonstrates the role phenolic compounds play in nature.

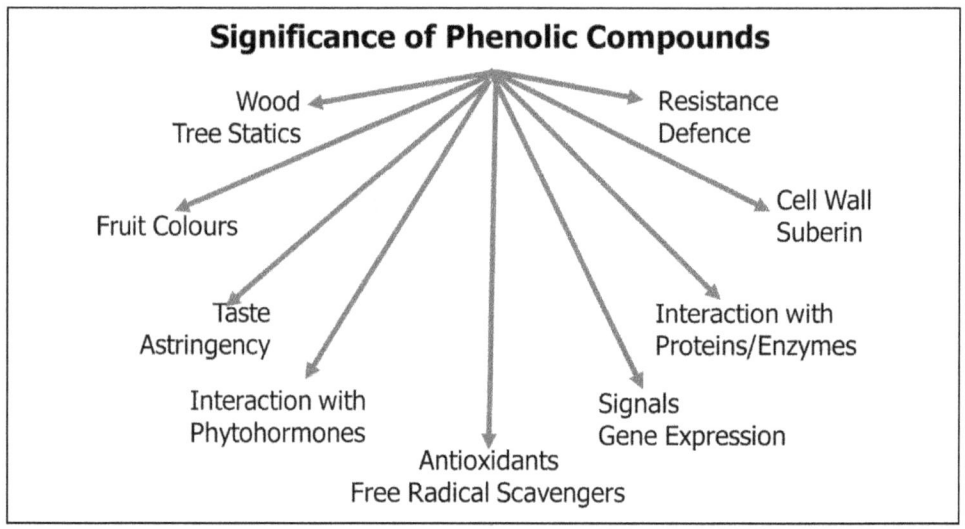

Robert W. Gardner, Ph.D. is a biochemist and professor emeritus of Animal Science at Brigham Young University and a pioneer in the study of phenolics. In his monumental work, **Chemical Intolerance: Physiological Causes and Effects and Treatment Modalities**, Dr. Gardner showed, with hundreds of trials, that a phenolic approach utilizing Homeopathic dilutions to desensitize was more effective than traditional allergy treatment.

Phenolics are essential to life as we know it, but when metabolized incorrectly, they can cause major and minor physical, mental, and emotional disturbances in a large number of patients. One example is Salsolinol, which is a product of natural fermentation in plants and alcohol. It is considered to be a derivative of dopamine, a neurotransmitter. When the body does not metabolize Salsolinol the result can be obsessive-compulsive behavior. It can also create a craving for sweets, carbohydrates and alcohol.

Cow's milk is ranked as one of the most allergenic foods in the entire human diet. If you look at the diet of a cow, substantial proportions of the diet contain phenolics. When coupled with fermentation, the cow excretes an enormous amount of phenolic materials. Milk is one of their main excretory routes; milk therefore contains a large array of very reactive 'allergenic' compounds. It is no wonder such a large portion of the population is allergic to milk and other dairy products.

The work of identifying the symptoms associated with common food phenolics led to the discovery of vast symptom pools that were previously denied to be associated with allergies or autoimmune responses. The fact that practitioners can now determine and negate the allergy is extraordinary in itself. The value is this therapy has the potential of creating a standard approach to the treatment of allergies.

The result of Dr. Gardner's work has been of great benefit to many people besides the successful treatment of his own severe allergies. Many patients who previously were unable to find relief from their symptoms now have a simple, inexpensive option to relieve suffering. Once the specific allergic phenolic compound is identified (by a practitioner) the patient is given a small dose daily of the offending compounded substance or combination of substances. Over time the body becomes desensitized and no longer reacts negatively. Proper dosage and length of treatment is specific to each person.

I was taught Phenolic therapy by Dr. Wagstaff and its use resulted in relief for many allergy sufferers we treated at our clinic. There are a few companies who specialize in the manufacture of phenolic compounds. The following detailed charts cross-reference the foods and conditions related to phenolic compounds. The charts are used with the permission of DesBio, manufacturers of phenolic substances. They can be accessed online.

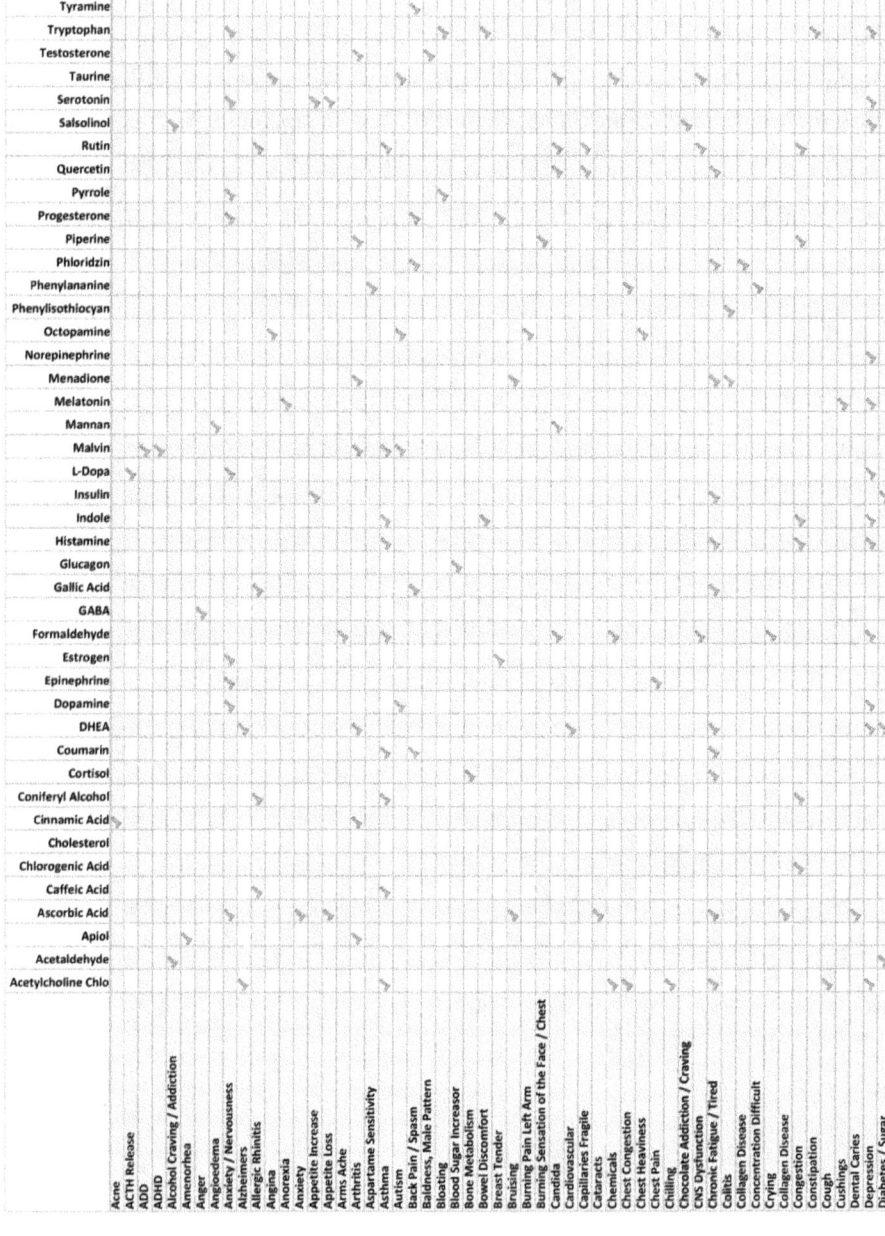

38 Elena Upton, Ph.D.

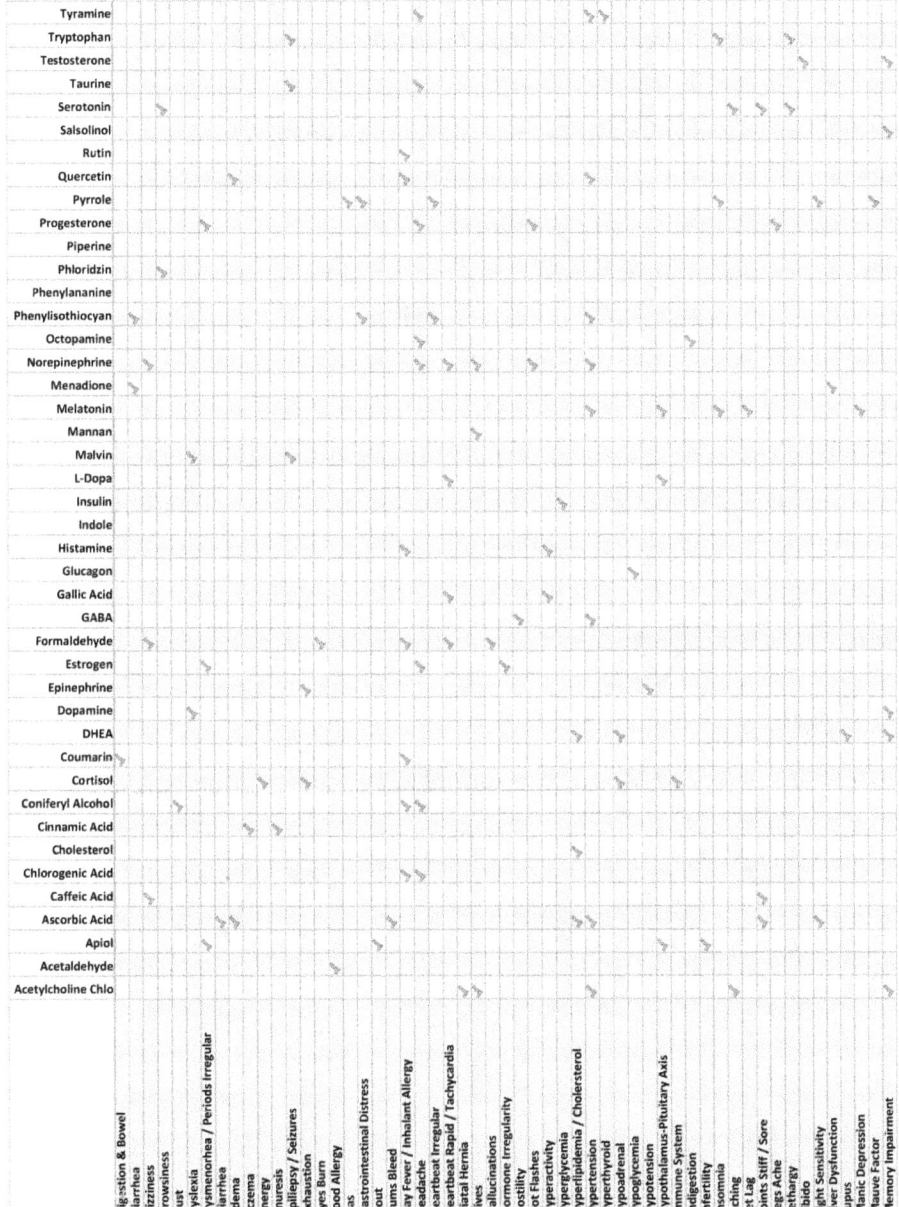

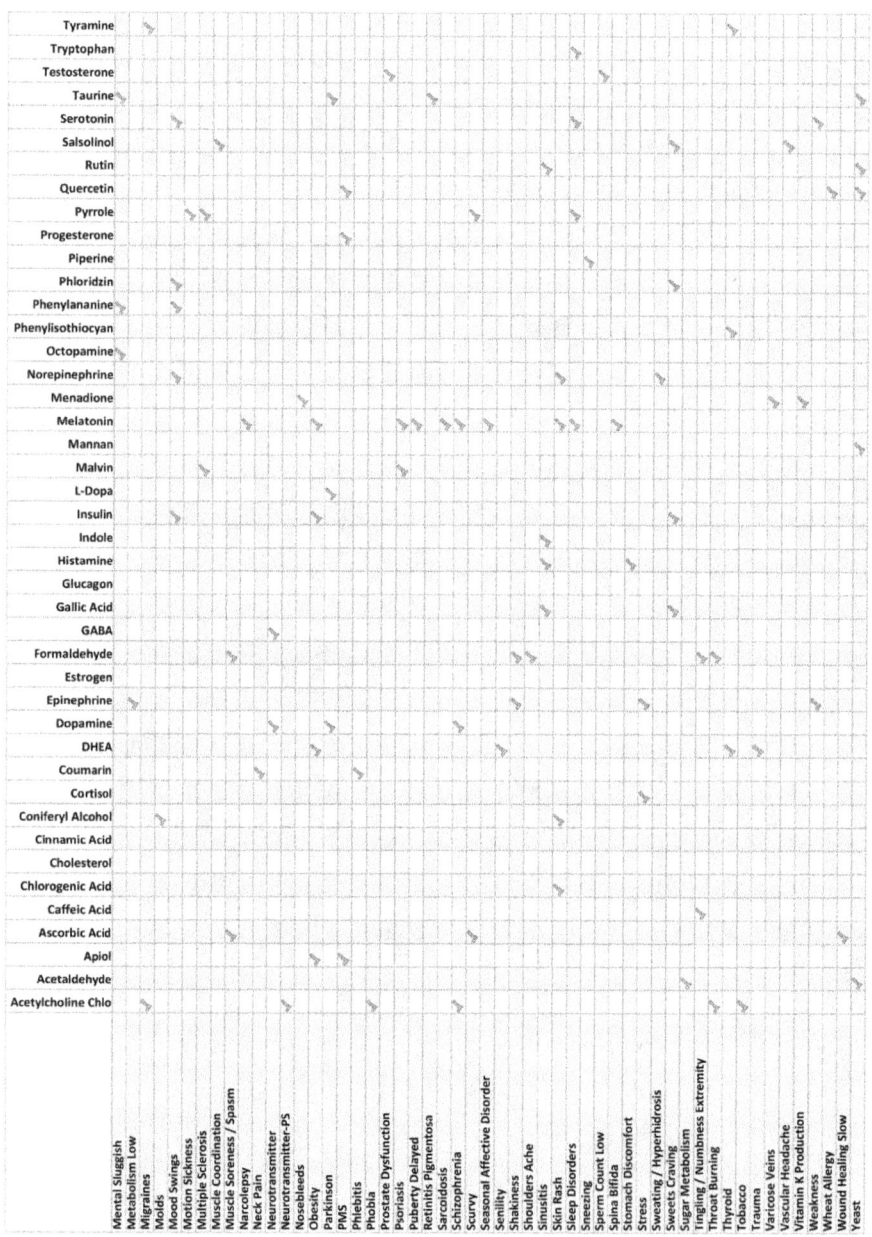

TRACE MINERAL THERAPY (OLIGOTHERAPY)

Trace Mineral Therapy, also known as Oligotherapy, is the use of trace elements or minerals to support healthy cells. Oligotherapy is from the Greek meaning "a very tiny quantity." The tiny traces of minerals are indispensable to the normal functioning of the body. These trace elements are necessary to the functioning of enzymes and basically act as a catalyst to speed up metabolism at the cellular level. The minute stimulus creates major reactions. Oligotherapy is NOT aimed at correcting nutritional deficits, but works by catalyzing chemical reactions, and hence assisting in the normalization of functions.

An excess of free radical activities, due to toxins in food and environmental pollutants, can cause disorders and malfunctions in the metabolism of humans and animals. Enzymes are the basic structure of the free radical scavenger system and enzymes need ionized trace elements for their chemical structure to function. Each mineral needs to be in a certain position to be catalyzed and activate enzyme activity.

Trace elements are necessary to keep the right concentrations of elements throughout the body for optimum enzymatic functioning. Without optimal enzymatic function many disorders can erupt without a physical cause to otherwise identify the abnormality. An example would be the use of the combination **Zinc-Nickel-Cobalt** for some cases of Endometriosis, since this combination of trace minerals affects estrogen receptor cites. In cases where there may be a lack of complete recovery from an illness the correct combination of trace minerals may be needed to increase metabolic function at the cellular level to complete the healing process. A combination of **Manganese-Cobalt, Zinc-Copper** and **Lithium** can reactivate a depleted, exhausted person. Another example is a thyroid issue that may need **Iodine,** as a trace mineral to correct the issue.

The combination of **Copper-Gold-Silver** can be used for the common cold and also used in recurrent viral and bacterial infection, psychological fatigue, loss of coordination, insomnia, memory loss, cardiovascular disease, poor concentration and even depression.

Another example is the combination **Manganese-Copper**, which can be helpful when treating allergies and upper respiratory infections, asthma, bronchitis, sinusitis, laryngitis, cystitis, diarrhea, hives, eczema, psoriasis, atopic dermatitis, arthritis, anemia, acne, headache, colitis and hypothyroidism.

Homeopaths, Naturopaths, Chiropractors and other natural health practitioners use trace mineral therapy. Trace mineral therapy remedies can also be found on the Internet and in some natural pharmacies.

TRACE MINERAL THERAPY- 'OLIGOTHERAPY' REFERENCE CHART

Trace elements are basic metal and mineral substances essential to the biochemical processes of metabolism in the body. Without them there can be no harmonious interaction between vitamins and enzymes. All trace elements are biologically significant and dynamic. Sometimes biochemical exchanges can be blocked or derailed and fortunately they can be re-ignited with the appropriate trace mineral supplementation. The following are examples of symptoms that occur as a result of trace mineral imbalance.

BISMUTH- Gastrointestinal ulcers, frontal headaches

COBALT- anemia, migraines, vegetative dysfunctions

COPPER- exhaustion, susceptibility to infection

CHROMIUM- blood sugar/insulin imbalance

FLUORIDE- weakness of connective tissue, osteoporosis

IODINE- glandular disorders, thyroid insufficiency

MAGNESIUM- neuritis, colitis, muscle spasms

MANGANESE- arthritis, allergies, gallbladder, anemia, asthma

MOLYBDENUM- premature aging, osteoporosis, hair loss, depression

POTASSIUM- muscle weakness, fatigue, tachycardia, chronic catarrhs

SELENIUM- immunodeficiency, impaired metabolism, rheumatism, cardiac risk

SULPHUR- acne, eczema, psoriasis,

ZINC- impaired brain function, compromised immune system

COPPER/GOLD/SILVER- antimicrobial, adrenal exhaustion, premature aging

ZINK/NICKEL/COBALT- disorders of the pancreas, imbalance of the endocrine

---

MANGANESE/COPPER/COBALT- anemia, chronic fatigu

Reference **THE ALTERNATIVE *CONTINUED,* Secrets to Success** for more in-depth information on the uses and protocols for therapies included in this chapter.

CHAPTER IV
WHY WE GET SICK & HOW TO PREVENT IT

All disease possesses the same characteristics; inflammation, hormonal imbalance, oxidative stress and mineral deficiency.

Sometimes when I dispense a remedy, a well-indicated remedy, it does not work. When this happens I know there is an over-riding condition, a condition that has a higher vibrational state. Meaning there is something wrong with the weakest link in the person's body that the remedy cannot reach.

Everyone's body works in the same way and this is our great hope, because if one person can heal, then everyone can heal. Disease is not selective it is a state of being.

All disease has some aspect of the four components listed above, but it is OXIDATIVE STRESS that drives disease. Oxidative stress is when there is damage to your cells through the oxidative process. Oxidation is a normal process that occurs in nature, including in our bodies.

You've heard the term *free radical*, an atom or molecule that has a single unpaired electron in its outer shell (valence shell). When a free radical looks to attach itself to another atom by stealing an electron, it damages the cell it stole it from. The results are toxic. The valence shell has to fill itself up to be neutral or stable so it steals electrons from healthy cells. When an "attacked" electron loses its charge, it becomes a free radical itself, beginning a chain reaction.

An example of this process outside of the body is rust. When metal is exposed to the elements it is oxidation that causes the rusting process. Free radicals that are missing a simple electron search for another molecule so that they can become electrically balanced. In this process they fire off charges that damage the other structures around them, which causes the rust.

You could say that aging is a form of 'rusting'. We rust on the inside and we rust on the outside (wrinkled, dried, spotted skin). Free radicals are running through your system throughout your life looking for a mate. The more free-radicals you have, the more damage and the faster aging can occur.

Where do the free radicals come from? They are everywhere.

- Toxic Chemicals
- Chemotherapy
- Cigarettes
- Rancid Oils
- Hydrogenated oils
- Air Pollution
- Herbicides
- Radiation
- Drugs
- Bad Diet

However, free-radicals aren't always bad. Even accelerated healing causes free-radicals. Sometimes the immune system will purposely create them to neutralize bacteria or a virus. This creates a cellular process referred to by researchers as lysing.

This is where antioxidants come into play. There is an abundance of electrons to satisfy the electron transfer to prevent the removal of any unbalanced atom at the valence shell orbit. An antioxidant is any substance that has an excess of electrons in its valence shell orbit so they can donate or be removed from its shell without damaging the donor atom.

The following two Chapters V & VI are a reference guide for First-Aid and Common Conditions. You will read in Chapters VI about drainage and detoxification. By explaining the concept of free radical damage the repetition will hopefully be of more value and with greater understanding as to why this process is crucial to your health. Only through the process of detoxification, whether it is through food, remedies or herbal formulas, free-radicals must be regularly flushed from the body in order to maintain vibrant health.

Cleansing the body has a specific order, since there is a natural order to healing. The following will accomplish gentle detoxification of the major organs.

13. Colon
14. Kidney
15. Skin
16. Lungs
17. Liver
18. Lymph

1. Colon Cleanse: if you have never done a colon cleanse, then it will take approximately *one month* for a complete cleanse. (Chronic conditions can take up to *three* months.) This creates a path of least resistance by affecting the other five organ systems, since they all drain into the colon. The colon has very distinctive nerve pathways to the other five organ systems. After the initial cleanse a *one week* cleanse is recommended *two times* per year at the change of seasons, spring and fall. It is important to take a pro-biotic during a colon cleanse.

Most health food stores and natural pharmacies carry colon cleanse kits. Your health care practitioner can make recommendations based on your particular needs. (My favorite colon cleane is *Emptiness*, by Chakra Food)

2. Kidney Cleanse: There are a number of herbal formulas that are effective to cleanse the kidney. You can also accomplish this task with herbal drainage remedies and with the foods and teas listed below.

- Cilantro
- Celery
- Chanca Piedra
- Dandelion
- Gravel root
- Juniper berries
- Nettle
- Parsley
- Watercress
- Watermelon

3. Skin Detoxification: The skin is the largest organ made up of protective layers, nerves and glands. Skin protects you from infection, helps to produce Vitamin D when exposed to the sun, interacts with your brain and plays a crucial role in whole body detoxification. Whatever touches the skin touches the liver, then the gallbladder, then the pancreas. This means there is a direct connection between skin health and the health of the other organs. This is a consideration when buying cosmetics, perfumes, skin creams, lotions and soaps. Also consider where you swim and the water you soak in. The skin is like a sponge and any chemicals placed on the skin are taken into the body and through to the organs.

The most efficient means of detoxification of the skin is by using a natural bristle brush (sold specifically for dry skin brushing). This method will help increase circulation; exfoliate your skin so it 'breaths' more efficiently; stimulates the lymph system; helps to diminish cellulite; can improve digestion and even help to relieve stress.

Always use brush strokes towards the heart. This helps to improve circulation and encourages lymph drainage. The best time is in the morning before a hot shower, bath or going into a sauna. Two times per day is even more helpful if you are actively involved in a detoxification program.

4. Lung Drainage: An efficient means of detoxification of the lungs is with *deep breathing*. We have unknowingly become a society of shallow breathers. There is actually more fluid in the breath than in the kidneys. There are many herbal formulas available to assist in lung detoxification, especially effective if you have had any type of pulmonary illness. However, remember to *breathe*.

5. Liver Detoxification: Herbal formulas are very effective for liver drainage and Acupuncturists use Chinese herbs. If you choose to do a liver flush on your own you can use the following ingredients.

- Olive oil
- Lemon juice
- Apple Cider Vinegar or Apple Juice

Combine 1 tsp. olive oil mixed into ¼ cup lemon juice + apple juice or apple cider vinegar. Repeat this process every 6 hours for a 24-hour period. The next two days will bring on a liver flush resulting in substantial evacuation.

Add cayenne capsules for increased circulation when you feel your level of health can handle it. You can also take the supplement milk thistle daily to protect your liver.

6. Lymph Drainage: Lymph drainage can be happening every day through dry skin brushing. Hot baths and showers also stimulate lymph glands to drain, as well as massage therapy. Other choices are herbal drainage and lymph message from a therapist trained in this specialty.

A castor oil pack can help to open everything up and move toxins through quickly. A castor oil pack is placed on the tummy to increase circulation and to promote elimination and healing of the tissues and organs underneath the skin. It is used to stimulate the liver, relieve pain, increase lymphatic circulation, reduce inflammation, and improve digestion.

Castor oil packs can be made by soaking a piece of flannel in castor oil and placing it on the skin. The flannel is covered with a sheet of cellophane and a hot water bottle is placed over the plastic, or heating pad, to heat the pack. Castor oil 'kits' can be purchased in health food stores and online.

WHOLE BODY CLEANSE

A whole body cleanse can be accomplished with food. An easy method is a juice cleanse. The following are the most efficient detoxification foods. (Buy organic, if possible.)

- Carrot
- Apple
- Beet
- Lemon

Juicing should be done under the guidance of a qualified health practitioner. This is *not fasting*, it is cleansing. Fasting can be dangerous.

HYDRATION

Hydration is an important issue for your health and wellbeing whether you are cleansing or not. In fact, hydration is the key to successful detoxification and healing. It is essential for toxins to be moving out of the cells regularly, especially in our industrialized existence.

The following is a formula sure to keep you hydrated and on the road to health.

- 1 liter of distilled or spring water
- 1 tsp salt
- 3 tsp of erythritol
- 3 tsp vegetable glycerin

Drink the mixture daily throughout your cleansing process. (Can be sipped through the day.) Always be sure your water is from a clean source. The salt is the electrolyte component and should be sea salt. (Not Pink Himalayan salt, it is rock salt – not from the sea and has a positive charge, rather than the negative charge needed.) The sugar takes the salt into the cells and the glycerin holds the water in the body so it is absorbed into the cells.

THINGS TO STAY AWAY FROM DURING DETOXIFICATION:

- **MAO Inhibitors-** MAOIs (monoamine oxidase inhibitors) are a class of medications used to treat depression. They interfere with the enzyme responsible for metabolizing serotonin, epinephrine, dopamine and norepinephrine.
- **Garlic-** acts like an anti-biotic killing intestinal flora.
- **Grapefruit juice** (except if it is a heavy metal detoxification) accelerates and amplifies the detoxification in the intestine. This can create achy joints.

While doing a Skin, Kidney and/or Lung detoxification add cayenne pepper. If there is inflammation and/or pain during the process add any of the following as a tea or in supplement form:

- Ginger root
- Turmeric
- Boswellia

During the detoxification process stay off ALL sugar, except in your hydrating water. You will want to preserve your insulin levels by not having a high carbohydrate diet.

If you follow the detoxification process and remove inflammation regularly, other remedies, supplements or therapies will respond much more efficiently.

Throughout Chapters V & VI are suggestions using the therapies mentioned in this chapter, whenever appropriate. They can always be utilized more extensively, but for the purposes of this book, I have kept their usage brief, while demonstrating how they can be effectively added to protocols.

PART II

PUTTING IT ALL TOGETHER

A MANUAL OF HEALTH CHOICES

"Don't just believe it because it sounds good, nor disbelieve it because it conflicts with your philosophy: go out and try it for yourself"

-The Kalama Sutta

FIRST-AID REMEDY REFERENCE CHART

First "Go-to" remedy for shock and/or trauma is Aconite
TOPICAL TREATMENT-Unbroken skin- Arnica; Broken skin-Calendula

Burns
Cantharis + Colloidal silver (topical)

Bites
Ledum + Pyrogenium

Bee Sting
Apis + Ledum

Bleeding
Phosphorus or Arnica

Sprains
Rhus Tox or Ruta

Concussion
Arnica + Nat Sulph

Puncture wound
Ledum

Eye Injury
Euphrasia + Arnica

Fractures
Symphytum

Heatstroke/Sunburn
Glonoinum

Dental Trauma
Hypericum
+
Hepar sulph Calc

Hangover/Overeating
Nux Vomica

Motion/Altitude Sickness
Cocculus

Food or Water Poisoning
Ars Alb

Copyright © 2018 Elena Upton, PhD

CHAPTER V FIRST AID A-Z
CONVENTIONAL WISDOM & NATURAL RELIEF

Are you prepared to handle an emergency before help arrives? Or for that matter, are you prepared to efficiently handle the everyday mishaps that we all encounter from time to time? Create a home pharmacy today by gathering simple, inexpensive supplies to have on hand and be prepared whenever the need arises. It may save your life or the life of someone you love.

Most of the first aid suggestions listed below call for the use of Homeopathic remedies. Having a Homeopathic kit at home, in your car and even at the office will prove to be of great assistance in many emergencies. Be prepared by understanding the basics of homeopathic prescribing.

Homeopathy provides a safe, effective, natural, nontoxic treatment for many acute and chronic illnesses. Homeopathy is safe for newborns, pregnant women, the elderly, and even animals. It uses natural substances that are gentle, yet extremely effective when used properly.

Be sure to have on hand at all times a sufficient supply of bandages, gauze, tape, tweezers, colloidal silver and hydrogen peroxide for disinfecting and Calendula cream and Arnica cream for topical use. (Calendula is for broken skin injuries and Arnica for bruises, abrasions, etc.)

CHOOSING THE CORRECT REMEDY

To make the correct choice of remedy, match the symptoms of the person (including their emotional state) to the symptoms of the remedy. Some acute remedies are basic to all injuries and are listed accordingly.

DOSAGE AND POTENCIES

First Aid A-Z addresses emergency and acute treatment, which is very different from chronic or constitutional Homeopathic treatment. For this reason, it is not crucial to be concerned about exact potencies (whatever you have on hand or can buy readily will suffice) and dosage is more frequent in emergency situations.

When the person is responding to a chosen remedy it can be re-dosed every 15 minutes for up to 6 doses. For example, if you've just smashed your finger with a hammer and it is throbbing, first submerge in cold water or apply an ice pack, then take 4-5 pellets of Hypericum. The Hypericum can be repeated every 15 minutes and stopped after a few doses if the throbbing has subsided. Then repeat the remedy every few hours throughout the day to help arrest swelling, bruising and pain.

DISPENSING REMEDIES

If a person is fully conscious and does not have any blockage of their airways, or breathing issues, dispense dry pellets directly under the tongue. If they are having difficulty, or you are uncertain if the person is fully conscious, dilute a few pellets in about an ounce of water, then rub into the skin a few drops on the inside of the elbow, behind the ear or on the wrist. It is preferable to do this on the left side of the body, if possible, since the body takes things in on the left.

For babies, dissolve a pellet in an ounce of water and dispense into the mouth using an eyedropper; or use topically as described above. An open bottle of the remedy can also be held under the nose in any situation. The nose is a powerful tool for absorption into the body. This method is called olfaction, and is the same method used with smelling salts.

When symptoms are resolved the remedy can be stopped. In some cases, the symptoms will change and the situation will call for a different remedy. This is not uncommon in acute cases.

The use of multiple remedies can cover the totality of symptoms. For example, your child has fallen off a swing and they have a bruised arm and cut knee. The child is frightened and crying uncontrollably. They may need Aconite or Chamomilla to calm them, Arnica or Bellis for the bruise and Calendula applied topically to the scrape.

BE CONFIDENT

Don't be afraid to make a choice and dispense. If there is little to no result, go on to the next remedy that fits a description of the circumstances. Homeopathic remedies are derived from plant, animal and mineral sources. They are made with a minimum of the original substance to give the body instructions, not to medicate or suppress symptoms. If the remedy you have chosen is not exactly correct, there is no harm, it will pass through the body unused. It is like a radio wave…when it is out of range there is no clear signal to connect to. The same is true with a Homeopathic remedy.

BASIC REMEDIES TO HAVE ON HAND

Many of the Homeopathic remedies suggested in this section are commonly used and can be found in most health food stores and natural pharmacies. Homeopathic kits are also available online and a few suggestions are listed in Chapter VII, What's In Your Home Pharmacy?

However, there are some rare remedies referenced that are not included in a basic kit, or sold over the counter in stores. Be prepared! For example, if you know you suffer from motion sickness and are planning on packing remedies for a boat trip look up in advance the medicines needed for motion sickness. Order them online or from a pharmacy in advance and you will be happy to have them with you when the need arises.

If you have a collection of remedies that you'd like to round out, or build your own first-aid kit, here are the basic 16 remedies every first-aid kit should include.

- **Aconitum napellus** 200C- panic, fear, shock, violent palpitations
- **Apis mellifica** 30C- Insect bites, bee stings, hydrocephalus
- **Arnica montana** 30C- Injuries, bruises, shock, muscle soreness, fatigue seizures from head injury
- **Arsenicum album** 30C- Food poisoning, gastroenteritis, severe burns, mountain sickness, asthma, shock
- **Belladonna** 30C- Congestive fever, sunstroke, migraine
- **Cocculus indicus** 30C- car sickness, sea sickness, exhaustion from lack of sleep
- **Calendula officinalis** 30C- wounds and abrasions (used as a disinfectant)
- **Cantharis** 30C- Burns with blisters (1st & 2nd degree), cystitis
- **Causticum** 30C- Internal and external burns, frostbite
- **Hypericum perforatum** 30C- Puncture wounds, if they are deep affecting nerves, any nerve injury
- **Ipecacuanha** 30C- Acute asthma, spastic coughing with nausea and vomiting
- **Ledum** 30C- Insect bites, all types of poisonous animal bites, puncture wounds
- **Rhus toxicodendron** 30C- Sprains and strains after Arnica
- **Ruta graveolens** 30C- Bone blows, fractures, sprains (ligament & tendon)
- **Symphytum** 30C- Broken bones and fractures, eyeball blows
- **Urtica urens** 30c- 1st degree burns, bites and hives

ALLERGIC REACTION (ANAPHYLACTIC SHOCK)

This occurs when someone is either stung, bitten or has eaten something that creates an allergic reaction. Pharmaceutical drugs can create this type of reaction. When we are exposed to something toxic to the system the body will react and attempt to shut down to minimize damage.

SYMPTOMS

- Difficulty breathing, wheezing, shortness of breath
- Tightness in the chest
- Consistent or uncontrolled coughing
- Swelling of the lips, tongue or throat
- Cyanosis, bluish color around lips or nail beds
- Respiratory failure
- Abdominal cramps
- Swelling on the skin
- Hives, itching, redness
- Extreme pain in area of injury
- Fainting

TREATMENT OPTIONS

This type of emergency calls for immediate medical response. Call 911 first and request ADVANCED life support.

Perform CPR if necessary.

Do you, or does the person have an EpiPen, if so use it. This is a prefilled auto-injector of epinephrine for use in life threatening allergic reactions. They are intended for immediate self-administration as emergency support when there is a severe reaction to allergens, excess exercise, or other known triggers.

These options are the product of conventional wisdom. Be aware that Homeopathy can be quite effective in an anaphylactic situation. The protocol calls for **Apis Mellifica****. The most effective potencies are 30c, 200c and 1M. The more intense the reaction, the higher the potency needed. However, always use whatever you have on hand. During an allergic emergency repeat the remedy as often as every 30 seconds. You may be surprised that by the time help arrives you have the situation under control.

**Warning: APIS MELLIFICA is not recommended for pregnant women.

BEE STINGS- Remove the stinger as soon as possible. A simple method is to scrape across the skin with a credit card. Do not offer food or drink, if the person loses consciousness they may vomit blocking their air passage.

SPIDER & SNAKE BITES- For all stings and bites do the following:

- Place an ice pack on the sting or bite
- Elevate the effected extremity
- Keep the person warm and comfortable

HOMEOPATHIC REMEDIES (REMEDIES CAN BE COMBINED)

- **ACONITUM-** **for shock or trauma, can be repeated first couple of hours.
- **APIS MELLIFICA-** **The 'go-to' bee sting remedy and other severe reactions- dose every 15 minutes, or until pain subsides (do not use if pregnant).
- **ARNICA MONTANA OR BELLIS PERENNIS-** for pain, swelling and bruising during recovery.
- **CARBOLICUM ACIDUM-** **A powerful antiseptic that can be given along with the Apis if there is heightened senses and terrible pain. Especially useful in chemical exposures.
- **CALENDULA-** Topical cream or gel to prevent infection and speeds healing.
- **HYPERICUM-** Useful in spider or snakebites with venom that may affect the nervous system.
- **LACHESIS-** For snakebites.
- **LEDUM-** For all puncture wounds, used as a substitute for tetanus.
- **PYROGENIUM-** If there is sepsis.
- **TARENTULA-** For spider bites.

The above is a representation of the most commonly used Homeopathic remedies for allergic reactions. Consult a Homeopathic Repertory for a more complete list of specific symptoms. Remedies can be combined, as needed.

Anaphylaxis is a serious medical situation and proper medical treatment is needed as soon as possible. However, Homeopathic remedies can be used until medical help arrives and will also hasten healing when used during recovery.

ALTITUDE SICKNESS

Altitude sickness is caused by traveling to high places, like the mountains, where there is a decrease in oxygen, low barometric pressure and dry air. Some people are affected at 5,000 feet and others not until 8,000 or 10,000 feet. The reason a person is affected, while another is not, has to do with liver function. Usually, optimum liver function can handle the stress to the body and adjust accordingly.

When I traveled to Peru the guides gave everyone Coca leaves to chew before climbing Machu Picchu. It is a very effective method for adapting to the change in altitude.

If you are traveling to a high altitude bring along a Homeopathic kit that contains the remedies that can prevent and/or reduce your symptoms.

HOMEOPATHY

ARGENTUM NITRICUM- dizziness or the sensation the mountains are closing in on you.

ACONITUM- shock, fear.

ARSENICUM ALBUM- nausea, diarrhea and vomiting.

BRYONIA- nausea and faintness when rising up.

CALCAREA CARBONICA- sour belching and/or vomiting.

CARBO VEGETABELIS- stomach upset, queasiness.

CHELIDONIUM- for nausea and/or gallbladder discomfort.

COCA- (This is a homeopathic remedy, not a drug.) Most effective remedy for the symptoms of dizziness, headache, shortness of breath, fainting, hoarseness, palpitations, anxiety, insomnia.

IPECACUANHA- nausea and vomiting, headache.

LYCOPODIUM- assists liver function, digestion.

NUX VOMICA- stomach upset, over-indulgence in food or drink, anxiety.

SILICA- vomiting after drinking, or swallowing food, chilliness, sour belching; feels like cold stone in stomach.

SPIGELLIA- nausea with sensation of a worm rising in throat, pressure in stomach, nausea on empty stomach.

SULPHER- great acidity, weak and faint, belching like bad eggs, worse at night.

BITES

Any type of animal bite can be dangerous, since domestic animals, as well as wild animals can have rabies. This is especially true with squirrels, skunks, raccoons, bats, and the fox. Even the neighbor's dog can be infected with rabies, which can account for the animals' violent behavior.

A human bite can be just as dangerous. Humans can transmit many types of diseases, such as HIV, AIDS or Hepatitis B. Humans also have hundreds of other germs in their mouths such as bacteria, fungus and even parasites.

Always seek proper medical treatment.

SYMPTOMS

- Some evidence of teeth marks
- Swelling
- Pain
- Skin Rash

If a poisonous bite:

- Cramping
- Sweating
- Nausea
- Vomiting
- Dizziness

TREATMENT

- Stop the bleeding with a dry sterile cloth and apply pressure to the wound.
- Flush the wound with clean water consistently for a few minutes (This is critical if it is an animal bite and you suspect rabies).
- Wash with soap and water (A turkey baster will further assist in flushing the wound).
- Pour Hydrogen Peroxide on the wound to further disinfect.
- Make a poultice with Sodium Bicarbonate (Baking Soda) before wrapping wound.
- Ice the area.
- Check for shock or if breathing is normal (If not perform CPR).
- Transport to the hospital if necessary.

Hydrogen peroxide is the first 'go-to' as a disinfectant. Colloidal Silver is also recommended for protection against infection. It is anti-bacterial, anti-fungal and anti-parasitic. Use a liquid form orally and a gel topically to hastening healing.

HOMEOPATHIC REMEDIES

- **ACONITUM-** For shock and trauma, usually one dose is sufficient.
- **APIS + ARSENICUM ALBUM-** if there is itching with extreme anxiety.
- **ARNICA MONTANA-** For bleeding, swelling, bruising- dose every 15 minutes up to 6 doses.
- **CARBO VEGETABILIS-** This remedy has antiseptic properties and is indicated if the person is having trouble breathing.
- **CALENDULA** cream- use topically on broken skin to help protect against infection and to hasten healing; I prefer cream to gel, since some gels contain alcohol and can burn when applied. Calendula tincture can be used in warm water to soak the bite.
- **FERRUM PHOS & KALI MUR,** one dose of each, every hour until pain is gone.
- **LEDUM-** Every 15-30 minutes for animal bites where there is puncture, this remedy can mimic tetanus.

BLACK WIDOW BITE

- **LACHESIS-** One dose every 15 minutes.
- **LACTRODECTUS MACTANS-** if Lachesis does not work, this acts as an anti-venom.
- **LEDUM-** If affected area is cold to the touch and the pain subsides with icing.

CORAL SNAKE BITE

Coral snake bites may be painless at first. Major symptoms may not develop for hours. Do NOT make the mistake of thinking you will be fine if the bite area looks good and you are not in a lot of pain. Coral snake bites are poisonous and can be deadly.

Coral snakes are not to be confused with King snakes. Coral snakes have red bands bordered by yellow or white, whereas King snakes have red bands bordered by black. Their venom is a poisonous neurotoxin that paralyzes the central nervous system. The antivenin is Micrurus fulvius.

EMERGENCY MEDICAL RESPONSE SYMPTOMS (CALL 911)

- Blurred vision
- Breathing difficulty
- Convulsions
- Drowsiness
- Eyelid drooping
- Headache
- Low blood pressure
- Mouth-watering (excess salivation)
- Nausea and vomiting
- Numbness
- Pain and swelling at site of bite
- Paralysis
- Shock
- Slurred speech
- Swallowing difficulty
- Swelling of tongue and throat
- Weakness
- Skin color changes
- Skin tissue damage
- Stomach or abdominal pain
- Weak pulse

TREATMENT

- Flush the area of the bite
- Wash with warm water and soap
- Splint to minimize movement
- DO NOT apply a tourniquet
- DO NOT try to remove venin by cutting or sucking
- DO NOT raise extremities above heart level
- Keep person warm
- Elevate lower extremities to eliminate shock
- Do not dispense anything by mouth
- Perform CPR if necessary

HOMEOPATHY

- **CEDRON-** (Rattlesnake bean) antidotes the effects of snake bite and stings of insects, there is a marked periodicity to symptoms, especially fever.
- **CROTALUS HORRIDUS-** Dispense one dose and wait 15 minutes to see if bleeding stops. If not, re-dose.
- **ELAPS CORALLINUS-** This is diluted coral snake venin and can be the most important remedy. One dose every 15 minutes, up to 6 doses, or until symptoms subside.
- **LACHESIS-** Assists in all types of sepsis.
- **PYROGENIUM-** After stabilization to prevent tissue destruction and to assist in clearing any sepsis.

BLEEDING

Some bleeding issues can be life threatening, while others are fairly mild and can be brought under control easily.

If there is bright red blood spurting out of a wound, then there is probably artery damage and it is necessary to call 911. This can be life threatening.

If the blood is a darker red color and flowing at a slower pace it is more likely to be a vein that has been torn. This is not as serious. An artery cut on an angle will repair itself fairly quickly. One that is a straight cut will close off and can become a bleeder. This type of injury needs immediate attention to stop hemorrhaging.

TREATMENT

- If a person is unconscious call 911.
- Make sure they are breathing, if not perform CPR.
- Observe the wound and locate the source of bleeding.
- With a clean compress, using the flat of the hand, apply pressure to the area. If it does not stop, apply another compress; do not remove the first one.
- Elevate the injured area.
- Indirect pressure points can also be used to stop bleeding. They are the bronchial artery on the upper inside of the arm (pinch between the bicep and triceps as tightly as you can with continuous pressure. The other is the femoral artery, which is where the leg connects to the body. Place the palm of the hand down firmly in this area. Apply pressure on the same side of the body as the bleeding. Continue this until help arrives.
- Use a tourniquet if necessary and DO NOT remove until help arrives and a professional can take over.

Hydrogen peroxide is the first 'go-to' as a disinfectant. Colloidal Silver is also recommended for protection against infection. It is anti-bacterial, anti-fungal and anti-parasitic. Use a liquid form orally and a gel topically to hastening healing.

YARROW has antispasmodic effects because of the flavonoids it contains. The herb also has salicylic acid (key ingredient in aspirin) that can reduce pain. Yarrow can be purchased as an herbal tincture and used on a cotton swab to slow bleeding.

HOMEOPATHY

After immediate treatment has been given, the following remedies can assist in slowing down and even stopping bleeding.

- **ARNICA MONTANA-** One dose every 15 minutes up to 6 doses for swift, spirting blood.
- **HAMAMELIS VIRGINICA-** bleeding is slow and a dark red.
- **MILLEFOLIUM-** liquid blood, dripping, painless.
- **PHOSPHORUS-** extremely effective and indicated especially if the patient is fearful of health and requesting cold drinks.
- **CALENDULA-** Used topically as a cream, assists in wound healing.

BLISTERS

Blisters can be annoying and painful, but usually not serious. They are fluid filled sacs that look like bubbles on the skin. They are caused by any number of situations, from burns, to shoes that are too tight, to doing yard work without gloves. Blisters can also be the result of viral outbreaks like Herpes, or from Impetigo, or frostbite. When using Homeopathic medicines, the remedy of choice is according to symptoms and sensations, rather than a disease diagnosis.

TREATMENT
- Remove source of irritation.
- Keep clean.
- Sterilize a needle with a match and puncture to release fluid.
- Apply calendula cream or colloidal silver gel.
- If you do not have the above, substitute a poultice of baking soda.
- Dress with the flannel type bandages or a water-based gel pad (like 2nd Skin).
- After properly dressing the wound Homeopathic remedies can help to speed up the healing process.

HOMEOPATHY
- **CALENDULA TINCTURE-** for soaking.
- **CANTHARIS-** If there is burning and itching.
- **ALLIUM CEPA-** if there is pricking and burning (heels).
- **BORAX-** if oozing.
- **RHUS TOXICODENDRON-** If there is redness, swelling and itching
- **CELL SALTS- FERRUM PHOS & KALI MUR** if pain is relieved by cold.
- **KALI PHOS-** If there is itching.

BRUISE (CONTUSION)

A bruise is when the skin has been injured by a blunt blow, but not broken, and the tissue beneath is damaged.

TREATMENT

- Place direct pressure to the area
- Elevate the extremity
- Ice the site of injury (do not put ice directly on skin) A bag of frozen peas works well if handy)

If a bone is fractured call for immediate medical response, 911, do not move the person.

Hydrogen peroxide is the first 'go-to' as a disinfectant. Colloidal Silver is also recommended for protection against infection. It is anti-bacterial, anti-fungal and anti-parasitic. Use a liquid form orally and a gel topically to hastening healing.

HOMEOPATHY

- **ACONITUM-** If the person is in shock from trauma, one dose.
- **ARNICA**** - To immediately slow down swelling and bruising and to address the pain take every 15 minutes along with **HAMEMELIS**, then 3 times daily until bruising has disappeared.
- **ARNICA CREAM-** Topically the use of Arnica will speed healing of the bruise and bring down swelling.
- **BELLIS PERENNIS-** Muscles, glands and highly innervated areas.
- **FERRUM PHOS-** Every 3-4 hours, a great anti-inflammatory.
- **LEDUM-** (After Arnica) older injury with large haematomas with cold skin.
- **SYMPHYTUM-** If there is a fracture, this remedy can address knitting the bone. Take one dose two times daily for three weeks.

BURNS

Burns can be minor or seriously life threatening, depending on if they are first, second, or third degree. Burns many times can be accompanied by shock or even breathing difficulties.

HEAT OR THERMAL BURNS
- **FIRST DEGREE-** Skin is inflamed, but does not blister.
- **SECOND DEGREE-** Blisters form on the burning, red skin.
- **THIRD DEGREE-** Burned area may be brown or charred, or chalk white Blood vessels may be seen clotting under the skin. There is no pain in the area, since the nerve endings have been destroyed Skin is leathery and dry.

TREATMENT

If the burn is first degree, it is important to take the "heat" out of the burn. Ice it (with a cloth between the ice and skin) or use a bag of frozen peas, or cool water it the skin is not broken.

If the burn is second degree and already has blisters DO Not Break Them. This causes scarring and also encourages infection. Gently take the heat out without breaking blisters.

If it is third degree, seek medical attention immediately.

There is another option that seems contrary, however it works. Dr. Ratera writes about this treatment in his book, *First Aid with Homeopathy*. Apply heated alcohol on a gauze (not hotter than 140°F/60°C) directly to the burn. Give the person a dose of Cantharis 30C and repeat every 10-15 minutes until pain is gone.

An efficient means and little known method of healing burns without scarring is with the use of an egg. Yes, you read that correctly. Scramble a raw egg and brush at least twice daily over the burned area. The egg contains the protein necessary to grow new skin. You will be amazed at the results.

Another more common method of healing burns is to use a compress dampened with colloidal silver changed frequently. It goes a long way to avoid infection and hasten healing. As an alternative, make a poultice from baking soda and water. This will ward off infection and reduce oxidative stress (free radicals) so the skin can heal more efficiently.

HOMEOPATHY
- **ACONITUM-** For shock and trauma, 1 or 2 doses should be sufficient.
- **APIS MELLIFICA-** To take out the "sting" or burning, use Cantharis if no result after 2 doses.
- **ARNICA MONTANA-** for pain relief, dose every 3-4 hours.
- **CALENDULA-** As a salve, topically will hasten healing.

- **CANTHARIS-** To take out the "sting", as needed if Apis has no effect and if there is relief from cold applications.
- **CAUSTICUM-** If there is weeping; every 15 minutes until there is change up to 6 doses.
- **HYPERICUM-** For third degree when there is nerve damage, 3 times per day until burns are healed.
- **KALI BICHROMIUM-** For second degree to bring down blisters, as needed.
- **URTICA URENS-** Helps with the burning and hastens healing, use as needed.
- **CELL SALTS- FERRUM PHOS & KALI MUR,** one dose of each, every 2 hours.

CHEMICAL BURNS

If chemicals containing acid or alkali have splashed onto your skin, there may be a reaction depending on the chemicals in question. If burning, redness and/or pain appear act quickly.

Wash the sight thoroughly and be careful not to splash into eyes. Gently pat dry with a clean dry dressing.

Take Aconitum if there is shock or trauma. Apis or Cantharis for the burning sensation and apply Calendula cream to hasten healing.

Seek medical attention immediately if it involves dangerous chemicals, or if the burns are severe. Use a baking soda and water poultice, since it will draw and neutralizes toxins. (and don't forget the egg, as mentioned above)

ELECTRICAL BURNS

Electrical burns can cause heart disruption and CPR may be necessary. Electrical burns occur when there is direct contact with high or low voltage. The most common home accident for this type of burn is children sticking things into electrical sockets.

There may be a small entrance point for the burn and it is important to look for an exit point. This type of burn can cause damage to muscles, but will not be readily noticeable. It may cause muscle contractions that could fracture a bone or compression fractures.

SYMPTOMS

- Unconsciousness
- Small entrance wound…large exit wound
- Fractures
- Dislocations

TREATMENT

- Call 911 IMMEDIATELY.
- DO NOT touch the person until electrical source is turned off (even if you are tempted to).
- When safe, perform CPR if the person is not breathing.
- Treat the shock with **Aconitum** every 15 minutes, up to six doses, until there is change.

CARBON MONOXIDE POISONING

Carbon monoxide (CO) is a gas that has no odor or color. But it is very dangerous. It can cause sudden illness and death. CO is found in combustion fumes, such as those made by cars and trucks, lanterns, stoves, gas ranges and heating systems. CO from these fumes can build up in places that don't have a good flow of fresh air and you can be poisoned by inhalation.

COMMON SYMPTOMS

- Headache
- Dizziness
- Weakness
- Nausea
- Vomiting
- Chest pain
- Confusion

It is often hard to tell if someone has CO poisoning, because the symptoms may be like those of other illnesses. People who are sleeping or intoxicated can die from CO poisoning before they have symptoms. A CO detector can warn you if you have high levels of CO in your home.

TREATMENT

This situation calls for EMERGENCY MEDICAL RESPONSE, CALL 911

- Protect yourself from the source of fumes first.
- Remove yourself, or the person, from the contaminated area.
- Perform CPR if necessary.

HOMEOPATHY

- **ANTIMONIUM TARTARICUM-** Helps to clear bronchi and lungs, one dose every 15 minutes up to 6 doses.
- **ARSENICUM ALBUM-** Relieves nausea and vomiting, one dose every 15 minutes until symptoms subside.
- **CAMPHOR-** Helps to bring subject back from shock, one dose every 15 minutes for up to 6 doses.
- **CARBO VEGETABLIS-** A powerful antiseptic that can reverse the symptoms of poisoning, one dose every 15 minutes, up to three doses.
- **PHOSPHORUS-** If there is paralysis; every 15 minutes, as needed. Continue 3 times per day for a week after exposure. It will help to drain toxins from the lymph system.
- **CELL SALT- KALI PHOS-** 1 dose every 3-4 hours until improvement.

CONCUSSION

A concussion is a type of brain injury. It's the most minor form. Technically, a concussion is a short loss of normal brain function in response to a head injury. But people often use it to describe any minor injury to the head or brain.

Concussions are a common type of sports injury. You can also have one if you suffer a blow to the head or hit your head after a fall.

Symptoms of a concussion may not start right away; they may start days or weeks after the injury. Symptoms may include a headache or neck pain. You may also have nausea, ringing in your ears, dizziness, or tiredness. You may feel dazed or not your normal self for several days or weeks after the injury. Consult your health care professional if any of your symptoms get worse, or if you have more serious symptoms.

SYMPTOMS

- Seizures
- Trouble walking or sleeping
- Weakness, numbness, or decreased coordination
- Repeated vomiting or nausea
- Confusion
- Slurred speech

Doctors use a neurologic exam and imaging tests to diagnose a concussion. Most people recover fully after a concussion, but it can take some time. Rest is very important after a concussion because it helps the brain to heal.

TREATMENT

If there is ANY indication of serious injury seek EMERGENCY MEDICAL RESPONSE, CALL 911. In all cases of head injury, better to be safe than sorry, since they can be fatal.

- Do not move the person.
- Make sure they are breathing, if not perform CPR.
- Do not move or elevate the head.

HOMEOPATHY

ARNICA MONTANA- One dose every 15 minutes for up to 6 doses, continue three times daily for up to a week for pain and swelling.

CICUTA VEROSA- For convulsions put bottle under the nose or dilute a few pellets in water and apply to the skin in the bend of the left elbow.

HELLEBORUS- If no result with Arnica and the head rolls with moaning; also if there is headache with vomiting; one dose every 15 minutes for up to 6 doses.

HYPERICUM- If there are shooting pains from brain and/or spinal cord, sensitive to touch dose every 15 minutes for up to six doses.

NATRUM SULFURICUM- If there is crushing or gnawing pain in the occipital region (back of the head), piercing pain in the ears, or a bursting feeling on coughing; One dose every 15 minutes for up to 6 doses. This remedy should be dispensed in a high dose after the injury. Consult a qualified Homeopath.

CUTS/ LACERATIONS/ WOUNDS

Cuts are injuries that break the skin or other body tissues. They include cuts, scrapes, scratches, and punctured skin. They often happen because of an accident, but surgery, sutures, and stitches also cause wounds. Minor wounds usually aren't serious, but it is important to clean them. Serious and infected wounds may require first aid followed by a visit to your doctor. You should also seek attention if the wound is deep, you cannot close it yourself, you cannot stop the bleeding or get the dirt out, or it does not heal.

SYMPTOMS

- Bleeding
- Swelling
- Bruising
- Pain

TREATMENT

Hydrogen peroxide is the first 'go-to' as a disinfectant. Colloidal Silver is also recommended for protection against infection. It is anti-bacterial, anti-fungal and anti-parasitic. Use a liquid form orally and a gel topically to hastening healing.

- Wash the site thoroughly with soap and water.
- Douse with Hydrogen Peroxide.
- Control the bleeding by applying pressure with a clean, dry cloth.
- Prevent further contamination.
- Immobilize the affected part.
- Apply a poultice made from baking soda and water.
- Bandage and splint if necessary.

HOMEOPATHY

- **CALENDULA-** as a tincture for flushing the wound.
- **CALENDULA CREAM-** applied before bandaging.
- **ARNICA MONTANA-** Assists in keeping down swelling, or bruising and slows bleeding.
- **HAMAMELIS-** Relieves pain and assists in slowing of bleeding.
- **HYPERICUM-** If the cut has caused nerve damage.
- **PHOSPHORUS-** Slows bleeding, especially if there is a desire for cold drinks.
- **CELL SALTS-** (If swelling is present) **FERRUM PHOS & KALI MUR;** One dose of each, every 2 hours.

DEHYDRATION

When you're dehydrated, your body doesn't have enough fluid to work properly. An average person on an average day needs about 3 quarts of water. But if you're out in the hot sun, you'll need a lot more than that. Most healthy bodies are very good at regulating water. Elderly people, young children and some special cases - like people taking certain medications - need to be a little more careful.

There are three stages of dehydration, *Mild*, *Moderate* and *Severe to Life threatening*. The stages define themselves as going from fatigued and thirsty with dark urine in the mild stage to very dry mouth, diminished urine and increased dizziness in moderate to swollen tongue and actual loss of consciousness in the severe stage.

SYMPTOMS

- Being thirsty
- Urinating less often than usual
- Dark-colored urine
- Dry skin
- Feeling tired
- Dizziness and fainting
- Nausea
- Either rapid or weak pulse
- Loss of consciousness
- Delirium

SYMPTOMS IN BABIES AND YOUNG CHILDREN

- Dry mouth and tongue
- Crying without tears
- No wet diapers for 3 hours or more
- A high fever
- Being unusually sleepy or drowsy

TREATMENT

- Call for EMERGENCY MEDICAL RESPONSE, 911 if the symptoms are severe.
- Check vital signs, if not breathing, perform CPR. If you are in sunlight, move to a shaded area.
- If you think you're dehydrated, drink small amounts of water over a period of time. Taking too much all at once can overload your stomach and make you throw up.

- For people exercising in the heat and losing a lot of minerals in sweat, drinks with electrolytes are helpful. Avoid any drinks that have caffeine or alcohol.
- DO NOT drink milk or other dairy products DO NOT take in solid foods.
- Coconut water is an excellent choice to rehydrate quickly.

HOMEOPATHY

- **BELLADONNA-** If the person is red and flushed in the face and has bright red ears, one dose every 15 minutes, up to 6 doses.
- **CALCAREA PHOSPHORICUM-** ailments from general loss of fluids.
- **CARBO VEGETABLIS-** Improves oxidation, one dose every 15 minutes up to 6 doses.
- **CHINA-** Vertigo, fainting, weakness, one dose every 15 minutes up to 6 doses.
- **CINCHONA-** If there is exhaustion and debility from loss of fluids (symptoms may include- bloating, headache, flushed face, sensitive scalp, buzzing in ears, pressure or a sensation of sand in eyes.)
- **PHOSPHORICUM ACIDUM-** Fainting, place bottle under nose.
- **VERATRUM ALBUM-** If there is extreme coldness, one to two doses should bring a response.

TO HELP TO AVOID OR RECOVER FROM DEHYDRATION

Utilize the following formula:

- 16 BIOPLASMA pellets
- ¼ cup yogurt with Bifidus or Kefir
- ¼–½ cup fresh lemon juice
- Maple syrup or honey to taste
- ¼ tsp salt (not Himalayan)

Combine and take a teaspoon as often as necessary until recovered.

DENTAL TRAUMA

I refer to dental trauma as any disturbance having to do with your teeth from a toothache to extractions to abscess. I have also included teething, since much can be done to relieve the pain and discomfort some children experience when teething. The effects of Homeopathy can be magical when it comes to dental issues. I have turned more than one dentist on to suggesting Homeopathy to their patients to assist them in getting through dental trauma. Below are remedy suggestions to help you to be prepared in the event you have to deal with painful dental situations. (See Gingivitis & Tooth Decay in the next Chapter for more suggestions)

Don't forget to use Baking Soda to wash out the mouth. It kills germs and hastens healing by balancing the pH of saliva and reducing free radicals.

Remedies can be repeated often (every 15 minutes) until there is improvement, and more than one remedy can be dispensed. As an example, Chamomilla can be given to a fussy child along with Arnica for pain or swelling.

HOMEOPATHY

- **ACONITUM-** to be given in advance of dental procedure if patient is fearful and traumatized.
- **ARNICA-** for extractions; slows bleeding, pain, bruising, swelling.
- **BELLIS PERENNIS-** helps to reduce bruising, soreness, boils, fever.
- **CHAMOMILLA-** the patient is fussy, irritable, quarrelsome, impatient, chilly but gets overheated easily.
- **COFFEA CRUDA-** pain and swelling can be brought down for patients that are highly excitable, nervous, pain is unbearable, do not want to be touched, restless and affected by noise and light, extremely restless and wants cold water in the mouth.
- **KREOSOTUM-** decayed teeth (black).
- **GELSEMIUM-** to be dispensed in advance of dental visits for anxiety and fear from anticipation.
- **HEPAR SULPH CALCAREA-** can drain abscesses quickly and relieve pain and swelling (antibiotic substitute).
- **HYPERICUM-** if there is nerve damage (do not use prior to treatment).
- **LYCOPODIUM-** if teeth are becoming loose.
- **MERCURIUS SOLUBILIS-** for infection, decay, abscess, loosening of teeth.
- **PHOSPHORUS-** slows bleeding and even hemorrhaging.

TEETHING

- **ACONITUM-** if there is fever, fear and the child seems traumatized.
- **CALCAREA CARBONICA-** if teething is late.
- **CALC. PHOS.-** 6X potency should be given as a cell salt preparation two times per day for an extended period during teething to assist in proper dentition and general easing of teething symptoms.
- **CHAMOMILLA-** if one cheek is red, child is irritable and fussy, wants to be carried.
- **PODOPHYLLUM-** if there is diarrhea.
- **SILICEA-** if teething is late.

DISLOCATED JOINTS

A dislocation is a separation of two bones where they meet at a joint. Joints are areas where two bones come together. The dislocated bone is no longer in its normal position.

Most dislocations can be treated in a doctor's office or emergency room. You may be given medicine to make you sleepy and to numb the area. Sometimes, general anesthesia in the operating room is needed. When treated early, most dislocations will not result in permanent injury. Once a joint has been dislocated, it is more likely to happen again, so care should be extended to the area.

CAUSES

Dislocations are usually caused by a sudden impact to the joint. This usually occurs following a blow, fall, or other trauma.

SYMPTOMS

- A dislocated joint may be:
- Accompanied by numbness or tingling at the joint or beyond it
- Intensely painful, especially if you try to use the joint or bear weight on it
- Limited in movement
- Swollen or bruised
- Visibly out of place, discolored, or misshapen

Nursemaid's elbow is a partial dislocation common in toddlers. The main symptom is refusal to use the arm. Nursemaid's elbow can be easily treated in a doctor's office.

TREATMENT

- Call 911 before you begin treating someone who may have a dislocation, especially if the accident causing the injury may be life-threatening.
- If there has been a serious injury, check the person's airway, breathing, and circulation. If necessary, begin rescue breathing or CPR, or bleeding control.
- Do not move the person if you think that the head, back, or leg has been injured. Keep the person still. Provide reassurance.
- If the skin is broken, take steps to prevent infection. Do not blow on the wound. Rinse the area gently to remove obvious dirt, but do not scrub or probe. Cover the area with sterile dressings before immobilizing the injury.
- Apply ice packs to ease pain and swelling.
- Take steps to prevent shock unless there is a head, leg, or back injury, lay the victim flat, elevate the feet about 12 inches, and cover the person with a coat or blanket.

ACUPUNCTURE

Acupuncture treatments can be very helpful after this type of injury, since the soft tissue may have been damaged.

OSTEOPATHIC OR CRANIAL SACRAL THERAPY

Both treatments can help to bring normal energy flow back to the injured area and prevent further injury.

HOMEOPATHY

- **RHUS TOXACODENDRON-** For shoulder dislocation, lameness in joint, coldness in limb, pain worse from first movement and/or sharp sudden pain.
- **RUTA GRAV-** Pain worse when lying down, if there is a bruised sensation.
- **CELL SALTS- FERRUM PHOS, MAG PHOS, CALC FLUOR, CALC PHOS-** three times daily, one dose of each

EYE INJURY

An eye injury can occur under any circumstance. Treatment is needed as soon as possible if the injury appears to be severe. The most pressing issue is retinal detachment. The retina is the light-sensitive layer of tissue that lines the inside of the eye and sends visual messages through the optic nerve to the brain. When the retina detaches, it is lifted or pulled from its normal position. If not promptly treated, retinal detachment can cause permanent vision loss.

In some cases, there may be small areas of the retina that are torn. These areas, called retinal tears or retinal breaks, can lead to retinal detachment.

SYMPTOMS OF RETINAL DETACHMENT

- Sudden or gradual increase in either the number of floaters, which are little "cobwebs" or specks that float about in your field of vision, and/or light flashes in the eye.
- The appearance of a curtain over the field of vision.
- A retinal detachment is a medical emergency. Anyone experiencing the symptoms of a retinal detachment should see an eye care professional immediately.

For less severe eye injury Homeopathy can help to alleviate symptoms.

HOMEOPATHY

- **ACONITUM-** For shock or trauma every 15 minutes to ½ hour up to 6 doses.
- **ARNICA-** For pain, bruising, swelling, every couple of hours initially.
- **CALENDULA-** Can be used as a tincture to rinse eye and encourage healing.
- **EUPHRASIA-** (Eyebright) For inflammation (also great for conjunctivitis) Can be used as a tincture to wash out the eye and also taken internally to encourage reduction of inflammation.
- **PHYSOSTIGMA-** flashes of light and/or if astigmatism is present.
- **CELL SALTS- CALC SUPLH & FERRUM PHOS, NAT MUR**

FAINTING

Fainting is a temporary loss of consciousness. If you're about to faint, you'll feel dizzy, lightheaded, or nauseous. Your field of vision may "white out" or "black out." Your skin may be cold and clammy. You lose muscle control at the same time, and may fall down.

CAUSES

Fainting usually happens when your blood pressure drops suddenly, causing a decrease in blood flow to your brain. Sometimes your heart rate and blood vessels can't react fast enough when your body's need for oxygen changes. This is very common among older people and in people who have certain health conditions, such as diabetes. Fainting can happen when:

- You stand up too fast.
- You work or play hard, especially if it's very hot.
- You begin to breathe too fast (called hyperventilating).
- You get very upset. Being upset can affect the nerves that control your blood pressure.
- You're taking medicine for high blood pressure.

Coughing, urinating and stretching can also get in the way of the flow of oxygen to the brain and may cause you to faint. If you faint once during one of these activities, it's probably not something to worry about. But if it happens more than once, tell your doctor about it.

If you faint when you turn your head to the side, the bones in your neck may be pinching on one of the blood vessels that leads to your brain. If this happens to you, be sure to tell your doctor about it.

A drop in your blood sugar may also cause you to faint. This can happen if you have diabetes, but it may also happen if you don't eat for a long time.

Some prescription medicines can cause fainting. Be sure to talk to your doctor if you think your fainting may be related to a medicine you're taking. Alcohol, cocaine and marijuana can also cause fainting.

More serious causes of fainting include seizures and problems with the heart or with the blood vessels leading to the brain.

SYMPTOMS

- Heat or dehydration
- Emotional distress
- Standing up too quickly
- Certain medicines
- Drop in blood sugar
- Heart problems

When someone faints, make sure that the airway is clear and check for breathing. The person should stay lying down for 10-15 minutes. Most people recover completely. Fainting is usually nothing to worry about, but it can sometimes be a sign of a serious problem. If you faint, it's important to see your health care provider and find out why it happened.

WHO IS AT RISK?

People who have certain medical conditions are more likely to faint. These conditions include:

- Heart problems such as an irregular heartbeat or blockages in or near the heart that block the blood from getting to the brain
- Diabetes
- Anxiety or panic disorders
- Dehydration
- Low blood sugar

WHAT TO DO IF I FEEL LIKE I'M GOING TO FAINT?

Before fainting, you may feel lightheaded, dizzy, like the room is spinning, sick to your stomach. You may also have blurry vision or a hard time hearing. If you feel like you're going to faint, lie down. If you can't lie down, sit and bend forward with your head between your knees. This helps get the blood flowing to your brain. Wait until you feel better before trying to stand up. When you stand up, do so slowly.

TREATMENT

If the fainting spell is serious call 911 for immediate medical response

- Secure the airway, perform CPR if necessary.
- Control bleeding if there is an injury.
- Elevate extremities, but keep person lying down.
- Keep the person warm.
- Do not dispense any food or drink.

HOMEOPATHY

When someone has fainted it is best not to put anything in the mouth. The remedies can be waved under the nose, or diluted in a little water and rubbed into the bend of the left elbow or behind the ear on the left side if possible.

- **ACONITUM-** One to two doses fifteen minutes apart should be sufficient to shift the shock and/or trauma.
- **ARNICA-** One dose every fifteen minutes if there is pain, up to 6 doses.
- **IGNATIA-** If the cause is grief. One to two doses fifteen minutes apart should be sufficient to shift the emotional state. Consult a professional Homeopath to treat with a higher dose if grief state lingers for an abnormal amount of time.
- **NUX MOSHATA-** fainting due to the sight of blood. One dose every 15 minutes until improvement.

FOOD & WATER POISONING

The National Institutes of Health report that each year 48 million people in the U.S. get sick from contaminated food. Common culprits include bacteria, parasites and viruses. Symptoms range from mild to serious.

SYMPTOMS

- Upset stomach
- Abdominal cramps
- Nausea and vomiting
- Diarrhea
- Fever
- Dehydration
- Weakness

Harmful bacteria are the most common cause of food borne illness. Foods may have some bacteria on them when you buy them. Raw meat may become contaminated during slaughter. Fruits and vegetables may become contaminated when they are growing or when they are processed. But it can also happen in your kitchen if you leave food out for more than 2 hours at room temperature. Handling food safely can help prevent food borne illnesses.

There are actually three specific pathogens that cause food poisoning. They are *Staphylococcus, Botulism* and *Ptomaine.*

STAPHYLOCOCCUS is the more common culprit, since it is from food left out too long without refrigeration. It is the food poisoning that happens at picnics from mayonnaise-based foods that linger too long in the sun. A bacterium develops toxins due to the warm conditions.

BOTULISM is the most severe form of food poisoning, since it attacks the nervous system. It is from the Clostridium bacteria and grows rapidly in food that is not kept heated (like chicken) or not cooked at a high enough temperature to kill off the bacteria that already exists. This type of bacteria can kill and emergency medical treatment is necessary as soon as possible.

PTOMAINE POISONING is from Salmonella. Salmonella is commonly found in eggs (and on their shells), lettuce and other greens contaminated by animal feces and is even carried by humans who can spread the bacteria to others.

TREATMENT

Emergency treatment may be needed for any type of food poisoning. It depends largely on the health of the individual. Someone in a robust healthy state can easily ward off a bit of food poisoning as the immune system kicks in. Small children or the elderly may not fare as well. It may also take up to 24 hours for symptoms to appear.

The treatment in most cases is increasing your fluid intake. For more serious illness, you may need treatment at a hospital. It is wise to drink ½ tsp. of baking soda in water every two hours to begin to kill off pathogens and to rebalance pH.

HOMEOPATHY

Homeopathy is extremely successful in the treatment of food poisoning. If symptoms do not subside in a fairly short period of time (1-2 hours) after taking remedies seek profession assistance.

- **ARSENICUM ALBUM-** treats anxiety with nausea or vomiting, burning stomach pain, diarrhea and dyspepsia, one dose every fifteen minutes up to six doses. Can continue to take two to three times per day for the next few days to continue to resolve infection.
- **CALCAREA PHOSPHORICA-** improves weak digestion, especially in babies. One dose 2-3 times per day for two to three weeks, or until improvement is seen.
- **LYCOPODIUM-** indigestion and nausea, effects from tainted oysters, one dose every 15 minutes until symptoms subside.
- **NUX VOMICA-** treats nausea, hiccoughs from overeating, weight and pain in the stomach, vomiting or the sensation to vomit, dizziness and feeling faint. One dose every 15 minutes until symptoms subside. Can be taken regularly for stomach disturbance and curbs handovers.
- **PYROGENIUM-** effects of bad meat, one dose every 15 minutes up to six doses.
- **CELL SALTS- KALI PHOS, NAT PHOS & CALC PHOS;** one dose of each every 2–4 hours for up to 3 days.

FRACTURES

A fracture is a break, usually in a bone. If the broken bone punctures the skin, it is called an open or compound fracture. Fractures commonly happen because of car accidents, falls or sports injuries. Other causes are low bone density and osteoporosis, which cause weakening of the bones. Overuse can cause stress fractures, which are very small cracks in the bone.

SYMPTOMS

- Out-of-place or misshapen limb or joint
- Swelling, bruising or bleeding
- Intense pain
- Numbness and tingling
- Limited mobility or inability to move a limb

Medical care is needed right away for any fracture. You may need to wear a cast or splint. Sometimes you need surgery to repair with plates, pins, or screws to keep the bone in place.

FRACTURES, COMPRESSION

Your backbone, or spine, is made up of 26 bone discs called vertebrae. The vertebrae protect your spinal cord and allow you to stand and bend.

A number of problems can change the structure of the spine or damage the vertebrae and surrounding tissue. They include:

- Infections
- Injuries
- Tumors
- Conditions, such as ankylosing spondylitis and scoliosis.
- Bone changes that come with age, such as spinal stenosis and herniated disks.
- Spinal diseases often cause pain when bone changes put pressure on the spinal cord or nerves. They can also limit movement. Treatments differ by diagnosis, sometimes doctors recommend back braces and/or surgery.

FRACTURES, SKULL

Chances are you've bumped your head before. Usually, the injury is minor because your skull is hard and it protects your brain. But other head injuries can be more severe, such as a skull fracture, concussion, or traumatic brain injury.

Head injuries can be open or closed. A closed injury does not break through the skull. With an open, or penetrating, injury, an object pierces the skull and enters brain tissue. Closed injuries are not always less severe than open injuries.

Some common causes of head injuries are falls, motor vehicle accidents, violence, and sports injuries.

It is important to know the warning signs of a moderate or severe head injury. Get help immediately if the injured person has:

- A headache that gets worse or does not go away
- Repeated vomiting or nausea
- Convulsions or seizures
- An inability to wake up
- Dilation of one or both pupils of the eyes
- Slurred speech
- Weakness or numbness in the arms or legs
- Loss of coordination
- Increased confusion, restlessness, or agitation

FRACTURES, RIB

It is important to take care of yourself when dealing with cracked ribs. Some common sense can go a long way to hastening the healing process.

- Get an x-ray to be sure it is not more serious than a hairline fracture. Shattered fragments can cause much more severe issues for lungs, kidneys or other organs.
- Ask for help, avoid any motions you don't have to make like reaching for objects or carrying heavy items (like children or animals).
- Avoid long car rides, especially on bumpy roads.
- Get lots of rest, pain can be exhausting.
- When rising, gently roll onto your side and raise yourself slowly using your arms, rather than abdominal muscles.

HOMEOPATHY

Skull fractures are dangerous and should be treated with proper medical help. While waiting for help acute remedies can be dispensed. There are also a number of remedies that assist in the healing of fractures.

- **ACONITUM-** initial remedy for shock and trauma.
- **ARNICA OR BELLIS-** pain, swelling, bruising.
- **HYPERICUM-** when the fracture is in an area rich with nerves, especially fingers, toes and spine.
- **BRYONIA-** if there is pain days after the fracture; any motion brings on pain and the person is irritable and wants to be left alone.
- **CALCAREA PHOSPHORICA-** if fracture is slow to heal, person is usually irritable and restless.
- **EUPATORIUM PERFOLIATUM-** when there is deep and aching pain, especially weeks later after the break; can also have body ache in unrelated areas.
- **MAGNESIUM PHOSPHORICUM-** works well for muscle spasms with fractured ribs.
- **NATRUM SULPHURICUM-** ill effects of falls or injuries to the head.
- **NUX VOMICA-** works well for fractured ribs if there are spasms.
- **RHUTA GRAVEOLENS-** when there is a bruised painful feeling that remains this remedy will work on bruising of the periosteum (fibrous material that covers the bone).
- **SILICEA-** helps to rebuild bone.
- **SYMPHYTUM-** known as "knit-bone" can be given immediately to heal or later if pain remains in an old injury.

FROSTBITE

Frostbite is an injury to the body that is caused by freezing. It most often affects the nose, ears, cheeks, chin, fingers, or toes. Frostbite can permanently damage the body, and severe cases can lead to amputation.

There are different levels of frostbite. The mildest version is Frostnip, where the skin surface is frozen but not the deeper tissue. Superficial Frostbite is when the skin is frozen and has turned white, yellow or bluish white. Deep Frostbite is when not only the skin is frozen, but the tissue beneath also.

SYMPTOMS

- A white or grayish-yellow skin area
- Skin that feels unusually firm or waxy
- Frostbitten surface is hard to touch
- Numbness
- Bluish skin and/or blisters with deep frostbite If you have symptoms of frostbite, seek medical care TREATMENT
- Get into a warm room as soon as possible.

Unless absolutely necessary, do not walk on frostbitten feet or toes. Walking increases damage. Put the affected area in warm - not hot - water. You can also warm the affected area using body heat. For example, use your armpit to warm frostbitten fingers.

Don't rub the frostbitten area with snow or massage it at all. This can cause more damage.

Don't use a heating pad, heat lamp, or the heat of a stove, fireplace, or radiator for warming. Since frostbite makes an area numb, you could burn it.

HOMEOPATHY

- **AGARICUS MUSCARIUS-** addresses symptoms of burning, itching, redness, swelling and sharp pain of frostbite; One dose every 15 minutes until symptoms subside.
- **APIS MELLIFICA-** takes the "sting" and swelling out of frostbite as it works on cellular tissue.
- **LACHESIS-** assists with capillaries, bluishness, blisters, redness and pain; one dose every 15 minutes until symptoms subside.
- **PETROLEUM-** assists with burning, itching, redness, raw and cracks that bleed easily; initially one dose every 15 minutes until symptoms subside, up to six doses. Can be used two to three times daily until frostbite is healed.
- **ZINC-** if frostbitten easily, for frostbitten nose or toes and ailments from frostbite; dispense as a low potency (6x) daily to improve tendency. Test for zinc deficiency.

The Alternative

HEAD INJURIES (SEE CONCUSSION)

HEAT EXHAUSTION (HEAT STROKE)

Your body normally cools itself by sweating. During hot weather, especially with high humidity, sweating just isn't enough. Your body temperature can rise to dangerous levels and you can develop a heat illness. Most heat illnesses occur from staying out in the heat too long. Exercising too much for your age and physical condition are also factors. Older adults, young children and those who are sick or overweight are most at risk. Drinking fluids to prevent dehydration replenishing salt and minerals, and limiting time in the heat can help.

Heat-related illnesses include:

- **Heatstroke-** a life-threatening illness in which body temperature may rise above 106° F in minutes. Symptoms include dry skin, rapid, strong pulse and dizziness
- **Heat exhaustion-** an illness that can precede heatstroke. Symptoms include heavy sweating, rapid breathing and a fast, weak pulse
- **Heat cramps-** muscle pains or spasms that happen during heavy exercise
- **Heat rash-** skin irritation from excessive sweating

Heat stroke, or Sunstroke is by far the most dangerous. Emergency Medical Response may be necessary, call 911. The person's level of consciousness rapidly decreases.

SYMPTOMS

- Change in behavior
- Decreased blood pressure
- Consciousness decreasing
- Rapid pulse
- Hot, dry skin

TREATMENT

- Remove person from the hot environment
- Cool down the person; remove clothing
- Apply cool towels
- Fan them
- Make sure airway is open; perform CPR if necessary

HOMEOPATHY

- **ACONITUM-** for shock, one dose every 15 minutes for 2 or 3 doses.
- **BELLADONNA-** from sleeping in the sun or body overheating, one dose every 15 minutes until symptoms improve.
- **BRYONIA-** especially if person is chilled, can repeat remedy every 5-10 minutes until improvement.
- **GLONOINE-** relieves throbbing headaches from exposure to the sun, one dose every fifteen minutes until pain subsides.
- **NATRUM CARBONICUM-** long-term effects from Sunstroke (Consult a professional).
- **VERATRUM ALBUM**- If there is chilliness after heat exposure; one dose every fifteen minutes until symptoms subside.
- **CELL SALTS- NAT MUR & FERRUM PHOS**; one dose of each every 15-30 minutes.

HEAT RASH

A heat rash, sometimes known as prickly heat, is just that, an area of the skin that has become irritated and possibly swollen from excess exposure to heat. They are quite common in babies and occurs when the pores of the sweat glands become blocked. This happens most often when the weather is hot or humid. As your infant sweats, little red bumps, and possibly tiny blisters, form because the blocked glands cannot clear the sweat.

During the hot season, dress your baby in lightweight, soft, cotton clothing. Cotton is very absorbent and keeps moisture away from the baby's skin. If air conditioning is not available, a fan may help cool your infant. Place the fan far enough away that there is only a gentle breeze drifting over the infant.

Avoid the use of powders, creams, and ointments. Baby powders do not improve or prevent heat rash. Creams and ointments tend to keep the skin warmer and block the pores.

NATURAL TREATMENT

The first step in improving heat rash is to remove the cause of the heat. The area can then be swabbed with Calendula diluted in water.

HOMEOPATHY

- **APIS-** sudden puffing of the area, or in some cases, the whole body. Skin is hot and raised.
- **ARSENICUM ALBUM-** there is itching, burning and restlessness with anxiety.
- **BELLADONNA-** for sudden intense symptoms of heat and redness that can alternate with paleness; painful.
- **URTICA URENS-** itching, burning, skin better from rubbing and from cold bathing.

HYPERVENTILATION

Hyperventilation is rapid or deep breathing that can occur with anxiety or panic. It is also called over-breathing, and may leave you feeling breathless.

When you breathe, you breathe in oxygen and breathe out carbon dioxide. Excessive breathing creates low levels of carbon dioxide in your blood. This causes many of the symptoms of hyperventilation.

Feeling very anxious or having a panic attack are the usual reasons that you may hyperventilate. However, rapid breathing may be a symptom of a disease, such as:

- Bleeding
- Heart or lung disorder
- Infection

Your doctor or nurse will determine the cause of your hyperventilation. Rapid breathing may be a medical emergency – unless you have had this before and have been reassured by your health care provider that it can be self-treated.

Often, panic and hyperventilation become a vicious cycle. Panic leads to rapid breathing, and breathing rapidly can make you feel panicked.

If there is frequent over-breathing you may have hyperventilation syndrome that is triggered by emotions of stress, anxiety, depression, or anger. Occasional hyperventilation from panic is generally related to a specific fear or phobia, such as a fear of heights, dying, or closed-in spaces (claustrophobia).

If you have hyperventilation syndrome, you might not be aware you are breathing fast. However, you will be aware of having many of the other symptoms, including:

- Belching
- Bloating
- Chest pain
- Confusion
- Dizziness
- Dry mouth
- Lightheadedness
- Muscle spasms in hands and feet
- Numbness and tingling in the arms or around the mouth
- Palpitations
- Shortness of breath
- Sleep disturbances
- Weakness

CAUSES

- Anxiety and nervousness
- Bleeding
- Cardiac disease, such as congestive heart failure or heart attack
- Drugs (such as an aspirin overdose)
- Infection such as pneumonia or sepsis
- Keto-acidosis and similar medical conditions
- Lung disease such as asthma, chronic obstructive pulmonary disease (COPD), or pulmonary embolism
- Panic attack
- Pregnancy
- Severe pain
- Situations where there is a psychological advantage in having a sudden, dramatic illness (for example, somatization disorder)
- Stimulant use
- Stress

CALL YOUR HEALTH CARE PROVIDER IF:

- You are experiencing rapid breathing for the first time. (This is a medical emergency and you should be taken to the emergency room right away.)
- You are in pain, have a fever, or notice any bleeding.
- Your hyperventilation continues or gets worse, even with home treatment.
- You also have other symptoms.

TREATMENTS

- If you are alone breath into a paper bag.
- Remain calm.
- If you are assisting another, have them breath with you.
- Breathe in through the nostril and out through pursed lips.

THE BUTEYKO METHOD

The Buteyko method is neither a medical treatment nor procedure. It does not involve any medication, homeopathy or herbs. It is series of lectures related to breathing that enables people to understand a concept of 'normal breathing' or breathing according to physiological norms. It contains simple breathing techniques and logical instructions to follow. It also gives the means of controlling breathing parameters without any technical appliances. Buteyko method brings the physiological parameters of the body to the norm. It can be easily incorporated into the daily life of any contemporary person. It does not require you to interrupt your everyday activities to perform any sophisticated procedures similar to yogi's 'asana'. You can use the concept of the method at any time in any situation.

HOMEOPATHY

- **ACONITUM-** to calm the effects of shock or trauma, one dose every 15 minutes until symptoms subside, up to 6 doses. Can put bottle under the nose, instead of ingesting pellets.
- **CHAMOMILLA-** if brought on by anger, one dose every 15 minutes until symptoms subside. Can use daily to balance anger and restlessness.
- **IGNATIA-** if brought on by grief, one dose every 15 minutes until symptoms improve.

INSULIN SHOCK (HYPOGLYCEMIA)

Hypoglycemia is a condition that occurs when your blood sugar (glucose) is too low. Blood sugar below 70 mg/dl is considered low. Blood sugar at or below this level can harm you.

CAUSES

- Your body's sugar (glucose) is used up too quickly
- Glucose is released into the bloodstream too slowly
- Too much insulin is released into the bloodstream

Insulin is a hormone that reduces blood sugar. It is produced by the pancreas in response to increased glucose levels in the blood. Low blood sugar is most commonly seen in people with diabetes who are taking insulin or other medicines to control their diabetes. Babies who are born to mothers with diabetes may have severe drops in blood sugar.

NON-DIABETIC CAUSES

- Drinking alcohol
- 'Insulinoma'- a rare tumor in the pancreas that produces too much insulin
- Lack (deficiency) of a hormone, such as cortisol or thyroid hormone
- Severe heart, kidney, or liver failure or a body-wide infection
- Some types of weight-loss surgery

SYMPTOMS

- Double vision or blurry vision
- Fast or pounding heartbeat
- Feeling cranky or acting aggressive
- Feeling nervous
- Headache
- Hunger
- Shaking or trembling
- Sweating
- Tingling or numbness of the skin
- Tiredness or weakness
- Trouble sleeping
- Unclear thinking

Sometimes your blood sugar may be too low, even if you do not have symptoms. If your blood sugar gets too low, you may:

- Faint
- Have a seizure
- Go into a coma

TREATMENT

Treatment depends on the cause. People with diabetes will need to learn how to treat and prevent low blood sugar levels. Diet is the easiest form of treatment for Hypoglycemia. Eating small amounts often helps, as well as balancing sugar intake. Fasting can bring on Hypoglycemia and must be undertaken responsibly.

If signs of low blood sugar do not improve after you have eaten a snack that contains sugar:

- GET A RIDE to the emergency room, or Call a local emergency number (911).
- DO NOT drive when your blood sugar is low.
- Get medical help right away for a person with diabetes or low blood sugar who:
- Becomes less alert.
- Cannot be woken up.

It is possible to be catapulted into a chronic hypoglycemic condition after the incidence of food poisoning. The event can change your gut chemistry, which in turn affects sugar metabolism.

HOMEOPATHY

Any physical constitution can fall victim to Hypoglycemia and should be treated by a professional Homeopath. The symptom particulars are numerous and fall under the category of a number of homeopathic remedy choices, too numerous to mention here.

The following suggestions are based on successful treatment by the Banerji Clinic:

- **CHELIDONIUM 6C-** two times per day, or
- **HELONIAS 200C-** two times per day, or
- **SYZYGIUM-** mother tincture, 5 drops two times per day

SUPPLEMENTS

- **FENUGREEK-** very effective as a tea, in seeds, or as a supplement to balance blood sugar levels.
- **CHROMIUM-** an essential trace mineral that can help to cut cravings for carbohydrates, fight body fat and control blood sugar levels
- **CINNAMON-** not only a spice for food, but can reduce fasting blood glucose, total cholesterol, triglycerides, and "bad" LDL cholesterol, while raising "good" HDL cholesterol.
- **VANADIUM-** a trace mineral that has the ability to lower blood sugar levels and improve sensitivity to insulin in people with type 2 diabetes.

MARINE ANIMAL STINGS

Bites from a Jellyfish, Corals, Anemones, Portuguese Man-O-War & Hydras.

SYMPTOMS

- Intense burning of skin
- Red, raised welt that appears suddenly
- Weakness
- Headache
- Muscle pain or spasms
- Sweating
- Change in pulse rate
- Chest pain and changes in breathing

TREATMENT

- Immediately come out of the water. Jellyfish and other marine stings can be very painful and can inhibit the ability to swim.
- Remove the stinger by applying shaving cream, or some other lubricant to skin and scrape the skin closely with a razor, knife blade or credit card. If you have none of these rub the area with sand to dislodge the stingers and rinse off with salt water.
- Deactivate the remaining stingers by pouring white vinegar or alcohol on the affected area.
- Sprinkle area with meat tenderizer to neutralize venom.
- Dust with baby powder.

ALTERNATIVE TREATMENTS

- Remove any venom by applying a paste of baking soda and water; reapply every 15-20 minutes.
- Ice the area.
- A hot shower can de-activate venom of some jellyfish, particularly Hawaiian box jellyfish.
- Take an antihistamine like Benadryl.

HOMEOPATHY

- **ACONITUM-** treats the shock and or trauma, one dose every 15 minutes.
- **APIS-** to take the "sting" out of the injury, one dose every 15 minutes until symptoms subside.

- **ARNICA-** main remedy for pain, repeat every 30 minutes, or as needed.
- **CALENDULA-** as a cream or gel to apply after treating area to inhibit infection.
- **HYPERICUM–** as a tincture to wash the area 2-3 times per day for a few days after injury.
- **LACHESIS-** an anti-venom, one dose every fifteen minutes until symptoms subside.
- **CELL SALTS- FERRUM PHOS, KALI MUR & CALC SULPH-** one dose of each, every hour, less often as severity is relieved.

MOTION SICKNESS

Motion sickness is the experiencing of unpleasant symptoms when in a setting of motion (like a boat, car trip or plane). The symptoms can vary from nausea to vomiting to headache to diarrhea. It is basically a form of dizziness. Motion sickness can also be confused with Meniere's Disease or Tinnitus, much more serious conditions that bring on similar symptoms.

For the purposes of this first-aid chapter we will be addressing common motion sickness. Homeopathy can be of great use if you find yourself experiencing motion sickness. Some of the remedies listed below are not common remedies easily obtainable, so if you anticipate a trip and expect these symptoms be prepared by ordering the medicines in advance.

HOMEOPATHY

- **COCCULUS-** Vertigo and dizziness with nausea and vomiting, exhaustion from lack of sleep.
- **NUX VOMICA-** Stomach upset, headache, irritable, worse from food.
- **PETROLEUM-** Prefers dry, warm weather, lung issues, diarrhea, fright.
- **TABACUM-** Feels faint, dizzy, nausea, finds cigarette smoke offensive.
- **CELL SALTS- CALC SULPH, FERRUM PHOS, KALI PHOS & NAT MUR;** one dose of each, every hour if the symptoms of nausea and dizziness are present.
- **NAT MUR & NAT PHOS-** if there are symptoms of headache, chills, worse from food or queasiness.

NOSEBLEED

A nosebleed is loss of blood from the tissue lining the nose. Bleeding most commonly occurs in one nostril only.

Nosebleeds are very common. Most nosebleeds occur because of minor irritations or colds. They can be frightening for some people, but rarely life threatening.

The nose contains many small blood vessels that bleed easily. Air moving through the nose can dry and irritate the membranes lining the inside of the nose, forming crusts. These crusts bleed when irritated by rubbing, picking, or blowing the nose.

The lining of the nose is more likely to become dry and irritated from low humidity, allergies, colds, or sinusitis. Thus, nosebleeds occur more frequently in the winter when viruses are common and heated indoor air dries out the nostrils. A deviated septum, foreign object in the nose, or other nasal blockage can also cause a nosebleed.

Most nosebleeds occur on the front of the nasal septum, the tissue that separates the two sides of the nose. The septum contains many fragile, easily damaged blood vessels. This type of nosebleed can be easy for a trained professional to stop. Less commonly, nosebleeds may occur higher on the septum or deeper in the nose. Such nosebleeds may be harder to control.

Occasionally, nosebleeds may indicate other disorders such as bleeding disorders or high blood pressure.

Frequent nosebleeds may also be a sign of hereditary hemorrhagic telangiectasia (also called HHT or Osler-Weber-Renlu Syndrome).

Blood thinners such as Coumadin, Plavix, or aspirin may cause or worsen nosebleeds.

CAUSES

- Allergic rhinitis
- An object stuck in the nose
- Blowing the nose very hard
- Chemical irritants
- Direct injury to nose, including a broken nose
- Nose picking
- Overuse of decongestant nasal sprays
- Repeated sneezing
- Surgery on the face or nose
- High Blood Pressure
- Taking large doses of aspirin or blood-thinning medicine

- Upper respiratory infection
- Very cold or very dry air
- Having a bleeder's disease (Hemophilia)

TREATMENT

- Pinch the bridge of the nose
- Hold a tissue up to your nose (don't blow nose)
- Sit up comfortably and lean slightly forward (do not lie down)
- Pinch the nostril shut for 10 minutes
- Apply a cold compress to bridge of nose
- Alternate with cold compress or ice to back of the neck

The use of apple cider vinegar on a cotton swab gently pressed into the bleeding nostril is an effective method to quickly slow the bleeding. If bleeding does not stop after 20 minutes, seek medical attention.

HOMEOPATHY

- **ARNICA-** if bleeding is due to an injury, one dose every 15 minutes until symptoms subside.
- **PHOSPHORUS-** one dose will usually stop bleeding fairly quickly. Dispense a second dose if necessary.
- **CALC PHOS 6x-** 3 times per day for a few days.
- **CELL SALTS- FERRUM PHOS 6x-** every 30 minutes until bleeding stops.

There are numerous remedies for specific symptoms of nosebleeds, consult a professional holistic practitioner. Chronic issues can be helped with the prescribing of a Constitutional remedy.

OPEN WOUND

Whenever the skin is cut open and exposed there is danger for infection.

TREATMENT
- Clean wound as soon as possible by clearing any debris, splinters or
- any other foreign objects from the site of injury
- Pour Hydrogen Peroxide over wound to disinfect or alcohol
- Clean with soap and water
- Cover with clean bandage

HOMEOPATHY
- **ACONITUM-** if there is shock or trauma, one dose.
- **ARNICA-** if there is pain or bruising, one dose every 15 minutes until symptoms subside, up to six doses. Can continue 2-3 doses per day for a few days after injury to further healing.
- **CALENDULA-** as a cream or gel to apply to broken skin to hasten healing and avoid infection.
- **HYPERICUM-** as a tincture to apply to open wound, especially if there is any nerve damage.
- **LEDUM-** if the wound is a puncture; known as a replacement for Tetanus, one dose per day for 3 days.
- **PHOSPHORUS-** to stop bleeding, one dose should suffice, repeat if bleeding persists after 20 minutes.
- **PYROGENIUM-** to avoid infection, take three times per day until wound closes.

If infection does occur, use **Hepar Sulph Calcarea**. Repeat at least 3 times per day until symptoms have cleared. It is a wonderful alternative to anti-biotics.

RIB FRACTURE

Rib fractures can be very painful and although they mostly heal on their own, there can be complications. Occasionally complications can occur if a broken rib perforates an internal organ. Therefore, you should know how to treat broken ribs to avoid further damage to your body.

SYMPTOMS

- Pain whenever you take a deep breath
- Headaches, dizziness
- Feeling tired
- Pain when you turn, bend or twist the body
- Increased pain when you press on the injured area
- Anxiety or fear sets in
- Deformity of a rib
- Favoring the injured side

Make an appointment with your doctor to confirm if the symptoms are from a fractured rib or if there is just bruising. A simple x-ray will confirm the situation.

TREATMENT

- Ice the area
- Wrap the chest to stabilize movement
- Take a mild pain medication, if necessary

HOMEOPATHY

- **ACONITUM-** if from an accident and there is shock or trauma; one dose every 15 minutes up to three doses.
- **ARNICA-** for swelling, bruising, pain; one dose every 15 minutes until symptoms subside. Continue to take for pain and swelling 3 times per day until healed.
- **BELLIS PERENNIS-** for swelling and bruising, injuries to deeper tissue if there are complications, can be taken with Arnica; one dose every 15 minutes until symptoms subside. Continue to take for pain and swelling 3 times per day until healed.
- **BRYONIA-** for injuries when there is stitching pain, tearing, worse by motion and better with rest. The person is aggravated by the least motion and is irritable. Repeat the remedy often until pain subsides, then adjust dosage accordingly.

- **CALCAREA PHOSPHORICA** (Calc Phos)- promotes ossification of bones. Take in a 6X potency for duration of healing period; 5 tablets 3 times daily.
- **RUTA GRAVEOLENS-** for injuries to muscles, tendons, or connective tissue. Symptoms are worse from movement. Take long term during recovery; 3-4 times daily until symptoms subside.
- **SYMPHYTUM-** this remedy is Comfrey or "knit bone"; it is specific to the healing of bones. Take 3-4 times daily until healing is complete.

SCRAPES (SEE CUTS)

SHOCK

Shock happens when not enough blood and oxygen can get to your organs and tissues. It causes very low blood pressure and may be life threatening. It often happens along with a serious injury.

There are several kinds of shock:

- **Hypovolemic shock** happens when you lose a lot of blood or fluids. Causes include internal or external bleeding, dehydration, burns, and severe vomiting and/or diarrhea.
- **Septic shock** is caused by infections in the bloodstream. A severe allergic reaction can cause anaphylactic shock. An insect bite or sting might cause it.
- **Cardiogenic shock** happens when the heart cannot pump blood effectively. This may happen after a heart attack.
- **Metabolic shock** is a loss of fluids caused by intense vomiting, diarrhea, hemorrhaging or too much urination.
- **Neurogenic shock** is caused by damage to the nervous system.

SYMPTOMS

- Confusion or lack of alertness
- Restlessness and anxiety
- Drop in blood pressure
- Loss of consciousness
- Sudden and ongoing rapid heartbeat
- Sweating
- Pale skin
- A weak pulse, or a rise in pulse
- Rapid breathing
- Nausea and vomiting
- Decreased or no urine output
- Cool hands and feet
- Thirst

Shock is a life-threatening medical emergency and it is important to seek help right away. Treatment of shock depends on the cause.

TREATMENT
- Gently lay the person down
- Do not move their head
- Do not remove them from the site, unless the area is dangerous
- Keep the person flat and still
- Check for signs of breathing; perform CPR if necessary
- Continue to check for breathing every 5 minutes
- Loosen clothing and keep person warm
- Do not give food or drink
- If there is vomiting, gently turn them on their side
- Treat any injuries that have occurred (bleeding, etc.)

HOMEOPATHY
- **ACONITUM-** anxiety, fright and shock, (they think they are going to die) pass under person's nose every 15 minutes until symptoms subside if there is decreased consciousness.
- **ARNICA-** trauma and its effects, especially if there is physical injury, pass under person's nose every 15 minutes until symptoms subside. Can continue oral dosage 3 times daily once trauma has passed for effects of physical injury.
- **BAPTISIA-** Septic shock, initially pass under nose every 15 minutes, or dissolve in a little water and rub into skin, bend of left elbow or behind ear; continued treatment; one dose three times per day until symptoms of sepsis resolve.
- **CARBO VEGETABLIS-** Respiratory shock, pass under nose every 15 minutes or dissolve in a little water and rub into skin, bend of left elbow or behind ear.
- **CHINA-** Metabolic shock, one dose every 15 minutes until symptoms resolve, up to 6 doses for weakness and decreasing consciousness.
- **CACTUS GRANDIFLORUS-** Cardiogenic shock, one dose every 10 minutes, pass bottle under nose if there is reduced consciousness.
- **DIGITALINUM (Digitalis)-** Cardiogenic shock, one dose every 10 minutes, pass bottle under nose if there is reduced consciousness.
- **HYPERICUM-** Neurogenic shock, when there is a spinal injury, one dose every 15 minutes until symptoms resolve.
- **IPECACUANHA-** Metabolic shock, to halt vomiting, pass under nose every 15 minutes until symptoms resolve.
- **PYROGENIUM-** Septic shock, one dose every 15 minutes, up to 6 doses. Continue 2-3 doses per day until sepsis is resolved.
- **CELL SALTS- KALI PHOS & NAT SULPH-** one dose of each, every 30 minutes.

SPRAINS

A sprain is a stretched or torn ligament. Ligaments are tissues that connect bones at a joint. Falling, twisting, or getting hit can all cause a sprain. Ankle and wrist sprains are common. Symptoms include pain, swelling, bruising, and being unable to move your joint. You might feel a pop or tear when the injury happens.

A strain is a stretched or torn muscle or tendon. Tendons are tissues that connect muscle to bone. Twisting or pulling these tissues can cause a strain.

Strains can happen suddenly or develop over time. Back and hamstring muscle strains are common. Many people get strains playing sports.

SYMPTOMS

- Pain
- Muscle spasms
- Swelling
- Trouble using limb

TREATMENT

- Ice (20 minute intervals) every hour or two
- Bandage to compress the area
- Keep weight off area
- Elevate
- Physical therapy may be necessary, depending on severity

HOMEOPATHY

- **ARNICA-** for swelling and bruising, initially one dose every 15 minutes until symptoms subside, continue one dose 3 times per day until healing is complete.
- **BELLIS-** if there is tissue damage and to bring down swelling and bruising, can be used with Arnica, initially one dose every 15 minutes until symptoms subside; continue one dose 3 times per day until healing is complete.
- **RHUS TOXICODENDRON-** after initial injury when discomfort is BETTER from movement.
- **RUTA GRAVEOLENS-** if pain is WORSE from movement, one dose every 15 minutes until symptoms improve; continue three doses per day until healing is complete, or as needed.
- **CELL SALT- FERRUM PHOS-** one dose every 2-4 hours depending on severity.

SUNBURN

Sunburn can be a minor inconvenience or a serious condition. Access the situation and choose the treatment that is in the best interest of the injured party. There can be mild skin redness and some exhaustion and dehydration or severe burns to the skin, blistering and lightheadedness. Seek immediate medical attention if the sunburn is severe.

TREATMENT

- Cover up or remove yourself from sun exposure as soon as discomfort begins
- Hydrate as soon as possible
- Replenish electrolyte imbalance
- Sooth affected skin with baking soda and water

HOMEOPATHY

- **APIS MEL-** for skin that is stinging.
- **ARNICA-** if there is swelling.
- **CALENDULA-** Cream or gel topically over burn area; repeat as needed. Can also take homeopathic pellets internally to encourage healing.
- **CAUSTICUM-** Every few hours for old burns that have not healed.
- **GLONOINUM-** If over exposure to the sun causes congestive headache. Feels like your head is throbbing. Take every 15 minutes initially until headache subsides.
- **URTICA URENS-** If skin feels itchy, prickly or stings.

TEETH (SEE DENTAL TRAUMA)

TICK BITES

Lyme disease is a bacterial infection you get from the bite of an infected tick. The first symptom is usually a rash, which may look like a bull's eye. The bite itself is painless. As the infection spreads, you may have other symptoms that appear at a later date. Many times it takes months to recognize a change in your level of health. It is important to seek treatment for a tick bite as soon as possible.

SYMPTOMS

- Fever
- Headache
- Muscle and joint aches (arthritic)
- A stiff neck
- Lesions
- Red spots with white centers
- Flu-like symptoms
- Nausea and/or vomiting
- Swollen lymph glands in neck, groin or under arms
- Backache
- Baker's cysts (large lumps under the skin)
- Fatigue (increases over time)

Be aware that symptoms come and go initially, which makes early diagnosis difficult.

Lyme disease can be hard to diagnose because you may not have noticed a tick bite. Also, many of its symptoms are like those of the flu and other diseases. In the early stages, your health care provider will look at your symptoms and medical history, to figure out whether you have Lyme disease. Lab tests may help at this stage, but may not always give a clear answer. In the later stages of the disease, a different lab test can confirm whether you have it.

TREATMENT

If you are aware of the bite remove the tick with tweezers by pulling straight out of the skin. It is especially important to remove the body as soon as possible, since it carries the infection.

Paint the area with disinfectant.

If possible save the tick (do not handle with bare hands) for analysis.

Conventional medicine will treat with anti-biotics, not everyone improves with this treatment. In fact, long-term use of anti-biotics can be dangerous to your health. The World Health Organization published a 257-page report in April 2014 putting forth the dangers of antimicrobial drug resistance with the overuse of anti-biotics.

Borrelia burgdorferi, the parasite transmitted by the tick, is actually a spirochete. To efficiently diagnose Lyme disease, which is transmitted by an infected tick, dark-field microscopy can be very helpful.

Dark-field microscopy must be used to view spirochetes. Dark field microscopy utilizes a special condenser that directs light toward an object at an angle, rather than from the bottom. As a result, particles or cells are seen as light objects against a dark background.

HOMEOPATHY

Initial treatment, if you suspect a tick bite is with the use of **Ledum 200c** (also known as a substitute for tetanus shot), one dose every three hours, then two times daily for one month. This is followed by continued treatment of one dose two times weekly for one month, then one time weekly for another month.

ADDITIONAL REMEDIES

- **ARNICA-** for swelling and pain, one dose every 15 minutes.
- **AURUM ARSENICUM-** if there is anxiety or depression.
- **PYROGENIUM-** if there is infection (sepsis), one dose every 15 minutes and seek medical attention as soon as possible.

CHAPTER VI COMMON CONDITIONS A-Z
CONVENTIONAL WISDOM & NATURAL RELIEF

The conditions listed in this chapter are just that. They are not seen as diseases within the philosophy of natural medicine, instead they are issues that develop from a disturbance in the body. Natural medicine shines in this category since there are no known side effects to their use and addresses issues that are not generally the focus of mainstream medical doctors. They are important issues, since many are signs and symptoms of deeper issues developing. Natural remedies do not palliate or suppress symptoms. Instead, they can go deep to resolve the root cause. Addressing problems as they arise can help to ward off more serious issues down the road. It is a means of preventative medicine.

Throughout this chapter you will encounter remedies referred to as the Banerji Protocols™. The Banerjis are four generations of medical doctors in Kolkata, India who have introduced a unique method of prescribing Homeopathic remedies. The Dr. Prasanta Banerji Homoeopathic Research Foundation (PBHRF) clinics use state of the art scientific testing methods along with non-traditional case taking. The Banerji's believe a modern diagnostic approach incorporates and assists in the selection of remedies so that specific medicines can be prescribed for specific diseases. Whenever you see remedies referenced as the Banerji Protocols™, know that they have been dispensed to thousands of patients for decades with great success.

ABSCESS

An abscess is a collection of pus in any part of the body that, in most cases, causes swelling and inflammation around it. Abscesses, boils and cysts are all the same issue with the infection affecting either soft tissue or hard tissue.

Abscesses occur when an area of tissue becomes infected and the body's immune system tries to fight it. White blood cells move through the walls of the blood vessels into the area of the infection and collect in the damaged tissue. During this process, pus forms.

Pus is the buildup of fluid, living and dead white blood cells, dead tissue, and bacteria or sometimes other foreign substances.

Abscesses can form in almost any part of the body. The skin, under the skin, and teeth are the most common sites. Bacteria, viruses, parasites, or foreign substances may cause abscesses. Inflammation surrounding hair follicles or sweat glands can lead to the formation of abscesses, as well.

Abscesses in the skin are easy to see. They are red, raised, painful and appear as a swollen area that is warm to the touch. Abscesses in other areas of the body may not be seen and may cause organ damage if untreated, especially in the brain, kidneys, lungs, liver, breast, neck or tonsils.

Dental abscesses are quite common. If a tooth has a crack and collects bacteria and/or fungus an abscess may form. Also root canals can collect pathogens forming an abscess. If a crown is capped over a tooth that has not been properly disinfected it is also cause for an abscess to form over time.

TESTS

A sample of fluid can be taken from the abscess and tested to see what type of germ is causing the infection.

CONVENTIONAL TREATMENT

Treatment varies depending on the circumstances. Some abscesses will open and drain spontaneously. Surgery is sometimes used to remove remaining infection.

NATURAL TREATMENT

There are a number of natural treatments to assist with skin abscesses, boils or cysts. The treatments can be used on pets, as well as humans. Remedies are easily administered to pets by melting pellets in their water bowl.

Warm compresses can help to bring the abscess to a head. The warm compress should be applied at least a few times per day for 5-10 minutes. Once the area is open and draining hydrogen peroxide can be used to disinfect the area and Calendula as a wound cleaner and to encourage healing.

A reliable "go-to" for any type of infection is Colloidal Silver. It can be taken orally and/or used topically on the affected area.

Further stimulate the immune system to remove infection with any of the following: Oregano Oil, Echinacea, Goldenseal, Elderberry, Turmeric and/or large doses of Vitamin C. Where there is infection, there is low pH, meaning an acidic environment. The use of Sodium bicarbonate (baking soda), ½ tsp. in 4-8 oz. of water twice daily on an empty stomach will quickly bring blood pH to an alkaline range.

Homeopathy is very effective in encouraging the draining and healing of an abscess. Given proper instructions, the body can reabsorb infected tissues at the site and filter them out of the body. Do not be afraid to use multiple remedies, covering all pertinent circumstances.

HOMEOPATHY

- **ARNICA-** taken orally is used for trauma and swelling and can help prevent an abscess at the time of injury.
- **LEDUM-** is used for puncture wounds and can help diminish the abscess from the start. It can also be used in place of a tetanus vaccine in emergency situations.
- **HEPAR SULPH CALCAREA-** is the number one remedy for draining an abscess. It is used especially when the puss has a foul smell and the area is particularly painful.
- **MERCURIUS VIVUS-** indicated in secondary stage of infection, when there is anemia, rheumatoid pains around joints, or ulceration of mouth or throat.
- **SILICEA-** is a great wound healer and can be given every day until the abscess disappears.
- **THUJA-** can be administered twice daily for spongy tumors, warty growths on mucus and skin surfaces, polyps and other soft growths.

BREAST ABSCESS

The Banerji Protocol™: In the case of acute abscess formation, with severe pain and suppuration give:

- **HEPAR SULPH CALC 6C + BELLADONNA 3C-** every 3 hours alternately; in acute pain dispense every hour.

If the abscess is already draining use the following:

- **HYPERICUM 200c + ARSENICUM ALBUM 200c-** Alternate every 3 hours with **HEPAR SULPH CALC 6c**.

DENTAL ABSCESS

- **HEPAR SULPH CALC 6C-** encourages abscess to drain and relieves pain; repeat remedy often for quick relief.
- **HECLA LAVA-** especially after tooth extraction and if jaw is affected, good for bone, teeth and jaw issues.
- **MERCURIUS VIVUS-** if there is great anxiety, increased saliva, metallic taste and mouth odor.
- **CAUSTICUM-** swelling at root of tongue, swelling in side of cheeks (bites inside of cheek when chewing), teeth may feel loose.

INTERNAL ABSCESSES

- **PYROGENIUM-** great remedy for septic states, especially when there is intense restlessness.
- **MYRISTICA SEBIFERA-** If there is indifference and lack of concentration this remedy can help to hasten the draining of an abscess and shorten duration.
- **CALCARIA SULPHURICUM-** is a blood purifier and can efficiently clear a wound that is slow to heal.

ANCIENT WISDOM

Clove Oil- (Eugenia aromaticum)- has been used effectively for centuries for its antimicrobial, antifungal, antiseptic, antiviral and stimulating properties. Clove oil is best known for its dental applications, but can also be effectively used topically on the skin, as well as diluted in small amounts and taken orally. It is an effectual means for many types of pain, including gout.

ACID-REFLUX

As we age the amount of acid produced dwindles, so it is not necessarily an excess of acid that produces acid-reflux, as is believed. When you are not digesting your food properly the acids begin to move up into the chest and there is a burning in the solar plexus (mid chest). If you are burping up what was eaten over an hour later it means you are not digesting properly and you have acid-reflux. Other reasons you may have this symptom is from a bacterial infection known as H. Pylori, or from a hiatal hernia.

Not too long ago I had a client with fairly severe acid-reflux. I suggested a particular homeopathic protocol that fit her symptoms. She should have had relief fairly quickly. When she did not, I suggested a Chiropractic exam. The exam revealed a hiatal hernia. The doctor worked to reposition her stomach to correct the hernia and together with the remedies she had complete relief.

TESTS

- Upper GI Tract X-Ray Upper GI Endoscopy
- Hour Esophageal pH Test

CONVENTIONAL TREATMENT

Many people can improve their symptoms by:

- Avoiding alcohol and spicy, fatty or acidic foods that trigger heartburn
- Eating smaller meals
- Chew your food well and eat slowly
- Not eating close to bedtime
- Losing weight if needed
- Wearing loose-fitting clothes

Conventional treatment is taking antacids or pharmaceutical prescription medicines that cause other side effects. This avenue will never cure the problem, but instead palliate symptoms and poor digestion will continue to create deeper health issues.

NATURAL TREATMENT

Beware of antacids! The issue with chewable antacids is that most of them contain just calcium. Taking calcium by itself has been shown to increase heart attack risk by as much as 31%! If you choose to use a chewable antacid be sure it contains calcium carbonate, which goes through the system quickly. Or buy an antacid that also contains magnesium with Vitamins D3 & K2. There needs to be three-parts magnesium to one-part calcium. This is a balanced combination of vitamins and minerals to keep the heart healthy.

Dr. Phil Salinsky wrote an eloquent description of what happens to the body when we ingest improper supplements such as antacids in his book, ***THE HUMAN MACHINE; A Trouble Shooter's Manual.*** Salinsky puts it this way, "Everything has a purpose and a reason and a function. There is a reason that the stomach is acidic and the mouth and small intestine are alkaline. To change that status arbitrarily would change the entire metabolic structure of the body...and change it detrimentally.

Acid in the stomach activates the digestive enzyme pepsin that breaks down protein. Acid also holds the protein in suspension so that it doesn't putrefy (rot). If that does not happen IN SEQUENCE, the protein (like any organic material) will rot before it gets to the place in the small intestine where it gets taken into the blood."

Jonathan E. Prousky, B.P.H.E., B.Sc., N.D. wrote in *The Journal of Orthomolecular Medicine* Vol. 16, 4th Quarter 2001, "When hydrochloric acid (HCl) secretion is insufficient, the gastric pH will not be sufficiently acidic, digestion will be impaired, and signs and symptoms of hypochlorhydria will be apparent. When taken with meals, vitamin B3 can markedly improve and possibly eradicate symptoms of hypo-achlorhydria."

HIATAL HERNIA

Dr. Salinsky also writes extensively about a condition called Hiatal Hernia. It occurs when the upper part of the stomach bulges through an opening in the diaphragm. Salinsky says, "Indigestion" followed by "heartburn", "lumps" in your throat, heart palpitations, shortness of breath, constipation/diarrhea, ileitis, colitis, irritable bowel, ulcerative colitis, low back pain, chest pain... any or all of these symptoms can point to hiatal hernia. Out of a random 100 people, 25 will have an acute, active hiatal hernia and 50 to 60 more will experience a "chronic" condition where symptoms come and go."

It is a condition frequently missed by medical doctors and has a simple fix. Most Chiropractors can work with relieving this condition by making simple adjustments to the stomach.

ACUPUNCTURE & TRADITIONAL CHINESE MEDICINE (TCM)

Diagnostics are made beginning with subjective intake of the patient's chief complaint and accompanying symptoms. Following the provider will incorporate observation, palpation, pulse and tongue diagnosis. Each individual organ and pattern is mapped in the tongue as well as the pulse. In addition, western diagnostics such as blood testing or ordering films may help the provider complete the current picture of a patient's present condition.

Gathering this information allows the practitioner to formulate a holistic individual diagnosis within Traditional Chinese Medicine. Treatment plan based on this diagnosis may utilize some of the more commonly known branches of TCM and may include acupuncture, herbal prescription, nutrition, exercise and 'tuina' (Chinese medical massage/manipulation).

Treating patterns of Acid Reflux/Gerd that form your individual diagnosis may be seen as Stomach fire with rising Stomach qi; or Liver qi stagnation. Some forms of TCM may be chosen singly or together for the best treatment plan and holistic response.

HOMEOPATHY

- **ABIES NIGRA-** relieves stomach pain after eating.
- **CALCAREA CARBONICA-** frequent loud, sour belching, cramping, gains weight easily.
- **CARBO VEG-** heartburn, sour stomach, constant belching, nausea, relieves stomach bloating with gas.
- **IRIS VERSICOLOR-** when there is nausea and sour vomiting, reflux and regurgitation.
- **LYCOPODIUM-** relieves bloated lower abdomen, gastric palpitations.
- **NUX VOMICA-** from excesses of alcohol, sweets, and/or greasy foods.
- **RAPHANUS SATIVUS-** relieves abdominal bloating with difficult gas.
- **ROBINIA PSEUDOACACIA-** relieves heartburn with acid indigestion.

THE BANERJI PROTOCOLS™ (FOLLOW FOR 13 WEEKS)

- **Acid Reflux (GERD)-** LYCOPODIUM 200c + IRIS VERSI-COLOR 200c, 2 times daily.
- **Bloating-** LYCOPODIUM 200c + ARSENICUM ALBUM 3C, 2 times daily.
- **Bowels, hard & dry-** LYCOPODIUM 200c + PLUMBUM METALLICUM 200c, 2 times daily.
- **Bowels loose with gas-** ARSENICUM ALBUM 6c + ALOE 200c, 2 times daily.
- **Bowels, prolapse-** RUTA GRAV 200c, 2 times daily or Lycopodium 200c + PLUMBUM 200c, 2 times daily.
- **Bloating from overindulgence-** with irritability and/or incomplete stool CHELIDONIUM 30c + NUX VOMICA 200c, 2 times daily.

ANCIENT WISDOM

Switching to a fresh food based alkaline diet is one method of bringing relief for symptoms of acid-reflux, indigestion and heartburn. Acid-reflux is completely unnecessary and is a modern, unnatural condition. It comes from eating processed foods that contain no enzymes, and what it does contain is completely unnatural to the body:

- Chemical preservatives
- Food colorings
- Pesticides
- Chemical fertilizers
- Fungicides
- Neonicotinoids
- Genetically Modified Organisms

This type of diet is the precursor to gall stones, kidney stones and many other health issues.

To quickly relieve acid-reflux add to your diet *apple cider vinegar*. Drink in the a.m. on an empty stomach in distilled water. A little honey to taste can be added if necessary (or stevia).

Another option for quickly balancing pH is the use of sodium bicarbonate (baking soda.) Start with ½ tsp. in 4-8 ounces of water. Drink on an empty stomach morning and evening. Monitor pH with pH strips or a pH meter to bring saliva within range (7.3-7.5). If you test urine, it should read slightly more acidic in a range of 6.8-7.0.

Acid-reflux can also be caused by not having enough salt. This concept is contrary to western medical belief; however, the body contains 70% salt water. Every cell in the body needs salt to function properly. Medications that deplete salt and increase potassium exacerbate the acid state in the body. A touch of natural sea salt can be added to the apple cider vinegar mixture. (not pink Himalayan salt).

THE ALKALINE DIET CONNECTION

The theory behind an alkaline diet is that because our body's pH level is slightly alkaline, with a normal range of 7.36 to 7.44, our diet should reflect this and also be slightly alkaline. An imbalanced diet high in acidic foods such as animal protein, sugar, caffeine, and processed foods tends to disrupt this balance. It can deplete the body of alkaline minerals such as sodium, potassium, magnesium, and calcium, making you prone to chronic and degenerative disease. Animal protein in moderation is important to the diet for many and its acidic base is balanced by eating green vegetables with your animal protein intake.

SYMPTOMS OF EXCESS ACIDITY

- Low energy, chronic fatigue
- Excess mucous production
- Nasal congestion
- Frequent colds/ flu
- Infections
- Nervousness, stress,
- Irritability, anxiety
- Weak nails, dry hair, dry skin
- Formation of cysts, such as ovarian cysts, polycystic ovaries, benign breast cysts (fibrocystic breasts)
- Headaches
- Joint pain or arthritis Neuritis
- Improved symptoms after detoxification
- Hives
- Leg cramps and spasms
- Gastritis, acid indigestion

Medical doctors try to test the acidity or alkalinity of the body tissues and cells by analyzing the blood. Pioneers Carey Reams, Harold Hawkins, and Emanuel Revici developed methods to measure urine pH and other factors such as saliva pH. Modern proponents of the alkaline diet look at the pH of blood, saliva, and urine, in addition to health symptoms and other factors.

An alkaline diet is composed of approximately 75-80% alkaline foods and 20-25% acid foods.

The human body is comprised of about 70% water. To be healthy all that water needs to have a healthy pH balance, not too acid, not too alkaline. The letters "pH" mean "potential of hydrogen" and simply measure how acid or alkaline the body is on a scale of 0-14. Optimum health is achieved when the body stays in a slightly alkaline environment at about 7.0-7.5 as measured by saliva.

Most drug stores carry pH strips to test saliva. Anyone experiencing acid-reflux will test below the neutral level of 7.0 which means digestion cannot function properly.

An alkaline diet that restores a healthy pH balance goes a long way to improve the symptoms of acid reflux, as well as bone loss, blood sugar imbalances, joint pain and deterioration of heart muscles.

A pH balanced diet consists of lots of fresh fruits and vegetables. In addition to providing vitamins and minerals, fruits and vegetables are rich in bicarbonate precursors the body needs to maintain normal alkalinity.

A team from the department of medicine and the General Clinical Research Center at the University of California, San Francisco, led by Anthony Sebastian, published research revealing that typical Western diets produce slight chronic systemic metabolic acidosis in humans. The research shows that such a diet accelerates aging; corrodes muscle and bone; and suppresses growth hormone secretion, while more alkaline diets have the opposite effects.

SIMPLE TIPS FOR INCREASING FRUIT AND VEGETABLE INTAKE

- Eat two to three servings (one cup or fist-sized portion each) of fresh vegetables or fruits at each meal.
- Make fruits and vegetables, not bread or cereal, the center of your breakfast.
- East more sweet potatoes, winter squash and baked whole potatoes. (less bread and rice).
- Have fresh, dried or cooked fruits for snacks or desserts.
- Favor fresh foods and avoid processed foods.

You may choose to add a plant-based digestive enzyme with meals to relieve acid-reflux and to replace the lack of enzymes missing from processed foods.

An easy, inexpensive method of improving acid reflux is to add sauerkraut to your daily diet. Sauerkraut contains all the necessary digestive enzymes, in their correct proportion, to break down foods properly. Through the process of lactic acid fermentation lactobacillus, among other natural bacteria are produced to aid in digestion. Not only that, but it delivers almost instantaneous relief.

Do not buy sauerkraut pre-made that includes vinegar and/or preservatives. This defeats the purpose of this natural digestive aid. Also, most brands are pasteurized and must say "raw" on the label to have any appreciable benefit. It is very simple and inexpensive to make your own sauerkraut.

EASY SAUERKRAUT RECIPE

Makes 1 – 1 1/2 quarts

- One medium head of organic green cabbage
- Distilled or filtered water
- 2 tbsp. Sea salt (not Himalayan or white table salt)
- Caraway seeds (optional for flavor)

Discard wilted leaves from outside of cabbage. Slice head into quarters, removing center core. Further slice quarters, if you like smaller pieces then slice each wedge crosswise into thin ribbons.

Transfer the cabbage into a large bowl and toss in salt, mixing thoroughly and massaging the cabbage until water begins to emerge. (If this seems like too much work you can go directly to your jar layering cabbage and salt) The cabbage will be a little crunchier.

Continue to press the cabbage into a large Mason jar, crock, or other glass container that has a tight seal. Keep compressing cabbage down with a wooden spoon, or the back of your hand, until the jar is filled. Fill with water to the very top.

Cover with an outer cabbage leaf or a piece of cheesecloth, secured by a rubber band. Leave out on counter to ferment for about a week. Keep away from sunlight and in a cool room temperature (65°-75°). Start tasting after 5 or 6 days, when it tastes fermented, remove the covering and replace with a tight lid. Store in the refrigerator for up to two months. Hopefully you will have eaten it long before this.

DIGESTION REMEDY REFERENCE CHART

Serious symptoms should be treated by a trained professional. However, many of the following Homeopathic remedies can greatly improve digestive issues.

Acid Reflux- Iris versicolor + Lycopodium

Celiac or grain intolerance- Bovista

Colitis- Ipecac + Merc sol

Constipation- Lycopodium + Plumbum

Dairy Intolerance- Aethusa

Diarrhea- Arsenicum album + Aloe

Diarrhea (chill)- Veratrum

Diverticulitis- Staphasagria, Lycopodium + Plumbum

Diverticulitis (bleeding)- Ferrum Phos

Heartburn- Lycopodium + Arsenicum alb

Hemorrhoids- Hamamelis

Indigestion (food allergies)- Ipecac + Merc Sulph

Indigestion (junk food, fats)- Nux Vomica

Irritable bowel- Lycopodium + Arsenicum album

Nausea- Arsenicum album or Ipecachuana

Bloating- Arsenicum album + Lycopodium

Parasites- Cina

pH Balance- Apple cider vinegar or fresh lemon in distilled water

Vomiting- Ipecacuanha or Arsenicum album

ACNE

Acne is a common skin condition that causes pimples. Pimples form when hair follicles under your skin clog up. Most pimples form on the face, neck, back, chest, and shoulders. Anyone can get acne, but it is most common in teenagers and young adults. The cause is usually due to a blocked pore that may get infected by skin bacteria causing inflammation and pustular acne. This is not serious, but may cause scars.

Hormonal changes, such as those during teen years and pregnancy play a role. Hormones increase the production of skin oils and the glands that make them, causing more opportunities for pores to clog.

There are many myths about what causes acne. Chocolate and greasy foods are often blamed, but there is little evidence that these foods have much effect on acne in most people. A high sugar and carbohydrate diet can however increase acne formation.

Another common myth is that dirty skin causes acne; however, blackheads and pimples are not caused by dirt. This does not mean that the skin shouldn't be kept clean. Stress can exacerbate an acne condition.

If you have acne:

- Clean your skin gently, twice per day, especially at bedtime
- Try not to touch your skin or to squeeze pimples, since this can cause scars

CONVENTIONAL TREATMENT

Anti-biotics- …antibiotics may do a spectacular job of clearing up acne initially, but relapses will occur due to the existence of non-microbial causes. Generally speaking, the various topical ointments available are relatively ineffective for the same reason. High dose anti-biotic treatment also has the disadvantage of destroying normal intestinal flora. Anti biotic treatment cannot discriminate between good bacteria and bad, so all can be destroyed in one fell swoop. Changing the chemical balance in the body in this way can be very dangerous and lead to a number of illnesses.

NATURAL TREATMENT

Keep skin clean using astringents. **Witch hazel** is an inexpensive, natural astringent. Another is **Tea Tree Oil**, but use sparingly, since it can be drying. After cleansing use a moisturizer so the skin will not go into overdrive creating new oils to replace what you have washed away. Be sure to read labels, since many skin creams contain chemicals and preservatives. *The skin is like a sponge and absorbs these chemicals into the body. The skin is the outside of the gut, just as the gut is the inside of your skin.*

Improve pH levels by drinking sodium bicarbonate (baking soda), twice daily. Add ½ tsp. to 4-8 ounces of water and drink on an empty stomach. Balancing your pH levels to bring you to an alkaline state will discourage oxidative stress (free radicals) and help to kill off fungal infection in the body. Fungus can contribute to acne as much as bacteria levels. Discontinue baking soda once pH is balanced and keep in check through dietary choices.

Fresh lemon squeezed into distilled water or apple cider vinegar can also efficiently help to balance pH levels.

IMPROVE GENERAL HEALTH

Acne, cystic acne, eczema, psoriasis and other skin conditions have a connection to liver issues. The liver can become damaged from pharmaceutical drugs, recreational drugs, excess alcohol, foods containing toxins and even a build-up of toxins absorbed into the body through the skin itself. Non- infectious hepatitis and numerous herpes viruses can also attack the liver.

When the liver is functioning properly the oil glands of the skin drain properly. A simple liver cleanse, also known as a liver, gall bladder flush, can be done with a combination of organic apple juice and olive oil. Gemmotherapy and German Biological Medicine can also be used to efficiently cleanse the liver.

Be aware of blood sugar levels whenever drinking large amounts of fruit juice. Eating foods high in fiber will balance blood sugars, as well as adding cinnamon to your diet and the supplement fenugreek.

Calendula cream or gel used topically, as well as orally in Homeopathic potency is an excellent natural acne remedy. Skin experts attribute the overproduction of skin oils, clogged and inflamed hair follicles and infection by the Propioni bacterium as the three main causes of acne. Calendula's astringent, anti-inflammatory and antibacterial properties can go to work on all three of the acne-causing factors.

Identify hormone levels. A simple hormone panel through your practitioner can reveal if there is an imbalance. If you prefer to order blood work directly many states allow the ordering of blood panels online at very reduced rates, then find a branch of their lab in your neighborhood to do the actual blood draw; they will then email the results.

HOMEOPATHY

- **ANTIMONIUM TARTARICUM-** 3-5 pellets, three times a day for purple scars.
- **ARSENICUM ALBUM-** when they are itchy; 2 times daily.
- **BERBERIS-** for cycle-related outbreaks; 2 times daily.
- **CHRYSAROBINUM-** hard, lumpy outbreaks, as needed.
- **ECHINACEA-** mother tincture- septic, pustular acne, 10 drops in warm water, apply 3 times daily.
- **EUGENIA-** acne before periods, as needed.
- **HEPAR SULPH CALC-** cystic acne, pustular; 2 -3 times daily.
- **HEPAR SULPH CALC 200C + ARSENICUM ALBUM 200-** an efficient combination, especially if there are digestive issues; 2 times daily.
- **KALI BROMATUM-** bluish-red, scars remain after outbreak.
- **PHOSPHORIC ACID 200C-** pimples, boils; every other day.

- **SELENIUM-** for blackheads; three times daily.
- **THYOSINOMINUM 6X-** for scarring (needed 3 times daily for a longer period of time).
- **CELL SALTS** can greatly improve acne, combine the following:
- **CALC FLUOR 6X + CALC SUPLH 6X + SILICEA 6X-**

SUPPLEMENTS

B5 Pantothenic acid- purchase 500 mg tablets; day one, take 1 tablet 3 times per day, day two take 2 tablets 3 times per day, day three, take 3 tablets three times per day, continue to titrate up until you are taking 7 tablets, three times per day. Continue at this level for 21 days (or until skin is clear) On the 22nd day begin to titrate down by 1 tablet each day until you are back to 1, 3 times per day. Continue at this level as needed.

CASTOR OIL (Ricinus communis) A secret to clearing skin issues is with the use of castor oil. Castor oil is one of the most ancient oils, known for its powerful therapeutic properties. It contains ricinoleic acid, which has antimicrobial properties enabling it to act as a disinfectant and as an anti-inflammatory. It has a high concentration of fatty acids, Vitamin E, proteins, minerals and antifungal properties.

Using castor oil topically will help to prevent further outbreaks. Because of its low molecular weight, it is absorbed easily into the skin. This stops the overproduction of sebum by the oil glands.

Vitamin A helps to dry the skin, hence the many skin creams with the ingredient Retin A.

Zinc is an excellent mineral to help repair damaged tissue and heal wounds. A zinc deficiency in men is sometimes signaled by unreliable erections. (Lasting too long, as well as too short).

Silica can help stimulate pimples to drain and to heal scars.

Selenium combined with **Vitamin E** serves as an excellent antioxidant.

TRACE MINERAL THERAPY- Copper-Gold-Silver; Zinc-Copper; Sulphur; or Phosphorus.

Treating hormone balancing Homeopathically is also an option. If blood panels show the need to increase a specific hormone they can be normalized individually with Homeopathic dilutions (i.e. Estrogen or Testosterone). Refer to phenolic therapy in Chapter III. (It is important to not self-treat hormonal issues.)

ACUPUNCTURE & TRADITIONAL CHINESE MEDICINE (TCM)

A treatment plan based on careful diagnosis may utilize some of the more commonly known branches of TCM and include acupuncture, herbs, nutrition, exercise and tuina (Chinese medical massage/manipulation).

With the expertise of the licensed provider of Chinese Medicine a correct pattern/s for your symptom/s is chosen from one of several that fall under a certain disease or condition category.

Treating patterns of Acne may be seen as toxic and damp heat accumulation. Some forms of TCM may be chosen singly or together for the best treatment plan and holistic response.

ACNE ROSACEA

Acne rosacea is different from juvenile acne. It is frequently found in women in their forties and fifties. They are usually Caucasian and fair skinned. These patients suffer from circulatory disorders characterized by a dilation of blood vessels in the face, especially the cheeks. This causes blotching, rashes and patchy redness, bumps and even pink and irritated eyes. It is not contagious or infectious. There can also be an imbalance of hormones, especially during menopause.

CONVENTIONAL TREATMENT

Western medicine does not consider acne rosacea as curable and suggests such treatments as topical anti-bacterial (even though it is not from a bacteria), laser therapy, pulsed-light therapies, a sulfa wash and even Accutane, a serious acne medication with many harsh and dangerous side-effects.

NATURAL TREATMENT

There are numerous methods of increasing blood circulation to improve rosacea. Exercise, massage, elevating legs and feet when you rest, eating fresh foods that are easy to digest, drinking lots of clean filtered water, eliminating smoking or excess alcohol, and adding supplements to your daily routine.

Important to look at hormone levels, once balanced, this condition will resolve. It is prudent to balance pH levels. This can be done by drinking apple cider vinegar or fresh lemon in the a.m. on an empty stomach. It can be mixed in water with a little honey or stevia. Another method of regaining an alkaline state is with baking soda. (See Acne)

Ginger can ease inflammation in the blood vessels and also improves digestion.

Vitamin E helps widen blood vessels and prevent blood clotting within vessels, which greatly improves circulation.

L-Arginine & L-Citrulline have been shown to be powerful natural vasodilators.

HOMEOPATHIC REMEDIES

SANGUINARIA CANADENSIS 30C + CARBO ANIMALIS 30C Alternate three pellets of each, three times daily.

The following is the Banerji Protocol™ for acne rosacea. Follow the protocol for a minimum of 13 weeks.

- **BOVISTA 200C**- one dose every 3rd day
- **ANTIMONIUM CRUDUM 6C**- two doses daily

ACUPUNCTURE & TRADITIONAL CHINESE MEDICINE (TCM)

Treating patterns of Acne Rosacea may be seen as yin deficiency and blood stagnation. Some forms of TCM may be chosen singly or together for the best treatment plan and holistic response.

ALLERGIES (SEASONAL)

Each spring, summer, and fall, trees, weeds, and grasses release tiny pollen grains into the air. Some of the pollen ends up in your nose and throat. This can trigger a type of allergy called hay fever.

SYMPTOMS

- Sneezing often with a runny or clogged nose
- Coughing and postnasal drip
- Itching or burning eyes, nose and throat
- Red and watery eyes
- Dark circles under the eyes

Your health care provider may diagnose hay fever based on a physical exam and your symptoms. Sometimes skin or blood tests are used. Taking medicines and using nasal sprays can relieve symptoms temporarily. You can also rinse your nose with distilled or sterilized water with saline. Conventional treatment recommends allergy shots that are believed to help make you less sensitive to pollen and may provide long-term relief. I have not nown them to be effective, based on reports from clients. The vaccines also contain other toxins and contaminants that may complicate health.

ALLERGIES (FOOD)

Food allergy is an abnormal response to a food triggered by your body's immune system.

In adults, the foods that most often trigger allergic reactions include fish, shellfish, peanuts, and tree nuts, such as walnuts and almonds. Problem foods for children can include eggs, dairy products, peanuts, tree nuts, soy, and wheat.

Symptoms of food allergy include:

- Itching or swelling in your mouth
- Vomiting, diarrhea, or abdominal cramps and pain
- Hives or eczema
- Tightening of the throat and trouble breathing
- Drop in blood pressure
- Diarrhea/ constipation
- Bloating/Acid reflux

CONVENTIONAL TREATMENT

Your health care provider may use a detailed history, elimination diet, and skin and blood tests to diagnose specific allergies. They may suggest allergy shots, steroids, inhalers, or any combination of the three. None of these methods cure allergies. They may provide temporary relief.

When you have food allergies, you must be prepared to treat an accidental exposure. Wear a medical alert bracelet or necklace and carry an auto-injector device containing epinephrine (adrenaline).

Within conventional thinking you can only prevent the symptoms of food allergy by avoiding the food. After you and your health care provider have identified the foods to which you are sensitive they must be removed from your diet.

TESTING

You can find an alternative method of allergy testing at http://www.elisaact.com/

NATURAL TREATMENT

Maintain a normal pH level to keep the body balanced. This is the first step to proper to digestion. Every person with allergies I have consulted with had acidic saliva. The most efficient means of correcting this is with sodium bicarbonate (baking soda.) Start with a ½ tsp. in 4-8 ounces of water twice daily on an empty stomach. Monitor your pH level with pH strips or a pH meter. Optimum level for saliva is 7.3-7.5 and urine is 6.8-7.0. Do not exceed 2 tsp. of baking soda in a 24-hour period.

You can also drink freshly squeezed lemon or apple cider vinegar in your water to obtain the same result.

It has been shown that we are not allergic to a food or pollen, but to the specific *phenolic* substance in that food or flower. Most allergy studies relate to proteins, but it was discovered by Dr. Robert W. Gardner, Ph.D., a biochemist and professor emeritus of Animal Science at Brigham Young University some years ago that phenolic compounds that exist both in protein and other substances are a major causes of substance intolerances.

Phenolics are essential to life as we know it, but when metabolized incorrectly, they can cause major and minor physical, mental, and emotional disturbances in a large number of people. Phenols are found in all foods and plants and their derivatives are commonly called aromatics.

For instance, the herb cinnamon contains the aromatic "Cinnamic Acid". Cinnamic acid is a phenol that may cause an allergic reaction for some. It is not however limited to cinnamon. It is also contained in 22 other foods including fruits, cheeses, lettuce and tomatoes. The phenolics are attached to proteins causing the reactions. It is essentially not the food itself causing the allergic reaction, but the phenol attached to its protein.

Phenolics administered Homeopathically can induce the body's immune system to protect itself from these phenols and learn once again to regard them as normal and not foreign or poisonous substances.

Dr. Abram Ber (1940-2014) published a paper in 1983 based on his clinical experience. Here are his comments on the phenolic preparation "gallic acid."

"Gallic Acid is found in some 70% of all foods, including food coloring agents and is, unquestionably, the most important of all phenolics. Neutralization of gallic acid is the basis of the Feingold Diet that eliminates salicylates. Instead of making a child's life miserable utilizing a restrictive diet, neutralization of gallic acid is less traumatic. Frequently, parents report a marked improvement in their child's school performance and a normalization of hyperactivity. It neutralizes the craving for sweets that is prevalent in so many of these dyslexic children. Gallic acid has effects upon the muscular skeletal system (14 out of 18 arthritics), the lower back, the main contributor to sciatica, and chronic severe chest pain which is non-cardiac and seems to originate in the thoracic wall and is non-cardiac in origin."

Reactions to phenolic substances may exacerbate, or perhaps cause conditions such as:

- Arrhythmias Enuresis
- Arthritis Fatigue
- Asthma Hyperactivity
- Autism Hypertension
- Colitis Insomnia
- Constipation Menstrual Disorders
- Depression Migraines
- Dyslexia
- Skin Problems

See Chapter III for a chart indicating symptoms and accompanying phenolic tinctures for treatment.

HOMEOPATHY AND FOOD ALLERGIES

The following remedies should be taken in a *200c potency* and continued long term. Remedies can be combined.

- **BOVISTA-** multiple food allergies (especially gluten) taken every other day.
- **AETHUSA-** for dairy allergies, taken twice daily; if there is bloating or gas add: **LYCOPODIUM 200C + ARSENICUM ALBUM 6C**, twice daily.

(Also refer to Chapter III, **Phenolic Therapy** for desensitization methods.)

NAET

In recent years a system of allergy-elimination acupressure has been developed in which the treatment is performed while the person is exposed to the allergen. Developed by Dr. Devi Nambudripad, this technique is called Nambudripad's Allergy Elimination Technique (NAET). The patient undergoes allergy testing to identify the allergen. Then acupressure and acupuncture techniques are used to clear the allergen while the patient is exposed to it. This treatment reprograms the body to accept the allergen without producing an allergic reaction. In some cases, the effects can be long-term.

My personal experience has been that some respond better than others, with children having a higher success rate.

ACUPUNCTURE & TRADITIONAL CHINESE MEDICINE (TCM)

A treatment plan based on careful diagnosis may utilize some of the more commonly known branches of TCM and include acupuncture, herbs, nutrition, exercise and tuina (Chinese medical massage/manipulation).

With the expertise of the licensed provider of Chinese Medicine a correct pattern/s for your symptom/s is chosen from one of several that fall under a certain disease or condition category.

Treating patterns of Allergies that form your individual diagnosis may be seen in Seasonal Allergies as wind cold with fluid congestion; damp-heat with fluid congestion; wind heat at skin level, heat in blood; toxic heat; lung heat; cold in lung phlegm accumulation; toxic heat accumulation upper jiao; spleen qi deficiency. Patterns from Food Allergies may be seen as Spleen and Stomach qi deficiencies accompanied many times by dampness/phlegm. Some forms of TCM may be chosen singly or together for the best treatment plan and holistic response.

HOMEOPATHIC REMEDY CHOICES

- **APIS-** the most important allergy remedy. Useful in anaphylactic reaction when repeated often (every 30 seconds, or as needed), as well as for the reactive symptoms to insect bites, sunburn, hives; hay fever, asthma with shortness of breath; swelling and puffiness and flu-like symptoms.

- **ALLIUM CEPA-** eyes tearing, nose running, but no burning sensation; clear nasal discharge that irritates the upper lip, violent sneezing, tickling cough, sharp sticking pain in the larynx; better from open air and worse in a warm room.
- **ARSENICUM ALBUM-** thin, watery, burning nasal discharge; also stopped up nose; sneeze from tickle and brings no relief; anywhere there is pain it is burning, relieved by heat or hot drinks; thirsty for small sips; anxiety, restlessness, needy and fearful; worse from midnight until 2 a.m. Can work at a deeper level to help eliminate the cause of allergies.
- **ARUNDO-** roof of mouth itchy, nostrils and base of nose, can also have burning sensation; eyes and ears may itch also with loss of sense of smell and sneezing.
- **EUPHRASIA-** eyes are red and inflamed with burning, itching and thick discharge, runny nose, worse daytime, better at night.
- **GALPHIMIA GLAUCA-** when there is sensitivity to change in temperature; runny nose and teary eyes; gastric issues; herpetic eruptions; urticaria and skin allergies
- **NATRUM MURIATICUM-** profuse runny nose that looks like raw egg white, can also become stopped up; dry chapped lips, dry mouth, tendency to cold sores; sneezing, averse to bright light; watery eyes when outdoors; can have depression and want to be alone.
- **NUX VOMICA-** nose runs all day, stopped up at night or when outdoors; irritable, chilly; over-sensitive to stimulation preferring quiet and dimmed lights; digestive issues, worse after eating.
- **SABADILLA-** prolonged sneezing, runny nose, frontal sinus headache; eyes are watery, red and burning; prefer warm food and drink.
- **SULPHUR-** watery, burning nasal discharge outdoors, plugged indoors, sinus blockage alternates from left to right.
- **WYETHIA-** may have itchy nose and throat (desire to scratch it with your tongue), possibly roof of mouth; throat may feel swollen and is dry, clearing brings no relief.

ALLERGIC RHINITIS & HOMEOPATHY

A specific medicine for building immunity against cold/allergy and a subsequent medicine for immediate relief are to be considered. The following are considerations for allergic rhinitis.

- **CALCAREA CARBONICA 1M** once per week for a number of months.
- **ARSENICUM ALBUM 6c** can be taken as needed if there is sneezing.
- **ALLIUM CEPA 30c** for sneezing, as needed, if Ars. Alb. does not bring needed relief.

ALLERGY REMEDIES

People who have allergies often are sensitive to more than one thing. Most allergic reactions are an immune response that is a false alarm.

CAUSES:

- Pollen
- Dust Mites
- Mold Spores
- Pet Dander
- Foods
- Insect stings
- Medicines

SYMPTOMS:

- Sneezing
- Runny Nose
- Itchy, watery eyes
- Headaches
- Rashes
- Asthma

ALLIUM CEPA:
hay fever with itchy eyes, thin, watery *irritating* nasal discharge, shooting pains in Eustachian tube

ARUNDO:
itchy palate and nose, sneezing, runny nose, burning and itching in ears and eyes

EUPHRASIA:
hay fever, eyes hot and irritated *bland* nasal discharge, sneezing, headache

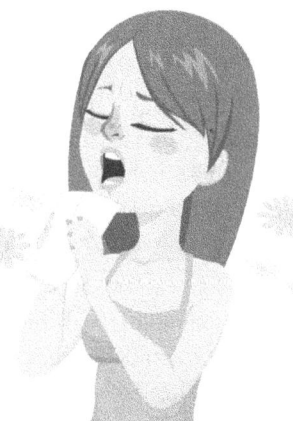

NUX VOMICA:
runny nose daytime and outdoors, stuffed at night, sneezing with crawling sensation in nose, acute sense of smell

NATRUM MURIATICUM:
watery or egg-white discharges, cold sores, watery eyes, swollen lids, headaches, nose alternates between runny and stuffed

SULPHUR:
watery, burning nasal discharge outdoors, plugged indoors, sneezing, blocked sinus alternates

SABADILLA:
violent sneezing attacks, watery nasal discharge, Itching and tickling in nose with irritating discharge

WYETHIA:
extreme itching in nose, palate and throat, itching at back of sinus, back of throat dry and irritated causing annoying cough

* During allergy attacks repeat remedies often, change remedy as symptoms change

Copyright © 2018 Elena Upton, PhD

ASTHMA & HOMEOPATHY

Best to consult a professional Homeopath for a Constitutional remedy since asthma often has an emotional component. The following remedies can be used for acute symptoms, including hay fever.

- **AMBROSIA-** can have itching of eyelids or nose, nosebleed, stuffed nose and head, whooping cough, diarrhea, sneezing, runny nose.
- **ALLIUM CEPA-** worse from dampness and cold; can have facial paralysis (Bell's Palsy), acrid nasal discharge, laryngitis, eyes burn and/or tear, hacking cough, especially breathing cold air; Bronchitis, hoarse cough, sneezing, bad breath.
- **ARSENICUM ALBUM-** anxiety and restlessness; air passages constricted from allergies; shortness of breath; wheezing; eyes burn and tear; darting pain through lung.
- **IODIUM-** anxiety when quiet; weakness and tickling in chest; Eustachian deafness; lungs have raw tickling feeling; croupy cough with difficult respiration; wheezy; nose red an swollen; sudden sneezing with dripping nose that feels hot.
- **NAJA-** wandering of the mind; tired, chest feels heavy and hot; asthmatic constriction, cannot expand lungs; stabbing pain from cough, followed by mucus; hay fever asthma with drainage from nose, then intense sneezing.
- **NUX VOMICA-** symptoms worse in early morning and from cold air; irritable; spasmodic constriction in chest; itching in ears; frontal headaches, cough brings on headache; asthma with fullness in the stomach; shallow, oppressed breathing; sneezing- feels like crawling in the nostril; smell from nose- like old cheese; digestion issues.
- **SABADILLA-** mental exhaustion from frightful thoughts; copious mucus from the nose; chilliness, sensitive to cold; diarrhea in children; cough; earache, tickling or burning itching in ears; headache; imaginary diseases; for children susceptible to tapeworm; eyelids red and burning; asthmatic breathing with itchy skin; wheezing; violent coughing attacks.

CHRONIC ASTHMA

- **STANNUM METALLIC 200c,** two times daily if there is great fatigue.
- **LACHESIS-** one dose every other day, asthma during menopause, assists with breathing difficulty.
- **KALI CARBONICUM 200-** twice daily for chest constriction.
- **NATRUM SULPH 200C-** if there is allergy to mold.
- **CALCARIA CARBONICA 200c-** if there is allergy to dust.

AILMENTS FROM ALLERGY SHOTS

- **CARCINOSIN-** anxiety over what might happen; if there are contradictory and alternating symptoms; multiple allergies and chronic fatigue; constriction in the chest; morning cough, bathing makes it worse; tickling in throat; symptoms worse from eating; whooping cough; recurring bronchitis.
- **SILICA-** has a deep, slow action to re-stimulate the body; for children with nutrition issues; likes to be warm, hates drafts; exhausts easily; sensitive to noise; feels like ears stopped up and clears on yawning or swallowing; child rubs ears; chronic colds that settle in the chest and bring on asthmatic attack; violent cough when lying down and can cough up thick yellow mucus.
- **THUJA-** for children (and adults) never well since vaccinations; mind becomes dull with fixed ideas; primarily works on the mucus membranes; better from dry weather, irritated by dampness; skin issues, especially after vaccines, warts, polyps, Condylomata; neuralgia; ear infections; asthma in children, dry hacking cough, cough worse during the day, however, asthma is worse at night.

ANCIENT WISDOM/TREATING POLLEN ALLERGIES

Source within your local area fresh *Raw Honey*, *Bee Pollen* and *Propolis*. Each day combine a little of the three together (about a tsp) and ingest. Over time you will build up the natural antibodies needed to no longer react to the pollens in your area.

TRACE MINERAL THERAPY- Manganese, Molybdenum

HAY FEVER & HOMEOPATHY

Alternate three pellets of each, three times per day on a regular basis during pollen season:

- **ARSENICUM ALBUM + HISTAMINUM +SABADILLA**

Or treat according to specific symptoms by adding any of the following:

- **APIS MELLIFICA-** if eyes are irritated.
- **NUX VOMICA-** sneezing.
- **IPECAC-** if accompanied by an asthma attack.
- **KALIUM IODATUM-** best used in a lower potency (6c), repeat often.
- **CALENDULA-** ointment can also be applied in each nostril before going outside, or spray Colloidal silver or REBOOST™ Decongestant spray.

Also refer to Chapter III, **Phenolic Therapy** for phenols that affect asthma.

ATHLETE'S FOOT

Athlete's foot (tinia pedis) is also known as ringworm of the foot. It is not a worm at all, but a fungal infection. It is contagious and can spread quickly. The fungus is transmitted in moist environments and typically communal areas such as gyms, pools or locker rooms, by sharing a towel used by someone with the disease, by touching the feet with infected fingers (such as after scratching another infected area of the body), or by wearing fungi- contaminated socks or shoes.

CONVENTIONAL TREATMENT

Over-the-counter creams and powders can help with tinea infections. For advanced cases your conventional doctor will prescribe anti-fungal medicine.

NATURAL TREATMENT

There are a number of natural remedies that quickly clear athlete's foot. The key is in keeping it clean and dry and to be careful not to recontaminate.

- **TEA TREE OIL** is a very efficient anti-fungal. Spread over affected area 2-3 times daily.
- **CLOVE OIL** is an ancient anti-fungal. Use multiple times per day and it will clear quickly.
- **ASAP Silver Biotics® Colloidal Silver Gel** topically 2-3 times daily.
- **SODIUM BICARBONATE** (Baking Soda)- soak the foot twice daily to re-establish normal pH and to help kill off fungus.

HOMEOPATHIC REMEDIES

The most effective Homeopathic remedies for ringworm fungal infections are:

- **CALCAREA CARBONICUM-** ulcerated wounds that do not heal readily, better by cold.
- **GRAPHITES-** slow to heal, worse from heat, moist, crusty, oozing eruptions.
- **NATRUM MURIATICUM-** dry eruptions, crusty, folds of skin and hairline, greasy skin.
- **PHYTOLACCA-** dry, harsh, itchy, best in early stages.
- **SEPIA-** ringworm in isolated spots, recurring in spring, itchy.
- **THUJA-** itchy or burns, worse from scratching, skin sensitive to touch.

BED-WETTING (ENURESIS)

Many children wet the bed until they are 5 or even older. A child's bladder might be too small. Or the amount of urine produced overnight can be more than the bladder can hold. Some children sleep too deeply or take longer to learn bladder control. Children should not be punished for wetting the bed. They don't do it on purpose, and most outgrow it.

Parents should be careful not to overdramatize the situation. Don't scold the child when an accident occurs, and don't offer praise when the bed stays dry overnight.

DO NOT use any kind of a device on children designed to shock or wake them when urinating in bed. The child is just as embarrassed about the situation as you are and there is no need for further emotional trauma.

CONVENTIONAL TREATMENT

- Therapy and anti-depressants

NATURAL TREATMENT

STRESS can be a major cause of bedwetting. Be sure to remove any unnecessary burdens from your child's life. If not within the family, look to a teacher at school, a dancing instructor, or any other person who may be traumatizing your child in any way.

Many bedwetting children and teenagers suffer nerve interference from spinal bones in their lower back where nerves exit the spinal column. A simple adjustment from a CHIROPRACTOR may just do the trick.

When nervous irritation is the cause of bed wetting, the irritation may be due to worms. My experience over the years has been that most children with bed wetting issues have worms (parasites.) An easy fix is the Homeopathic remedy Cina 30c taken twice daily for at least a month to six weeks.

CONSTIPATION can also cause bedwetting. Be sure your child has regular bowel movements daily. A little prune juice can help or eating a combination of walnuts and raisins for their nighttime snack, or an apple can improve the situation. (See CONSTIPATION for Homeopathic constipation remedies.)

APPLE CIDER VINEGAR can also be used for preventing bedwetting in small children. Drop a pinch of it in one glass of water, add a touch of honey and have your child drink it.

CORNSILK is a safe and gentle herb to use in the treatment of bedwetting. Use the tea or tincture during the day (up until about 4 or 5 hours before bed) to help strengthen a weak urinary system. You may want to combine it with plantain or yarrow for more effect.

CRANBERRY JUICE can encourage more urination during waking hours and help to clear any possible infection.

CINNAMON has been shown to stop bedwetting in children. Mix some powder with sugar and sprinkle of buttered toast. Do this each morning, or as a bedtime snack. Also add cinnamon to other foods and recipes.

HOMEOPATHIC REMEDIES

Constitutional Homeopathic treatment can help greatly with bedwetting. In the meantime, the following are remedies for specific symptoms. Suggested dose: four pellets, three times daily until improvement.

- **ARGENTUM NITRICUM-** sporadic occurrence.
- **BELLADONNA-** restless sleep, when child talks in their sleep, or when has dreams of urinating.
- **BENZOICUM ACIDUM-** if urine has a strong smell.
- **CAUSTICUM-** early in the night, sensitive children, cry easily.
- **CHINA-** in children, weekly.
- **EQUISETUM-** Soothes nervous dispositions and also when there are no remarkable symptoms, or there is no tangible cause.
- **HEPAR SULPH CALC-** if there has been infection.
- **HYOSCYAMUS NIGER-** if the bowels are released with urine.
- **KALI PHOSPHORICUM-** restless, easily startled, urine can be yellow/ orange.
- **KREOSOTUM-** difficult to wake child.
- **LAC-CANINUM-** bedwetting in adolescence.
- **NATRUM MURIATICUM-** close family ties, fear of robbers.
- **PHORPHORUS-** when child has fears.
- **PULSATILLA-** weepy, whiny children.
- **SEPIA-** if urination happens early in the evening.
- **SULPHUR-** can cover for no reason other than a bad habit.
- **TUBERCULINUM-** night sweats, restless sleeper.

BRONCHITIS

Bronchitis is an inflammation of the bronchial tubes, the airways that carry air to your lungs. It causes a cough that often brings up mucus, as well as shortness of breath, wheezing, and chest tightness. There are two main types of bronchitis: acute and chronic.

The same viruses that cause colds and the flu often cause acute bronchitis. These viruses spread through the air when people cough, or through physical contact (for example, on unwashed hands). Being exposed to tobacco smoke, air pollution, dusts, vapors, and fumes can also cause acute bronchitis. Bacteria can also cause acute bronchitis, but not as often as viruses.

Most cases of acute bronchitis get better within several days. But your cough can last for several weeks after the infection is gone. If you think you have acute bronchitis, see your healthcare provider.

CONVENTIONAL TREATMENT

Conventional treatments include rest, fluids, and aspirin (for adults) or acetaminophen to treat fever. A humidifier or steam can also help. You may need inhaled medicine to open your airways if you are wheezing. You probably do not need antibiotics. They don't work against viruses - the most common cause of acute bronchitis. If your healthcare provider thinks you have a bacterial infection, he or she may prescribe anti-biotics.

NATURAL TREATMENT

Coughing during and after can actually be good for you. It's the body's way of eliminating the infection that causes bronchitis. Instead of stifling a cough with an over-the-counter suppressant, help it along by using a warm- or cool-mist humidifier to add moisture to the air. The added humidity will help bring the sputum (matter that's coughed out of the body) up and out. Standing in a steamy shower with the bathroom door closed, keeping a pan of water at a slow boil on the stove (never leave it unattended!), and using a tea kettle to shoot out warm, moist air can also help loosen and bring up phlegm. And if you have a few drops of peppermint or eucalyptus oil to add to the water, these can be quite soothing. The use of a warm compress on the chest can also be helpful.

Drink as much fluids as possible, especially hot fluids like lemon water, medicinal teas or soup. Gargling with saltwater may provide a double dose of relief by soothing the inflammation in the throat and by cutting through some of the mucus that may be coating and irritating the sensitive throat membranes. It only takes one teaspoon of salt in a glass of warm water; too much salt causes burning in the throat, and too little is ineffective. Gargle as often as needed, but be sure to spit the salty water out after gargling.

Monitor pH of the body to ward off infection. A way to correct this in those over 6 years-old is with sodium bicarbonate (baking soda.) Start with ¼- ½ tsp. in 4-8 ounces of water twice daily on an empty stomach. Adjust pH levels with the use of pH strips or a pH meter. Optimum level for saliva is 7.3-7.5 and urine is 6.8-7.0. Do not exceed 2 tsp. of baking soda in a 24-hour period.

Fresh lemon tea or apple cider vinegar also help to balance pH levels.

HOMEOPATHIC REMEDIES

Chronic Bronchitis and recurring Bronchitis can be effectively treated with Constitutional Homeopathy. When my son was a teenager he suffered from seasonal Bronchitis. After dispensing the remedy Lachesis, which was a match for his health profile and personality, he was completely relieved from a re-occurrence. Seek the advice of a professional Homeopath for Constitutional Therapy.

The following are some remedies specific to acute Bronchitis: (remedies can be combined)

- **ANTIMONIUM TARTARICUM-** deep congested sounds in the chest, a feeling of being suffocated by mucus, drowsiness.
- **BRYONIA ALBA-** Bronchitis with a small, dry cough.
- **CHINA SULPHURICUM-** oppression of the chest, pain across chest, pressure on left, heart palpitations.
- **FERRUM PHOSPHORICUM-** if fever is present.
- **IPECACUANHA-** wheezing in the chest.
- **KALI BICHROMICUM-** cough that produces lumps of greenish/yellow phlegm.
- **KALI CARB-** intolerance of cold weather, sharp stitching pain, whole chest very sensitive.
- **MERCURIUS SOL OR VIV-** Bronchitis with large lumps of yellow phlegm.

ACUPUNCTURE & TRADITIONAL CHINESE MEDICINE (TCM)

A treatment plan based on careful diagnosis may utilize some of the more commonly known branches of TCM and include acupuncture, herbs, nutrition, exercise and tuina (Chinese medical massage/manipulation).

With the expertise of the licensed provider of Chinese Medicine a correct pattern/s for your symptom/s is chosen from one of several that fall under a certain disease or condition category.

Treating patterns of Bronchitis may be seen as rebellious Lung qi, Lung heat; Lung cold; accumulation toxic heat and/or Lung qi and yin deficiency. Some forms of TCM may be chosen singly or together for the best treatment plan and holistic response.

OTHER TREATMENT CHOICES

Pelargonium- is a South African herb, also known as black geranium. It has been known to help soothe acute bronchitis, according to a 2008 report published in 'Phytomedicine.' In their analysis of six clinical trials testing pelargonium's efficacy as an acute bronchitis treatment, the report's authors found that pelargonium significantly improved symptoms of acute bronchitis without causing any serious side effects.

Oregano Oil- contains a compound called carvacrol, which has been shown to help break through the outer cell membranes that help protect bacteria from the immune system. Studies have shown that oil of oregano is effective at killing bacteria, and could also help the immune system take action against viruses, fungi and parasites.

To help relieve respiratory congestion, allergies, coughs, chronic bronchitis, and sinusitis, add a few drops of the oil to a diffuser or vaporizer and inhale deeply for a few minutes.

The diluted oil should be avoided when pregnant or nursing and on babies and children. It should not be used on sensitive or damaged skin and it is not recommended for use if you have high blood pressure or a heart condition. Wise consumers should be cautious of adulterated oils or oils that are made from Spanish oregano, thyme, or from cultivated oregano. These do not produce the same medicinal benefits as the wild Mediterranean herb.

Colloidal Silver- a natural anti-bacterial, anti-fungal, anti-viral and anti- parasitic. ASAP by Silver Biotics is the only patented colloidal silver product presently on the market. It is formulated with an extra bond of hydrogen allowing the silver particles to efficiently flow through and out of the body.

Clove Oil- used by Ancient China & India it is known for its anti-infectious, analgesic and anti-inflammatory properties. Its anti-infectious properties include: anti-viral, anti-bacterial and anti-fungal.

CANDIDA (CANDIDIASIS)

Candida is the scientific name for yeast. It is a fungus that lives almost everywhere, including in your body. Usually, your immune system keeps yeast under control. If you are sick or taking antibiotics, it can multiply and cause infection.

Candida also develops from an over burden of *heavy metals*. If your body has been contaminated by the removal of metal amalgams from your teeth, or other exposures, the body's natural defense is for the immune system to increase fungal levels to protect cells against the metal poisoning. Other common causes of yeast overgrowth are atrophy of intestinal mucus membrane, digestive disorders, chemotherapy, radiation therapy and/or hormone therapy. Yeast infections affect different parts of the body in different ways:

Thrush is a yeast infection that causes white patches in the mouth

Candida esophagitis is thrush that spreads to the esophagus, the tube that takes food from your mouth to your stomach. It can make it hard or painful to swallow and feel pain behind the breastbone.

Women can get *vaginal* yeast infections (Vaginitis), causing itchiness, pain and possibly a cottage-cheese type discharge and pain with intercourse.

Yeast infections of the *skin* (Coetaneous) cause small to large patches of red, itching, moist, rawness and rash.

Yeast infections in your *bloodstream* can be serious and cause many symptoms.

CONVENTIONAL TREATMENT

Antifungal medicines can reduce yeast infections in most people. If you have a weak immune system, treatment might be more difficult. Using prescription drugs usually brings *temporary* relief only. Complete relief needs further natural intervention.

NATURAL TREATMENT

There are a number of effective anti-fungal treatments, but they must be taken while following a Candida Diet. If not, the very foods you eat will continue to feed the Candida faster than the remedy is able to bring it into balance. For further dietary information, a book written about human health and nutrition, including Candida, is by Dr. Weston A. Price, **Nutrition and Physical Degeneration**.

- **Candida Diet** – Remove from diet all of the following for a minimum of 4 weeks:
- **Sugar** all types: brown, white, syrup, molasses, honey, fructose, lactose, maltose, dextrose etc. Check all ingredients. Also eliminate Agave, since it is another form of fructose.
- **Yeast** products: bread, pizza, buns, breadcrumbs, gravy mix etc. flavored foods i.e. crackers, and foods containing citric acid.

- **Refined grains** white flour products, cakes, biscuits, pasta, corn flour, cereals etc. all prepared breakfast cereals except Shredded Wheat, Oatmeal and Buckwheat cereal.
- **Cured and smoked** products: bacon, meats, kippers etc.
- **Fermented** products, vinegar, pickles, chutney, soy sauce, alcohol.
- **Black Tea** (carries mold) Ovaltine and all **malted** products.
- **Cow's milk** all cheese products, cream cheese (except yoghurt and cottage cheese).
- **Fruit juice** from concentrate or dried fruits (berries such as raspberries, blueberries and blackberries are OK.)
- **Mushrooms** they are fungi.
- **Peanuts** and peanut products- they can be contaminated with mold.

ENJOY THE FOLLOWING FOODS (EAT AS MUCH ORGANIC AS POSSIBLE)

- **Onions** and **garlic**
- **Fresh vegetables** and their juices, especially dark, leafy greens (beware of carrot juice, it is high in sugar)
- **Rainbow salads** (multi-color greens)
- **Meats** unprocessed preferably organic or free-range
- **Almond milk**, **Hemp** and other nut milks
- **Butter** (never margarine)
- **Herbs** mild spices
- **Freshly cracked nuts** seeds (less mold contamination)
- **Cold pressed oils** Olive oil, Sunflower, Safflower (never Canola)
- **Coconut oil** and coconut butter
- **Brown rice** and flours, nut flours (use for baking)
- **Oats** (porridge makes an excellent breakfast – make with water and serve with nuts and seeds and natural sweeteners (Stevia & Xylitol)
- **Fish** preferably unprocessed, oily fish, *wild caught* is best
- **Eggs** lentils, peas and beans,
- **Sourdough bread** made from a culture (no yeast)
- **Natural sweeteners** Stevia & Xylitol, (never Agave, since it is a form of fructose)
- **Fruit and herbal** teas
- **Distilled water** (helps with detoxification)

MONITOR YOUR pH LEVELS

Candida thrives in an acidic environment. The main purpose of making dietary adjustments is to bring the body into a more alkaline state. It is important to keep the pH of the body balanced to be able to ward off fungal infections. Every person with candida I have consulted with had acidic saliva.

One way to correct this is with *sodium bicarbonate* (baking soda.) Start with a ½ tsp. in 4-8 ounces of water twice daily on an empty stomach. Monitor your pH level with pH strips or a pH meter. Optimum level for saliva is 7.3-7.5 and urine is 6.8-7.0. (Do not exceed 2 tsp. of baking soda in a 24- hour period.)

Fresh *lemon* water or *apple cider vinegar* are also an efficient means of raising pH levels.

Baking soda can also be used topically as a soothing swab for vaginal infections. Sometimes it is your sexual partner who may need to be treated, since candida is passed through bodily fluids enabling the infection to be passed back and forth.

HOMEOPATHIC REMEDIES

A Constitutional Homeopathic Remedy can help to strengthen the immune system which will assist in keeping natural fungus balanced. Consult a professional Homeopath.

- **General Fungal Infections**: Hepar Sulph, 200C, every other day
- **Nail Fungus**: GRAPHITES 200C, every 3rd day
- **Fungal patches on skin** (white): MERCURIUS SOL 200C, every other day
- **Ringworm**: TELLURIUM 200C, every other day

The following Homeopathic remedies treat fungal overgrowth:

- **CALCAREA CARBONICUM–** recurring illness
- **CANDIDA-** (as a homeopathic remedy) covers many symptoms
- **HELONIAS-** worse from sugar
- **LYCOPODIUM-** digestive issues
- **MERCURIUS SOL-** especially if there is a cheesy odor
- **PULSATILLA-** if worse from fats
- **SEPIA-** vaginal infection
- **THUJA-** skin issues
- **CELL SALT; KALI MUR 6x-**   for thrush or eruptions around the mouth, 2-3 x's daily

ACUPUNCTURE & TRADITIONAL CHINESE MEDICINE (TCM)

Treating patterns of Candida may be seen as damp heat in lower jaio Liver channel. Some forms of TCM may be chosen singly or together for the best treatment plan and holistic response.

GEMMOTHERAPY- There are a number of antifungal Gemmo's and a choice of protocol is dependent on accompanying symptoms.

Elm, Cowberry, Olive, Walnut, Black Currant, Black Elder, Grape Vine are the most active anti-fungal. They should be accompanied by Juniper and Rosemary to flush the liver and kidneys after infection.

SUPPLEMENTS

CAPRYLIC ACID- Caprylic Acid is one of the three fatty acids (along with capric acid and lauric acid) that are found in coconut oil. It is a potent antifungal that kills Candida cells, as well as restoring your stomach acidity to its normal levels. It is available in gel capsules, which will allow the caprylic acid to infiltrate the intestinal tract and start killing off Candida cells.

Natural antifungals like caprylic acid work best in combination, as this prevents the Candida yeast from adapting to a single treatment. So you can combine caprylic acid with other natural antifungals like oregano oil, garlic and grapefruit seed extract.

GARLIC- Garlic is another extraordinary anti-fungal. Garlic contains many different substances with anti-bacterial and anti-fungal properties, including allicin, alliin, and S-allylcysteine. Due to the variety of substances, Candida will not develop a resistance to garlic like it does with many pharmaceutical drugs. Chop garlic and add it to food or use garlic capsules.

OREGANO OIL- Wild Oil of Oregano contains powerful antifungal agents that eliminate Candida effectively and safely. Take 1-3 drops under the tongue or with juice 3 times daily. Some cases may need more aggressive treatment by filling a gel cap or vegi cap with 5-8 drops of the Oregano oil and taking that once a day with a meal. Continue treatment until all symptoms have cleared.

CLOVE OIL- cloves are a powerful anti-fungal agent often used to treat athlete's foot and other fungal infections. Clove oil's use as an antifungal is well supported by research. The constituents of clove oil are eugenol, eugenyl acetate, caryophyllene and iocaryophyllene, of which eugenol is the active ingredient. Its antiseptic properties allow it to kill the Candida yeast, while it also boosts your immune system.

GRAPEFRUIT SEED EXTRACT- for many years grapefruit seed extract was touted as an effective antifungal treatment. In recent years a number of studies have revealed that many grapefruit seed extract products are adulterated and contain benzethonium chloride, a synthetic antimicrobial often used in cosmetics and other topical preparations, as well as the preservatives triclosan and methylparaben. For this reason, it would be prudent to use this product with caution.

COLLOIDAL SILVER- a powerful antifungal

DIGESTIVE ENZYMES- an overgrowth of candida albicans in the intestinal tract compromises digestion; the addition of a digestive enzyme will support rebuilding of the immune system. Digestion is the most important function of the body.

LEMON GRASS- (Cymbopogon citratus) Stimulates cell regeneration and soothes and treats intestinal infections, as well as pathogenic intestinal flora such as Candida albicans. It has known antibacterial and antifungal properties and can help to repair intestinal walls that have been damaged by Candida overgrowth.

PRO-BIOTICS- fungal infections greatly disrupt the balance of natural bacteria vs. natural fungus in the gut and bowel tract. It is important to re-introduce healthy bacteria back into the body.

CANKER SORES

Canker sores are small, round sores on the inside of the cheek, under the tongue, or in the back of the throat. They usually have a red edge and a gray center. They can be quite painful. They are not the same as cold sores, usually caused by herpes simplex.

Canker sores aren't contagious. They are mouth ulcers and caused by a disruption of oral mucosa. They may happen if you have a viral infection. They may also be triggered by stress, food allergies (such as gluten), lack of vitamins and minerals, hormonal changes or menstrual periods. In some cases, a simple case of broken skin in the mouth can turn into a canker sore or mouth ulcer.

CONVENTIONAL TREATMENT

In most cases, the sores go away by themselves. Some ointments, creams or rinses may help with the pain. Avoiding hot, spicy food while you have a canker sore also helps.

Conventional medicine treats severe canker sores with prescription anti-inflammatory ointments (such as Aphthasol or Kenalog in Orabase) applied directly to the sore. These agents don't cure the sores, but they may prevent them from becoming irritated and more painful when you eat, drink or brush your teeth.

NATURAL TREATMENT

Zinc lozenges, Vitamin C, Vitamin B complex, or a Lysine supplement can help shorten the duration of the sore.

Mouth sores usually occur because the saliva pH is too acidic. It is important to keep the pH of the body balanced to ward off infections. One method of correcting this is with sodium bicarbonate (baking soda.) Start with a ½ tsp. in 4-8 ounces of water twice daily on an empty stomach. Monitor your pH level with pH strips or a pH meter. Optimum level for saliva is 7.3-7.5 and urine is 6.8-7.0. (Do not exceed 2 tsp. of baking soda in a 24-hour period.)

Fresh lemon water and apple cider vinegar also help to raise pH levels.

HOMEOPATHIC REMEDIES

- **BORAX-** (sodium borate) is a powerful remedy for painful mouth sores. Taking a dose at the earliest onset, followed by a dose one hour later, then three times per day will help to alleviate pain and shorten the duration. If caught soon enough, the sore will recede before manifesting completely. Ulcers are very painful on contact, especially with acid or salty food and may bleed easily. Good for babies or children teething.
- **ARSENICUM ALBUM-** if the person tends to be chilled, has fears (especially about health), is irritable and has burning pain.
- **KALI BICHROMICUM-** large ulcers with a border; circled in redness, can have yellow or yellow-green coating.

- **MERCURIUS SOL OR VIV-** person is thirsty with excess salivation; bad breath and even a metallic taste; tongue margins have tooth imprint, pain is burning and worse at night.
- **MERCURIUS CYANATUS-** ulcerations that are grey, sores after antibiotics.
- **NITRIC ACID-** mouth ulcers that are red and bleeding with pricking pain.
- **SULPHURIC ACID-** ulcers are white or yellowish; bleed easily, bad breath, excess saliva; feels weak and hurried.
- **GEMMOTHERAPY-** Canker sores are caused by a virus, any anti-viral Gemmo's can be used to reduce the level of viral infection in the body.

ACUPUNCTURE & TRADITIONAL CHINESE MEDICINE (TCM)

Treating patterns of Canker sores may be seen as stomach heat. Some forms of TCM may be chosen singly or together for the best treatment plan and holistic response.

CARPAL TUNNEL SYNDROME (CTS)

Tendons located at the passageway, also known as the carpel tunnel, between the forearm and the hand become inflamed, a build-up of pressure occurs. This is due to the limited space at the juncture of the carpel tunnel. The median nerve gets compressed at the wrist, causing pain and weakness to both the forearm and hand. This will result in numbness and tingling sensation in the thumb, index finger and even the ring finger. It is usually found to be as a result of repetitive motion that causes the stress.

Proper diagnosis is important, since other conditions can mimic carpal tunnel syndrome. Besides physical examination you may need x-rays, ultrasounds, MRI and electro-diagnostic tests.

CONVENTIONAL TREATMENT

Treatment can include both non-operative and surgical options. This depends on the severity of the condition and how long it has persisted. Non-operative treatment could include medication, splinting, hand therapy, ergonomic modifications, and lifestyle changes.

NATURAL TREATMENT

If you are looking to repair cartilage, the following is an easy formula:

- 1 packet of unflavored gelatin
- Liposomal Vitamin C (at least 1,000 mg)
- Multi minerals or fulvic acid

Combine ingredients in a smoothie daily. Results will start to be felt after six weeks.

ACUPUNCTURE & TRADITIONAL CHINESE MEDICINE (TCM)

Acupuncture can be very effective in treating this condition. Diagnostics are made beginning with subjective intake of the patient's chief complaint and accompanying symptoms. Following the provider will incorporate observation, palpation, pulse and tongue diagnosis. Each individual organ and pattern is mapped in the tongue as well as the pulse.

A treatment plan based on your diagnosis may utilize some of the more commonly known branches of TCM and may include acupuncture, herbs, nutrition, exercise and tuina (Chinese medical massage/manipulation).

HOMEOPATHIC REMEDIES

The following remedies are a Banerji Protocol™. If the first line does not bring the desired results after 12-13 weeks move on to the second line and then the third.

FIRST LINE MEDICINES (COMBINE)
- **SYMPHYTUM OFFICINALIS 200C**; two times daily
- **HYPERICUM PERFORATUM 200C;** two times daily

SECOND LINE MEDICINES
- **RHUS TOXICODENDRON 30C,** two times daily
- **HYPERICUM PERFORATUM 200C,** two times daily

THIRD LINE MEDICINES
- **RUTA GRAVEOLENS 200C,** two times daily
- **CALCAREA PHOSPHORICA 3X**, two times daily

ARNICA can be added to any of the protocols to improve pain and swelling, topically, as well as pellets.

GEMMOTHERAPY- A combination of Gemmo's can be very powerful treatment. As with most natural therapies, it takes time for the internal damage to be repaired and can take a minimum of three months and as long as six months. Combining Gemmo's is recommended.

- **ASH-** anti-inflammatory for ligaments
- **BLACK CURRANT-** an anti-inflammatory for tendons and ligaments
- **GIANT REDWOOD-** ligaments and tendons
- **MOUNTAIN PINE-** chronic inflammation, pain and can regenerate tendons and ligaments
- **VIRGINIA CREEPER-** rebuilds tendons and ligaments

SUPPLEMENTS
- **LECITHIN-** 1200 mg, 1 cap, 3 times daily
- **CLOVE OIL-** pain relief, topically as needed

CAVITIES, DENTAL CARIES (SEE TOOTH DECAY)

CHOLESTEROL

It was a difficult decision how to approach the topic of 'cholesterol'. Cholesterol is not a disease, since it is an important, integral part of the normal workings of the body. It is only a 'condition' for a small percentage of the population. In fact, it is a health concern only for those with severe heart conditions. Unfortunately, in the age of statin drugs people now believe it is a rampant 'dis-ease' that afflicts most of the population. This could not be further from the truth.

Cholesterol is a waxy, fat-like substance that occurs naturally in all parts of the body. Your body needs cholesterol to work properly. If you have too much in your blood, it may combine with other substances in the blood and stick to the walls of your arteries. This is called plaque. Plaque can narrow your arteries or even block them.

Plaque is not however exclusively a product of cholesterol. Other plaque producers are type 2 diabetes and high blood pressure. Also, being pre-diabetic and having pre-hypertension can contribute to the creation of plaque.

High levels of cholesterol in the blood is said to increase your risk of heart disease. There is not an abundance of research to corroborate this, but it seems to have become deeply imbedded in the theories of western medicine. Cholesterol levels rise as you get older. There are usually no signs or symptoms that you have high blood cholesterol, but it can be detected with a blood test. Doctors say you are likely to have high cholesterol if members of your family have it, but it is just as likely to be the result of subscribing to the same lifestyle, rather than genetics.

An unnaturally decreased blood cholesterol level can be the cause of depression, joint pain and sleeplessness. Compounds that contain Cholesterol like progesterone, estradiol and testosterone increase serotonin receptor activity. A low cholesterol level decreases serotonin receptor activity, which in turn can cause depression.

Statin drugs were initially meant to help lower cholesterol in those who already had heart disease. AstraZeneca, however, received permission from the FDA to sell Crestor® to a potential new market of 6.5 million people, none of whom actually have cholesterol or heart problems, as a preventive measure.

This means, even though only a very small portion of the population would ever need a statin drug, it is now believed by doctors that everyone should have reduced levels of cholesterol. That's like saying we should all take chemotherapy, just in case!

There is little to no evidence in any of the industry sponsored trials that warrants the mass distribution of statin drugs. Lowering your natural cholesterol levels is dangerous to many and causes serious side-effects.

You can lower your cholesterol to your healthy normal level by exercising and eating a proper diet with more fruits and vegetables. Finding the correct cholesterol level that is right for you is very important, especially since the brain, which is made up of 70% fat, and the liver, which needs cholesterol to function properly can be at risk with lowered fat levels. Healthy cholesterol should have a spread of approximately 100 points between your HDL and LDL (without concern for the actual numbers themselves.)

CONVENTIONAL TREATMENT

- Statin drugs

NATURAL TREATMENTS

Proper diet and exercise; even walking 20 minutes a few times per week can help. Do not subscribe to LOW FAT diets, they are dangerous and can exacerbate your health issues. The body needs fat to operate properly, but it needs the correct mono-unsaturated fats. Coconut oil, olive oil, avocado oil, sunflower seed oil and hemp oil are examples of healthy fats. Grass fed meats are also a healthier choice. When the body is fed good fats there is a feeling of satiation and appetite can be normalized. Always choose butter over margarine.

Statin drugs may be a quick fix for reducing cholesterol levels, but they come with a price. A healthy lifestyle creates optimum health and longevity.

HOMEOPATHY

There are many remedies that can assist with cholesterol balance, most being dispensed as a constitutional remedy. This is done with the assistance of a qualified Homeopath. The following are a few remedies to be considered.

- CALCARIA CARBONICA
- CORTISOL
- DULCAMERA
- LYCOPODIUM
- SULPHUR
- **GEMMOTHERAPY-** Hawthorn, Hazel, Maize, Olive

Combine any of the above with *Juniper* and *Rosemary* for efficient detoxification through the liver and kidneys.

COLDS AND FLU

Colds and flu share some symptoms, but each have their own specific symptoms that can help to differentiate.

A fever, headache, body pain, fatigue, weakness, chest discomfort, and cough and sinus issues usually accompany flu.

A cold is rarely accompanied by a fever or body ache, but may include a stuffy or runny nose, a sore throat and mild chest discomfort. Many colds are also accompanied by a cough; however, many times this cough is actually due to allergies. The symptoms of seasonal allergies mimic a cold and a further diagnosis may be necessary.

CONVENTIONAL TREATMENT

Anti-biotic use should be avoided with most colds and flu, since they are generally not driven by a bacterial strain and are ineffective. They can further erode the immune system by killing off much needed natural bacteria.

NATURAL TREATMENTS

Hydrogen peroxide- will bring amazing results for symptoms of cold and flu. An inexpensive bottle of 3% hydrogen peroxide sold at any drugstore is surprisingly effective, as well as inexpensive. Use to gargle, put a drop in each ear, dilute and use as a sinus spray.

Put a few drops into the ear, let it bubble and wait 5-10 minutes. Empty ear and repeat on opposite side. This process can be repeated every few hours until discomfort has passed.

Baking Soda- it is important to keep the pH of the body balanced to be able to ward off infections. One way to correct this is with sodium bicarbonate. Start with a ½ tsp. in 4-8 ounces of water every few hours as soon as symptoms arise. Monitor your pH level with pH strips or a pH meter. Optimum level for saliva is 7.3-7.5 and urine is 6.8-7.0. (Do not exceed 2 tsp. of baking soda in a 24-hour period.)

Fresh **lemon** water or **apple cider vinegar** also help to quickly increase pH levels.

A Soothing Tea- combine elderflower, yarrow, boneset, linden, peppermint and ginger; drink it hot and often for combating a cold or flu. It causes you to sweat, which is helpful for eradicating a virus from your system.

For a sore throat gargle with **Calendula** or make a tea of honey, lemon and fresh ginger.

HOMEOPATHIC REMEDIES

One of the areas where Homeopathy shines is in abbreviating and even stopping in its tracks a cold or flu. It is important to treat immediately, as symptoms first appear and repeat remedies often initially. This insures speedy results. The following are some of the more widely used remedies. If you are unsure of which remedy or have a number of symptoms, combining or alternating remedies can work for you.

- **ACONITUM-** at the slightest sign of a cold or flu take one dose and repeat in 30 minutes, if necessary take any of the following depending on symptoms (Combine with **Bryonia** for quick results.)
- **ALLIUM CEPA-** for clear watery nasal discharge.
- **ARSENICUM ALBUM-** if there is restlessness, headache, darting pain in upper lung; shortness of breath, as in asthma; watery discharge from nose; nausea, vomiting and/or diarrhea.
- **BELLADONNA-** fever exhibited by red cheeks and/or ears; throbbing headache; tickling, short cough, worse at night; nosebleeds; sore throat, red, dry and hot.
- **BRYONIA-** mucous membranes are dry; better from rest; bursting, splitting headache, worse from motion; dry hacking, painful, dry hard cough; excessive thirst; buzzing in ears; swelling of tip of nose.
- **CHAMOMILLA-** whining, restless, irritable; children want to be carried; sensitive to pain; earache with soreness; dry tickling cough.
- **GELSEMIUM-** drowsiness, apathy; dry cough with sore chest and fluent mucus; can lose hearing for a short time; heavy, droopy eyelids; acute bronchitis; feels chilled.
- **HEPAR SULPH CALCAREA-** if there is infection with green discharge **(anti-biotic substitute)**.
- **HYDRASTIS-** for nasal discharge that is lumpy and yellow.
- **DROSERA-** spasmodic cough resembling whooping cough; easily angered, does not want to be alone; asthma, bronchitis, nausea, fears, cough worse lying down.
- **FERRUM PHOSPHATE-** anemic, nervous, sensitive people; affects circulation, increases hemoglobin; gets colds easily; for the first stages of otitis (ear infection); for the first stage of fevers.
- **KALI BICHROMIUM-** greenish/yellow nasal discharge, coughs up stringy mucus.
- **MERCURIUS SOL or VIV-** cold moves to eyes, ears and throat; yellow irritating discharges; cough is dry at night; profuse perspiration with a strong odor; gets chilled easily; raw sore throat with difficulty swallowing **(antibiotic substitute)**.
- **NUX VOMICA-** if sneezing a great deal; nose is stopped up at night and runny during the day. Can be irritable and sensitive to all stimulation.
- **OCSILLIOCOCCINUM-** this is my first go-to remedy at the first sign of flu-like symptoms; 3 doses 12 hours apart. You will be amazed at the result.
- **PHOSPHORUS-** desires company, especially in the evening; intense thirst; pulmonary congestion; laryngitis, cough, fearful about health.

- **PULSATILLA-** yellow, non-irritating nasal discharge; loss of sense of taste and smell, earaches in children.
- **RHUS TOX-** when there is *body ache* combine with **BRYONIA**.
- **SAMBUCUS-** if the nose is stopped up and dry.
- **SULPHUR-** flu-like symptoms with diarrhea; good go to when other remedies don't work; burning and itching of skin, worse from water; eyes burn; offensive discharge from ears; difficult respiration, better from cool air. Use when cold symptoms linger.

ACUPUNCTURE & TRADITIONAL CHINESE MEDICINE (TCM)

Treating patterns of Cold/Flu may be seen as wind-heat; Lung heat; Lung cold; accumulation of toxic heat and/or wei qi deficiency. Some forms of TCM may be chosen singly or together for the best treatment plan and holistic response.

GEMMOTHERAPY- European Alder, Black Currant, White Birch.

SUPPLEMENTS

- **ECHINACEA-** helps to support the immune system and is many times paired with the herb goldenseal.
- **ELDERBERRY-** an antioxidant that boosts the immune system; an anti-bacterial and anti-viral; great for colds, coughs and flu; used in 1995 flu epidemic in Panama.
- **GOLDENSEAL-** a strong antimicrobial, a mild anti-inflammatory and is usually combined with Echinacea.
- **LEMON BALM-** a powerful anti-viral, make tea from fresh leaves and drink throughout the day.
- **LICORICE ROOT-** can help to keep virus from replicating, a tea can be made by steeping the raw root and drinking throughout the day.
- **NETTLE LEAF-** jam packed with vitamins and minerals this all-purpose medicinal herb is great to help stay hydrated and to carry the toxins out of the body.
- **OLIVE LEAF EXTRACT-** anti-viral and widely known as a natural, non-toxic immune system builder.
- **OREGANO OIL-** a great natural anti-bacterial and anti-viral. For a sore throat, put a few drops in water and gargle. Follow individual manufacturer's directions for dosages.
- **PROPOLIS-** collected by bees from the conifer and poplar buds, a resin to help form their hives and keep them germ free. It is one of the most broad-spectrum antimicrobial compounds in the world; propolis is also the richest source of caffeic acid and apigenin, two very important compounds that aid in immune response.

- **VITAMIN C-** a very potent anti-oxidant, use in large amounts during bouts of cold or flu. Children can take up to 2,000mg per day and adults 2,000-5,000mg per day. Purchase a liposomal Vitamin C if your tummy is sensitive to C. It is coated and does not cause stomach distress. It is also protected from stomach acids that interfere with absorption. *(See Chapter VII, What's In Your Home Pharmacy for my favorite brand.)*
- **UMCKA-** is a remedy that shortens the duration, speeds recovery and reduces the severity of the common cold, nasal, throat and bronchial irritations. It is made from the African Geranium and works with the immune system to help support the body's own natural defense mechanisms.
- **YARROW-** this herb is used for colds, flu and measles, as well as to clear gastric excess mucus and dyspepsia.
- **ZINC-** Taking zinc, either as a syrup or lozenge, through the first few days of a cold may shorten the misery of an upper respiratory infection, a new research review shows. The review also found that zinc cut the number of days that kids missed school because of being sick and reduced the use of antibiotics by cold sufferers. It also appeared to prevent colds in people who used it over the course of about five months.

COLD AND FLU REMEDIES

At the earliest onset of cold or flu symptoms reach for:

- **OSCILLIOCOCCINUM** OR **ACONITUM + BRYONIA**
- To shorten duration and severity use **UMKA** drops
- If symptoms linger add **SULPHUR**
- If depression sets in after flu, **AURUM METALLICUM**

The following remedies address *specific symptoms* if condition continues to progress. Not all symptoms need be present.

BELLADONNA:
quick, violent onset, high fever, flushed face, red throat, tickling short, dry cough < night

FERRUM PHOSPHORICUM:
early stages when there are no clear symptoms beyond fever, red cheeks or pale face, nosebleeds, sore throat

HEPAR SULPH CALC:
yellow, or green smelly discharge, heat alternating with chilliness, loose rattling (choking) cough, < in a.m.

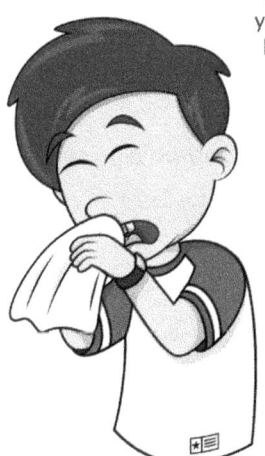

ALLIUM CEPA:
itchy, tearing, burning eyes, clear runny nose, cough from cold air, lump in throat, sneezing

MERCURIUS SOL OR VIV:
sore throat, swollen glands, foul breath, chest pain, < coughing or sneezing, sensitive to heat or cold, green/yellow mucous

KALI BICHROMICUM:
sticky, ropey discharge, post-nasal drip, loss of smell, great weakness, anxiety from chest

GELSEMIUM:
chills up spine, drowsy & droopy, trembling, muscular weakness

PHOSPHORUS:
Heightened senses, tightness in chest
Craves cold drinks, sneezing, cough,
Nosebleed, sore throat, Bronchitis

As symptoms change, remedies change. Repeat remedy often initially, if not enough improvement move on to next appropriate remedy. (< means worse by)

Copyright © 2018 Elena Upton, PhD

COLIC

The US National Library of Medicine describes colic as a condition that affects up to one third of infants in their first 3 months of life. It was defined in the mid-1950s as "the rule of three": healthy, well-fed infants with paroxysmal irritability and crying lasting a total of 3 hours a day and occurring more than 3 days a week. Colic is a "noisy phenomenon" that manifests as excessive and inconsolable crying, usually in the evening. Episodes of crying sometimes occur in clusters during which babies can have increased body tonus and be excessively alert. While the etiology of colic is unknown, it is clear that this self-limiting condition resolves in up to 90% of infants by the age of 4 months.

PRESENTING SYMPTOMS

- Inconsolable crying – typically, high pitched and occurring frequently in the afternoon and evening
- The crying or fussing most frequently begins suddenly and often after a feeding
- The baby cries for more than 3 hours on at least three occasions per week over the course of at least 3 weeks, but is otherwise healthy
- Baby kicks a lot, pulls his legs up close, and makes tight fists
- Baby's abdomen seems to be distended, prominent or hard
- Baby burps and passes gas often
- The crying sounds as if the baby is in great pain
- Baby spits up frequently after feeding
- There may be flushing of face

Amongst all colicky babies there are factors that may worsen the colic symptoms:

- Overfeeding in an attempt to lessen crying
- Feeding certain foods, especially those with high sugar content (undiluted juices) may increase the amount of gas in the intestine and worsen the situation
- The presence of excessive anger, anxiety, fear, or excitement in the household

There are certain features that indicate a need for concern:

- Elevated temperature
- History of breathing problems
- Poor weight gain

Red flags that indicate a need to rule out organic causes and may need further investigations:

- Vomiting (green or yellow, bloody or occurring more than 5 x's day)
- Change in stool (constipation or diarrhea, especially with blood or mucous)
- Abnormal temperature (a rectal temperature less than 97.0 °F (36.1°C) or over 100.4 °F (38.0 °C)

- Irritability- crying all day with few calm periods in between
- Lethargy, excess sleepiness, lack of smiles or interested gaze, weak sucking lasting over 6 hours
- Poor weight gain- gaining less than 15 grams a day

MANAGING COLICKY BABIES:

Managing colicky babies can be stressful for parents. Such parents always require support, as they will be anxious and worried about the cause of crying and their inability to help the baby. It's important that the physician should be caring and compassionate and offers reassurance. Main line management is through conservative means. Certain calming measures may be of use to console the crying baby:

- Swaddle your baby with legs flexed.
- Hold the baby on its sides or stomach.
- Swing the baby side to side or back and forth while supporting the head.
- Try giving him more time in a front baby carrier (the type worn over your chest).
- Make eye contact, talk, hold the baby.
- Take your baby for a ride in the car (but not when you are sleepy).
- Use "white noise" (such as static on the radio or the vacuum cleaner), classical music, or a "heartbeat tape" next to the crib, or make a shushing sound. Adding a small fish tank in the room with the motor running replicates the sound of being in the womb. (No fish needed).
- Try infant massage.
- Put a warm water bottle on your baby's belly.
- Have baby suck on a pacifier.
- Soak baby in a warm bath.
- Try an infant swing.
- Increase or decrease the amount of stimulation in the environment, like light, noise, heat, cold, etc.
- Watch out for over-stimulation or increased fatigue.

You've heard that babies only cry for three reasons; they are *wet, hungry* or *in pain*. The pain is usually from 'gas' and the gas is most times what is commonly referred to as 'colic.' It is important to look at the health and dietary habits of the mother. Is she eating foods that have been shown to cause distress to a baby, such as garlic, spicy food, chocolate or even dairy products. A deeper look into the mother's health might reveal that her state of health produces milk with a pH lower, more acid than the baby can tolerate. If this is the case the mom can adjust her own acidic state through an alkaline diet and/or supplements such as pro-biotics.

There is no specific evidence for restricting certain foods or changing over to certain foods. However, some infants benefit from modifications in the diet:

- Change from one cow's milk formula to another.
- Change from a cow's milk formula to a home-made formula (see below).
- Change from a regular formula to a "pre-digested," hypoallergenic formula.
- If you're breastfeeding, avoid eating certain foods such as caffeine, excessive use of milk products, certain vegetables like cabbage, broccoli, cauliflower; nuts, too much animal protein and taking herbal supplements.
- If breastfeeding, nurse whenever your baby seems hungry, usually every 2–3 hours.
- Elevate your infant's head during and after feedings.
- If bottle-feeding, ask your baby's pediatrician to recommend a formula that is not based on cow's milk and that is not iron-fortified.
- Keep the baby in a sitting position when feeding, and massage their back to get rid of gas bubbles.
- Burp after every ounce or two of milk.
- Try the "colic-carry"– Place your baby, chest down, on your extended forearm, with his head supported by your hand and his legs on either side of your elbow. Use your other hand to provide additional support and walk around with the baby.
- If bottle feeding, try to limit milk intake, and if that doesn't work, avoid limiting milk intake.
- If your baby is spitting up, keep him upright after he feeds.

As for the baby, there are a number of natural solutions. One such solution that can improve colic in some babies is the use of a pro-biotic. Probiotics for babies are specifically designed for infants, since they have a very different chemical balance in the gut than adults. The *'bifidobacterium infantis'* strain is the friendly bacteria most prominent in infants. Infant specific brands promote proper digestion and absorption, encourages the formation of antibodies against undesirable bacteria, viruses and allergens, especially important for babies delivered by caesarean, and is recommended for both breast-fed and formula-fed babies.

Your baby's pH may be too acidic, causing excess gas. You can easily test their saliva with the use of a pH strip. The results should be between 7.3-7.5. If it is lower, then you know it is acidosis contributing to the colic. This can be rectified by dissolving a little baking soda in water and putting a few drops on their tongue. Repeat this a few times per day on an empty stomach. Continue to monitor pH until in normal range.

MAKING FORMULA FROM SCRATCH

Recipes for baby formula can be sourced from **Nourishing Traditions** by Sally Fallon & Mary Enig, **Wise Traditions Journal** by the Weston Price Foundation and at:

http://www.realmilk.com/how-to/recipes-for-whole-foods-baby-formula/.

The ingredients can be sourced at www.radiantlifecatalog.com

HOMEOPATHY

There are a number of Homeopathic remedies that work swiftly to ease the pain of colic. It might be helpful to ask your doctor for a specific diagnosis. Do not be afraid to repeat remedies often (every 15 minutes). If there is not enough improvement after the first 3 doses, move on to the next appropriate remedy. Remedies can also be combined. Sugar pellets can be dissolved in a little water and given to the child orally with a syringe.

ABDOMINAL COLIC

- **COLOCYNTHIS-** relieves cramping and intestinal spasms, baby is irritable and restless, better with firm pressure to the abdomen as when laying them over knee or shoulder, pain better after passing gas, baby prefers to fold legs up to the chest, pains may occur after the nursing mother has become angry.
- **MAGNESIA PHOSPHORICUM-** Can be combined or alternated with the Colocynthis. This remedy relieves spasmodic pains when baby prefers gentle pressure like rubbing tummy gently. Pain is also improved by applying warmth to the abdomen.
- **ARNICA MONTANA + BELLADONNA-** when there is sudden onset of intense, spasmodic pains, pains come and go suddenly, flushing of the face, bending forward may relieve pain, baby prefers lying on abdomen and from pressure.
- **BERBERIS VULGARIS + CALCAREA CARBONICA + LYCOPODIUM-** dissolve together and repeat as often as needed. The Lycopodium helps to relieve excess flatulence with much rumbling in the abdomen. Baby is usually worse from 4 P.M-8 P.M. Baby is irritable and cross and abdomen is distended and firm. They cannot bear pressure on the abdomen and prefer a loose diaper. They may prefer to lay on their right side if given the opportunity.
- **BRYONIA-** is the remedy of choice when pain is worse from least movement, motion or jarring. Baby seems to be more comfortable by lying still with legs drawn up. They are irritable and prefer to lie alone in a cool, quiet, dark room without being disturbed.
- **CHAMOMILLA-** bloated, distended tummy, tight like a drum. This baby has the highest degree of irritability. They appear angry and distressed with screaming and howls. They may kick the mother and be oversensitive to light, noise and touch. They prefer to be held and rocked slowly.

- **COLOCYNTHIS-** cramping, dysenteric stool renewed by food or drink (combines well with **Nux Vomica**).
- **IPECACUANHA-** baby does not like to be moved, copious saliva, belching, pleased by nothing.
- **NUX VOMICA-** Irritable, straining, ineffectual urging to defecate, worse after eating, in a.m. and if chilled or tired, startled easily by noise and light.
- **SECALE-** bloated like in Chamomilla, but with watery diarrhea and/ or discolored stools.
- **SENNA-** for flatulent colic when baby is full of wind, there is constipation that leads to colic.
- **STAPHYSAGRIA-** dislikes being touched, may throw things, mother suffering from emotional indignation.

CONSTIPATION

The US library of Medicine website, Medline Plus defines constipation as a person having three or fewer bowel movements in a week. The stool can be hard and dry. Sometimes it is painful to pass.

As a consulting health care practitioner my experience has been that healthy people have at least one to two bowel movements per day. If not, the toxins in stools, while impacted in the colon and large intestine are reabsorbed into the blood.

There are many reasons this condition occurs. One of the most prevalent is that the intestinal and bowel chemistry has changed. This may have been through antibiotic use or other pharmaceutical drugs. Other reasons can be dehydration, poor circulation chemical sensitivities or food allergies.

There are many things you can do to prevent constipation. They include:

- Eating more fruits, vegetables and grains, which are high in fiber
- Drinking plenty of clean spring or filtered water
- Getting enough exercise
- Taking time to have a bowel movement when you need to
- Monitor your pH levels

NATURAL TREATMENTS

There are many different types of natural treatments that can successfully rebalance the bowel tract.

- *Pro-biotic* use
- *Digestive Enzymes*
- *Boric acid* or *baking soda* if pH of saliva and urine are too acidic
- Drainage remedies can rebalance body chemistry if there are pathogens present

The first step is proper diagnosis by a qualified health practitioner.

HOMEOPATHY

There are literally dozens of Homeopathic remedies that can assist with constipation. Most are symptom specific and can be prescribed by a trained Homeopath. The following are the Banerji Protocol™ remedies.

Very Hard Stools

- **LYCOPODIUM 200C + PLUMBUM METALLICUM 200C,** two times daily

Stool is Soft and cannot be passed to one's full satisfaction
- **MERCURIUS VIVUS 200C + CHELIDONIUM 30C,** two times daily

If neither is completely effective
- **NUX VOMICA 30C,** two times per day

An effective remedy for constipation accompanied by hemorrhoids is **COLLINSONIA**

ACUPUNCTURE & TRADITIONAL CHINESE MEDICINE (TCM)

Treating patterns of Constipation may be seen as heat in Large Intestine; Liver qi stagnation; Kidney yang deficiency; blood deficiency; blood stagnation and/or Stomach yin deficiency. Some forms of TCM may be chosen singly or together for the best treatment plan and holistic response.

COUGH

Coughing is a reflex that keeps your throat and airways clear. Although it can be annoying, coughing helps your body heal or protect itself. Coughs can be either acute or chronic. Acute coughs begin suddenly and usually last no more than 2 to 3 weeks. Acute coughs are the kind you most often get with a cold, flu, or acute bronchitis. Chronic coughs last longer than 2 to 3 weeks.

CAUSES

- Chronic Bronchitis
- Asthma
- Allergies
- COPD (chronic obstructive pulmonary disease)
- GERD (gastroesophageal reflux disease)
- Smoking
- Throat Disorders such as croup in young children
- Pharmaceutical Drugs

Water can help ease your cough, whether you drink it or add it to the air with a steamy shower or vaporizer.

CONVENTIONAL TREATMENT

- Antihistamines
- Allopathic cough medicine

Children under four should not have cough medicine. For children over four, use caution and read labels carefully. OTC cough medicines are not all safe for children. Allopathic cough medicines can stop the cough, but leave mucus trapped inside bronchial tubes.

NATURAL TREATMENT

Make a tea with honey and lemon juice, cinnamon or ginger can also be added.

Other useful choices:

- Clove oil
- Elderberry
- Slippery Elm
- Thyme
- Zinc lozenges

HOMEOPATHIC REMEDIES

Coughing sometimes is a good sign because it can eliminate bronchial mucus and germs. It can also be uncomfortable and unpleasant. Homeopathy helps to remove cough when it is no longer useful, first by eliminating secretions and then when the cough no longer plays a useful role. Sometimes this method takes longer, but is much more beneficial and helps to prevent relapses. In other words, Homeopathy does not suppress the cough and assists through the healing process.

The following are common symptom specific cough remedies. When choosing a remedy all symptoms do not have to fit and move on to the next closest fit if there is not enough improvement. As symptoms change the remedy may need to be changed.

- **ACONITUM-** tickling, starts suddenly.
- **ANTIMONIUM TART-** rattling cough with mucus.
- **ARSENICUM ALBUM-** wheezing.
- **BRYONIA-** dry cough, feels like it originates in the stomach, painful hacking, worse moving around and going into overheated room.
- **CAUSTICUM-** bronchial passages feel paralyzed, no mucus coughed up, sensation chest is full of mucus, soreness in chest.
- **CHAMOMILLA-** dry worse at night, especially in children.
- **DROSERA-** worse lying down, non-stop coughing fits, hoarse voice, laryngitis, bleeding nose, chest aches, worse at night.
- **GELSEMIUM-** mostly in children, dry at night.
- **HEPAR SULPH CALC-** dry at night, yellow, loose and suffocating in the morning, hoarseness.
- **HYDRASTIS-** dry, hawking with yellow ropey phlegm.
- **IPECACUANHA-** sensation of irritation and itching in the trachea, nausea, relentless, wrenching (works well for cough from allergies).
- **KALI BICHROMIUM-** heavy cough with stringy mucus, thick, ropey, sticky phlegm, clogged sinus.
- **LACHESIS-** worse during sleep, set off by touching larynx, cough with a sensation of a crumb in the throat.
- **PHOSPHORUS-** racking cough, can be harsh.
- **PULSATILLA-** worse after exertion, heavy productive cough during the day, dry at night.
- **RUMEX-** worse going into the cold, breathlessness, coughing spasms, tickling behind top of sternum.
- **SANGUINARIA-** repeated burping and/or passing gas.
- **SPONGIA TOSTA-** worse eating or drinking, hoarse cough like a barking dog, painful vocal cords.
- **STANNUM METALLICUM-** worse speaking or laughing.

- **WYETHIA-** dry, tickling, hacking cough.
- **TRACE MINERAL THERAPY-** If cough and colds are chronic, Potassium, Manganese-Copper.

ACUPUNCTURE & TRADITIONAL CHINESE MEDICINE (TCM)

Treating patterns of Cough may be seen as Lung heat; Lung cold; wind-heat; Lung and Kidney deficiency; phlegm accumulation; toxic heat and/or Lung yin deficiency. Some forms of TCM may be chosen singly or together for the best treatment plan and holistic response.

COUGH REMEDIES

A nagging cough is annoying and disruptive. Cough remedies are specific to symptoms. Many coughs are the result of post-nasal-drip and the cause, Rhinitis and/or Sinusitis may also need treating.

BRYONIA ALBA:
cough feels like it originates in the stomach or chest, dry cough, <moving around or in heated room, thirsty for cold water

IPECACUANHA:
allergic cough, shortness of breath cough may bring on nausea and vomiting, loose rattle in chest with great constriction, no expectoration

DROSCERA:
non-stop coughing fits, hoarse voice, constriction of chest, < lying down and talking

LACHESIS:
cough set off by touching throat, sensation of crumb in throat or plug cough during sleep

KALI BICHROMICUM:
cough with pain in sternum extended to shoulders and back, stringy, sticky, ropey mucous from cough or sinus

RUMEX:
cough from incessant tickle in throat pit and bronchial tubes, mucous discharge, rawness & burning in chest, < from inhaling cool air

SPONGIA TOSTA:
hollow cough like a barking seal (croupy), spasmodic, constrictive pains in chest painful vocal cords
> eating & drinking
rawness and burning in chest dryness of mucous membranes

PULSATILLA:
heavy productive cough during day, dry cough at night smothered feeling on lying down thick, yellow discharge, child wants to be carried slowly

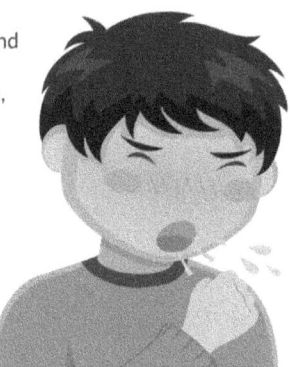

> better by
< worse by

Copyright © 2018 Elena Upton, PhD

DEPRESSION

Depression can be a serious medical illness or a temporary situation due to a sad experience, too much stress, or trauma. If sadness is new to you and not debilitating, you may be able to treat the situation with a number of natural remedies. If the feelings do not go away and interfere with your everyday life seek the help of a healthcare professional.

SYMPTOMS

- Sadness
- Loss of interest or pleasure in activities you used to enjoy
- Change in weight
- Difficulty sleeping or oversleeping
- Energy loss
- Feelings of worthlessness
- Thoughts of death or suicide

If you feel you need temporary relief from an acute bout of depression seek the help of a holistic practitioner who may suggest any of the following therapies.

NATURAL TREATMENT

Many holistic modalities can be utilized in the treatment of depression. Psychotropic drugs are habit forming and difficult to wean off.

HOMEOPATHIC REMEDIES

Homeopathic remedies are extremely effective in the treatment of depression. A qualified practitioner can access your situation and dispense a constitutional remedy. The following are the more common remedies that affect acute depression with common causes.

- **ACONITUM-** for shock and trauma, sudden or old.
- **ARNICA-** I'm OK, I'm tough.
- **ARGENTUM NITRICUM-** needs recognition and respect for their efforts.
- **ARSENICUM ALBUM-** anxiety, fears about health.
- **AURUM METALLICUM-** hopelessness, grief, feels future looks dark, hypersensitive to noise. Works especially well for men who are fatigued and depressed.
- **CALCAREA CARCONICUM-** overworked and exhausted, overwhelmed by life, worries about responsibilities and worries.
- **CAUSTICUM-** ailments from long-lasting grief, hopeless, despondent, overly sympathetic to others, cries easily.
- **CONIUM-** fear of loss of independence, dependent on others.

- **GELSEMIUM-** bad effects from fright, fear, stage fright, dread of failing, fear of doctors, dentist, etc.
- **HYDRASTIS-** over responsibility toward others, guilt over not having prevented a harmful occurance.
- **HYPERICUM-** (ST. JOHN'S WORT) devastated by loss, sympathetic to underdogs.
- **IGNATIA-** grief, disappointment, sighing and sobbing; internal conflicts with self.
- **LACHESIS-** nervous, excitable, talkative, suspicious and jealous of others.
- **LEDUM-** inability to let go and move on.
- **NATRUM MUR-** depressed and introverted, *disappointed love*, chronic effects of grief.
- **PULSATILLA-** timid, emotional, tearful, changeable moods, cries easily, fear of abandonment.
- **STAPHASAGRIA-** violent outbursts of passion, angry, gloomy, humiliation, deep guilt, past sexual abuse.
- **THUJA-** fixed ideas, dullness of mind, feels like mind and body separated.
- **VERATRUM ALBUM-** melancholy, nerves, coldness, effects are sudden and violent, sullen, indifferent, worse from drinking alcohol.

GEMMOTHERAPY

- **FIG-** anxiety, anguish, anger, stress, facial neuralgias, neuro-sensorial balancing, psychosomatic afflictions, existential depression; contains the element lithium.
- **BLACK CURRANT-** an effective Monoamine oxidase inhibitor that has been associated with depression.
- **CHASTE TREE-** menopausal depression associated with insomnia.
- **HAWTHORNE-** Depression, Existential depression, sympathetic, balances the vagus-sympathetic, anti-anxiety, anguish, central nervous system & cardiac sedative.
- **BEECH-** following a shock, grieving, sadness.
- **HAZEL-** Depression associated neuro-vegetative state, anger with liver conditions; can help to increase serotonin.
- **OAK-** depression with sexual frigidity.

ACUPUNCTURE & TRADITIONAL CHINESE MEDICINE (TCM)

Treating patterns of Depression may be seen as stagnation of phlegm, qi blood and food. Some forms of TCM may be chosen singly or together for the best treatment plan and holistic response.

PHENOLIC THERAPY

If you have had testing and know which neurotransmitters are out of balance and causing your depression it can be treated by taking a homeopathic version or phenol. Examples would be Dopamine, L-dopa, Serotonin, Gaba, Melatonin or a combination of homeopathically prepared neurotransmitters. (See Phenolic Charts in Chapter 3)

SUPPLEMENTS

- **Gaba-** (Gamma-aminobutyric acid) a neurotransmitter that helps send messages between the brain and the nervous system.
- **SAMe-** (*S-adenosylmethionine*) helps with mood regulation, immune function and pain.
- **St John's Wort-** (*Hypericum*) can elevate moods, helps depression, PMS and menopause symptoms.
- **Valerian-** (*Valeriana officinalis*) Can help with sleep issues.
- **5-HTP-** (O*xitriptan*) naturally occurring amino acid, can help to synthesize serotonin.
- **B6-** helps with neurotransmitter synthesis.
- **Omega-3** fatty acids (*Pharmaceutical grade) hormonal balance.
- **TRACE MINERAL THERAPY-** Copper-Gold-Silver, Zinc-Nickel-Cobalt.

DERMATITIS

Rashes are a symptom of many different medical problems. Causes include irritating substances, allergies and even a pH level that creates an acid environment in your body. A nursing baby can even get diaper rash from a mother's milk being too acid.

Contact dermatitis is a common type of rash and a catchall work for many different kinds of skin irritations. It causes redness, itching, and at times small bumps. You get the rash where you have touched an irritant, such as a chemical, or something you are allergic to, like poison ivy or pollens. Candida can also cause skin rashes.

CONVENTIONAL TREATMENT

Because rashes can be due to a number of different causes, it is important to determine the underlying cause before you treat. If it is a bad rash, spreading quickly, or if you have other symptoms you should see your health care provider. Treatments may include moisturizers, lotions, baths, cortisone creams that relieve swelling, and antihistamines that can relieve itching. Cortisone and antihistamine can bring relief fairly quickly, but do not reach the cause of the problem. The symptoms will most likely reappear and with continued suppression the issue becomes more difficult to treat.

NATURAL TREATMENTS

If your 'dermatitis' is caused by a fungal infection, known as Candida, you will need a Candida cleanse. (See Candida)

The skin is the largest organ of the body and liver is the organ directly connected to the skin. You may need a liver cleanse. Drainage and detoxification can go a long way to clearing skin issues, since the body will naturally push toxins out of the body through the skin. This is why Candida infection will sometimes show itself at the skin level.

Skin issues can be contributed to poor diet. Always look to any offending foods that might be causing the problem. A poor diet can also contribute to establishing an acid pH in the body. Refer to (pH Balance) for suggestions on re-establishing an alkaline environment in the body.

When there are skin issues you will also find pH imbalance, specifically acidosis. To rectify, use sodium bicarbonate (baking soda) to raise pH levels. You can purchase pH strips in the drug store to monitor progress. Begin with ½ tsp. of baking soda in 4-8 ounces of water. Repeat twice daily on an empty stomach. pH level should read 7.3-7.5 for saliva and 6.8-7.0 for urine. (Do not exceed 2 tsp. of baking soda per day.)

Fresh lemon water or apple cider vinegar can also efficiently raise pH levels.

SUPPLEMENTS & OINTMENTS

Supplements can help to relieve the irritation of skin symptoms, but the cause is internal and needs to be addressed for long term healing to occur. The following supplements can assist in the process.

- **ACIDOPHILUS-** helps to restore natural bacteria in the gastrointestinal tract.
- **ALOE VERA-** soothes and helps to heal inflamed skin, can use topically or internally.
- **APPLE CIDER VINEGAR-** can help to restore the proper pH to the skin.
- **BIOTIN-** a B vitamin, sometimes referred to as Vitamin 'H'; essential for the formation of fatty acids and blood sugar; aids in the metabolism of carbohydrates, fats and proteins as well. Has been shown to work well in conjunction with **Primrose oil** and **Acidophilus**.
- **CALENDULA** cream or gel- Calendula is a Homeopathic preparation that sooths and heals the skin. Some brands of gel contain alcohol, which can sometimes burn the skin so if you are sensitive you may want to choose cream.
- **CLOVE OIL-** has antifungal and anti-viral properties.
- **EVENING PRIMROSE OIL-** a good source of omega 3 and works well when used in conjunction with Biotin and Acidophilus.
- **GRAPEFRUIT SEED EXTRACT-** if this is effective for you then fungus is the cause of your skin irritation.
- **TEA TREE OIL-** a potent anti-fungal and anti-bacterial; can also clear ringworm on the skin.

HOMEOPATHIC REMEDIES

The following remedies are Banerji Protocols™ from the Banerji Clinic for relief from various skin issues that fall under the category of dermatitis. Repeat remedies twice daily for 3 months, or until issue is cleared.

- Shingles- **ANTIMONIUM CRUDUM 6C + RHUS TOX 200C**
- Skin rashes- **ANTIMONIUM CRUDUM 6C**, as needed
- Oozing eczema- **HEPAR SULPH CALCAREA 200C**
- Itching at night- **COFFEA CRUDA 200C** at bedtime

BANERJI PROTOCOLS™

- Dry, cracked skin- **PETROLEUM 200C**, 2 times daily
- Eczema- **ANTIMONIUM CRUDUM 200C** mixed with **ARSENICUM ALBUM 200C**, 2 times daily
- Fungal Patches- **MERCURIUS SOLIBUS 200C**, every other day
- Fungal Infections- **ANTIMONIUM CRUDUM 6C** with **ARSENICUM ALBUM 200C**, 2 times daily

- Hives- **APIS 6C** or **URTICA URENS 30C**, every 3 hours
- Itching during change of seasons- **ANTIMONIUM CRUDUM 6C**, 2 times daily
- Pioson Ivy/Oak- **ANACARDIUM 30C**, 2-4 times daily

ACUPUNCTURE & TRADITIONAL CHINESE MEDICINE (TCM)

Treating patterns of Dermatitis may be seen as wind-heat or damp-heat at wei (Skin) level; toxic heat or excess heat accumulation. Some forms of TCM may be chosen singly or together for the best treatment plan and holistic response.

GEMMOTHERAPY

The Gemmo tinctures that work well for skin drainage are:

- **CEDAR OF LEBANON-** Fountain of youth for skin. Affects dryness, is anti-inflammatory, can affect eczema, psoriasis, dermatosis and can also help to improve wrinkles by working on the elastin of the skin.
- **BLACK CURRENT-** High in Vitamin C, known to stimulate the endocrine system. As a result, the skin benefits from improved hormonal balance.
- **ELM-** An anti-inflammatory and detoxifier. For this reason works on diaper rash and jock itch, as well as eczema, blistering, acne, boils and dermatitis. Can also help to expedite outbreaks from Herpes.
- **EUROPEAN ALDER-** Has been used to settle down *allergic skin reactions* to drugs, stings, exposure to toxic plants, or food reactions.
- **FIG-** Assists with sensitivity to the sun, warts and necrotic issues.
- **GRAPE VINE-** Allergic dermatitis, warts, herpetic outbreaks (since it is anti-viral), and works to improve collagen.
- **GREY ALDER-** Can be used topically on poison ivy/oak, or orally for eczema, pustular acne, and boils.

SKIN REMEDY REFERENCE CHART

ABSCESS
Silicea + Clove Oil

ACNE
Hepar Suph Calc

BOILS
Hepar Sulph Calc

DRY, CRACKED SKIN
Petroleum or Graphites

ECZEMA
Antimonium crudum

HERPES
Antimonium crud + Mercurius

HIVES
Apis or Urtica urens

IMPETIGO
Antimonnium crudum
+ hepar Sulh Calc

ITCHY SKIN (SEASONAL)
Antimonium crudum

POISON IVY
Anacardium

SHINGLES
Antimonium crud
+ Rhus tox

STRETCH MARKS
Thiosinominum
+ Calc Fluor

Copyright © 2018 Elena Upton, PhD

DIARRHEA

Diarrhea, in and of itself is not a disease, but can be a symptom related to disease such as Irritable Bowel Syndrome or Crohn's Disease.

Diarrhea means that you have loose, watery stools regularly. You may also have cramps, bloating, nausea and an urgent need to have a bowel movement.

Causes of diarrhea include bacteria, viruses, fungal infection (Candida) or parasites; certain medicines, food intolerances and diseases that affect the stomach, small intestine or colon. It can also be the result of food poisoning, especially during or after travel. Drinking tainted water, or even brushing your teeth with contaminated water can cause diarrhea.

Although usually not harmful, diarrhea can become dangerous or signal a more serious problem. You should talk to your doctor if you have a strong pain in your abdomen or rectum, a fever, blood in your stools, severe diarrhea for more than three days or symptoms of dehydration. If your child has diarrhea, do not hesitate to call the doctor for advice. Diarrhea can be dangerous in children.

NATURAL TREATMENTS

There are many natural treatments that work efficiently to normalize bowel issues and proper diagnosis is necessary. Blood and urine testing can determine the evidence of pathogens and a stool sample taken during a full moon can reveal the infestation of parasites. (Parasites hatch during the full moon cycle.)

Allergy testing also applies, especially if you notice the condition after eating certain foods. The cause might be as simple as a symptom that accompanies the flu. Sometimes bowel function becomes abnormal after having received numerous prescriptions of anti-biotics. If this is the case, only natural means can rebuild proper body chemistry.

Investigate the emotional aspect of the incidences. If the abnormality occurs after trauma, in the presence of anxiety, restlessness or exhaustion, remedies that address specific emotional issues can help to resolve the problem.

Once you have determined the cause choices can be made for treatment. In acute situations natural remedies can afford great relief.

HOMEOPATHIC REMEDIES

- **ARSENICUM ALBUM-** the number one go-to remedy for relief from diarrhea caused by food poisoning, flu symptoms, anxiety and overeating; symptoms show as nausea, sudden urgency, vomiting, burning and cramping pain.
- **ALOE-** if accompanied by mucus in stool.
- **CAMPHORA-** one dose can many times stop vomiting and watery stools quickly.
- **GELSEMIUM-** usually emotionally based, from grief or fright, bad news, anticipation and even stage fright.
- **IPECACUANHA-** diarrhea with persistent nausea and vomiting (also during pregnancy), nausea does not improve after vomiting, head hot while legs cold, frothy expulsion.
- **LYCOPODIUM-** during pregnancy, while away from home, from cold drinks, alternates with constipation.
- **MERCURIUS-** severe diarrhea, food poisoning, can be bloodstained, green in children; usually painful before, during and after; constant urging, never feel done.
- **NUX VOMICA-** top remedy after excess of drinking and eating, especially greasy or spicy foods, can be chilly and irritable.
- **PODOPHYLLUM-** sudden urgency, profuse, offensive smelling, gurgling and rumbling in abdomen, cramping between stools, prefers cold drinks.
- **PULSATILLA-** diarrhea after eating too much fruit, children who are worse at night or had exposure to cold, or from eating rich foods.
- **SULPHUR-** great acidity, morning diarrhea on waking, hurried in early morning; gets weak about 11 a.m., overheated individuals with lax hygiene.
- **VERATRUM Album-** accompanied by vomiting and fatigue, cold sweats, weakness and may collapse, wanting cold food and drinks.
- **CELL SALTS; NATRUM MURIATICUM 6X + KALI PHOS 6X** given every 3 hours to avoid dehydration.

ACUPUNCTURE & TRADITIONAL CHINESE MEDICINE (TCM)

Treating patterns of Diarrhea may be seen as spleen deficiency; damp- heat in Intestines or toxic heat. Some forms of TCM may be chosen singly or together for the best treatment plan and holistic response.

EAR INFECTION (OTITIS MEDIA)

Ear infections are the most common reason parents bring their child to a doctor. Three out of four children will have at least one ear infection by their third birthday. Adults can also get ear infections, but they are less common.

The infection usually affects the middle ear and is called Otitis media. The tubes inside the ears become clogged with fluid and mucus. This can affect hearing, because sound cannot get through all that fluid.

If your child isn't old enough to say "My ear hurts," here are a few things to look for:

- Tugging at ears
- Crying more than usual
- Fluid draining from the ear
- Trouble sleeping
- Balance difficulties
- Hearing problems

Your health care provider will diagnose an ear infection by looking inside the ear with an instrument called an Otoscope.

CONVENTIONAL TREATMENT

Your health care provider may recommend pain relievers. (This will mask the issue causing the pain.) Severe infections and infections in young babies are usually given anti-biotics.

You may find that children who get infections often are recommended to have surgery to place small tubes inside their ears. The tubes are to relieve pressure in the ears so that the child can hear again. This method is not usually necessary if the child is treated properly by instead getting to the cause of the fluid buildup.

NATURAL TREATMENT

Natural treatment of ear infections goes beyond the symptoms and investigates the cause. Ear infection in children is many times attributed to dairy sensitivity. A bottle fed baby may also be allergic to the formula they are being given. Also be aware of ear infections after vaccinations. Consult a Naturopath or Homeopath to explore the causes of your child's ear infections, especially if they are reoccurring.

Holistic practitioners do not recommend tubes in the ears and can usually arrest an infection before the need for anti-biotics. They can also stop the chronic syndrome by rebalancing with natural remedies and dietary adjustments.

Ear infection in adults is usually a result of a sinus infection or dental issues. Dental and jaw infections are often times overlooked. An infection coming from a decayed tooth, root canal or crown will drain into the thousands of vessels in the jaw and travel to the ear canals. Consult a biological dentist if you believe the problem may be dental related.

Sinus drainage can also back up into the ears. Using an antibacterial and or an antifungal remedy can clear both.

- **HYDROGEN PEROXIDE-** is an amazing natural antibacterial. For sinus infection tilt your head back and spray into nostrils with your 50/50 mixture of 3% whenever you have plugged sinus. It will bubble and help to kill the bacteria. Hold for a few minutes and blow your nose into a tissue. Place a few drops into each ear, waiting for the bubbles; hold for 5-10 minutes.
- **SODIUM BICARBONATE** (Baking Soda)- if there is ear infection, there is an acidic environment. pH strips can easily give you your answer. Normal alkaline range for saliva is 7.3-7.5 and urine, 6.8-7.0. For adults, ½ tsp. in 4-8 ounces of water on an empty stomach, twice daily with work to rectify. For children under 6, dispense a few drops of the mixture. Continue to monitor with the pH strips. You can even put a drop of the mixture in each ear.
- **COLLOIDAL SILVER-** is a safe, anti-viral, anti-fungal and bacteria-killing liquid that boosts the immune system in fighting off sickness and disease.

HOMEOPATHY

A qualified homeopathic practitioner can prescribe a Constitutional remedy to improve overall health and wellbeing. Using suggested remedies, along with any number of the referenced supplements can improve the issues related to ear infections. If there is no improvement after repeating the first choice remedy two or three times, recheck symptoms and move on to the next remedy.

- **BELLADONNA-** one of the main remedies for ear infections; sudden onset, usually fever is present red cheeks and red ears, pain extends down neck, sore throat and even facial pain, irritable, even angry.
- **CHAMOMILLA-** patient is irritable; babies want to be carried, but scream and push away, extreme pain, earache during teething, better by warmth, clear discharges.
- **FERRUM PHOSPHORICUM-** not as sudden onset as Belladonna, but used in early stages of illness; fever, radiating pain, can have humming in ears.
- **GRAPHITES-** offensive discharge, sticky, the color of honey; child is cold, aversion to sweets, can be constipated; bold and forward children.
- **HEPAR SULPH CALC-** sharp, severe pain, usually accompanied by colored discharge from nose, ears or from cough; usually irritable, chilly, wants to be covered; worse from the cold and at night. (*antibiotic substitute*)
- **MERCURIUS SOLUBUS OR VIVUS-** usually used in the presence of pus, worse at night and from warmth, head sweats, bad breath and foul smelling discharges. (*antibiotic substitute*)
- **MERCURIUS DULCIS-** for children with ear fluid and closure of the Eustachian tube, may have temporary deafness. *Can prevent having to put tubes in child's ears.*

- **PHOSPHORUS-** nervous fears, desires company, pleasant disposition.
- **PULSATILLA-** one of the main remedies for ear infections, the child will say it hurts to hear (they mean to listen); mild disposition, affectionate, can have yellow or green discharge; worse at night and from warm room; desires fresh air and has little thirst.
- **SILICEA-** sometimes for later stages of ear infection; can have roaring in ears, children rub ears, pain behind ear, sweating on head, hands or feet; whimpering disposition, chilliness, long history of infection and chronic abscess, cracking around ears.

SUPPLEMENTS

- **CLOVE OIL-** an amazing pain reliever, rub externally to help relieve earache pain.
- **ECHINACEA-** helps to support the immune system and is many times paired with the herb Goldenseal.
- **ELDERBERRY-** an antioxidant that boosts the immune system; an anti-bacterial, good for children to take daily during the winter months and change of season.
- **GOLDENSEAL-** a strong antimicrobial, a mild anti-inflammatory and is usually combined with Echinacea.
- **NETTLE LEAF-** jam packed with vitamins and minerals this all-purpose medicinal herb is great to help stay hydrated and to carry the toxins out of the body.
- **OREGANO OIL-** a great natural anti-bacterial and anti-viral. If earache is accompanied by a sore throat, put a few drops in water and gargle. Follow individual manufacturer's directions for dosages.
- **VITAMIN C-** a very potent anti-oxidant, use in large amounts during bouts of illness. Children can take up to 2,000 mg per day and adults at least 2,000-5,000mg per day. Children love *Suffient C*™. Great tasting form of Vitamin C made into a lemonade. (See Chapter VII, What's In Your Home Pharmacy)
- **UMCKA-** great immune builder, speeds recovery and reduces the severity of the common cold, nasal, throat and bronchial irritations. It is made from the African Geranium and works with the immune system to help support the body's own natural defense mechanisms.
- **ZINC-** Taking zinc, either as a syrup or lozenge, through the first few days of illness may shorten the misery of infection, a new research review shows.

ACUPUNCTURE & TRADITIONAL CHINESE MEDICINE (TCM)

Treating patterns of Ear Infection may be seen as damp-heat Liver and Gallbladder channels and/or accumulation of toxic heat. Some forms of TCM may be chosen singly or together for the best treatment plan and holistic response.

EAR INFECTION REMEDY REFERENCE CHART

CAUSES:
Inflamation of the lining of the mucosa the middle ear. Can be caused by viral or bacterial infection, traumasuch as diving or injury.

SYMPTOMS:
- Pain
- Fever
- Chills
- Noises in ear
- Discharge
- Deafness

ACONITE: sudden onset, pain, anxiety and restlessness increased thirst, skin dry and hot

BELLADONA: sudden onset, throbbing pain, anger, redness and burning, high fever

CHAMOMILLA: teething children, wants to be carried, irritable, screams with pain, fever, thirst

HEPAR SULPH: splinter-like pain, fever with chills, cheesy yellow/green discharge, faint with pain

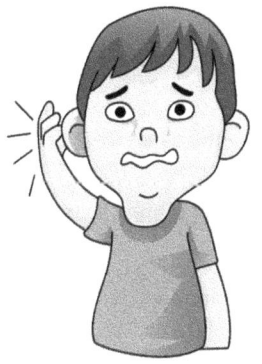

MERC DULCIS: for children with ear fluid and closure of Eustachian tube, temporary deafness

PULSATILLA: pain with weeping, fever with chilliness, green/yellow discharge from ears, no thirst

MERC SOL OR MERC VIV: salivation with fever and chills, boils in ear canal, blood-stained offensive ear discharge

SILICEA: low energy, foot odor, swollen lymph, offensive smelling pus in eardrum

Copyright © 2018 Elena Upton, PhD

ECZEMA (SEE DERMATITIS ALSO)

Eczema is a term for several different types of skin rashes. Eczema is also called dermatitis. It is not dangerous, but most types cause red, swollen and itchy skin. Factors that can cause eczema include other diseases, irritating substances and allergies. Eczema is not contagious.

The most common type of eczema is atopic dermatitis. It is an allergic condition that makes your skin dry and itchy. It is most common in babies and children.

The above are allopathic statements describing the causes of eczema. Eczema is most often caused by a chemical imbalance in the gastrointestinal tract that shows itself on the skin and can be treated with Homeopathy, Gemmotherapy, Chinese herbs or other forms of natural medicine to rebalance the gut.

An acidic environment will also exist. Test pH levels with pH strips or a pH meter. Normal saliva is 7.3-7.5 and urine is 6.8-7.0. To balance quickly, dissolve ½ tsp. of sodium bicarbonate (baking soda) in 4-8 ounces of water. Drink on an empty stomach twice daily. Continue to monitor levels until they normalize. A baking soda solution can also be used topically to sooth the skin and encourage healing.

Fresh lemon water or apple cider vinegar also work to help raise pH levels efficiently.

HOMEOPATHIC REMEDIES

- **ANTIMONIUM CRUDUM 200C+ ARSENICUM ALBUM 200C-** take daily for 2-3 months.
- **GRAPHITES-** cracked skin, eruptions ooze and itch, thick yellow fluid that dries into golden crystals on the skin, worse from heat of the bed, scratches to the point of bleeding.
- **HEPAR SULPH CALCAREA 200c + ARSENICUM ALBUM 6c-** twice daily, if there is oozing.
- **PSORINUM-** tremendous itching, worse at night, worse from being overheated, scratches until it bleeds.
- **MEDORRHINUM-** usually starts in childhood, worse from thinking about it, skin cold but blood feels hot, yellow/copper color spots.
- **MEZEREUM-** intolerable itching, worse heat of bed, ulcers itch and burn surrounded by vesicles, shiny and red. Herpes zoster with burning pain.
- **PETROLEUM-** deep cracks in folds of skin, nipples, finger tips; itching with burning, skin gets raw and does not heal; cracks worse in winter, cracks bleed.
- **SULPHUR-** eruptions usually moist and itchy, worse bathing, worse from heat, painful and usually recurrent tendency.

GEMMOTHERAPY-DRY ECZEMA
- BLACK CURRANT
- CEDAR OF LEBANON
- HOLLY
- WEEPING ECZEMA
- ELM
- WALNUT
- BLACK CURRANT

OTHER GEMMOS FOR SKIN
- GREY ALDER
- HAZEL
- HORSETAIL
- OLIVE
- ORIENTAL PLANE TREE
- WALNUT
- WAYFARING TREE

ACUPUNCTURE & TRADITIONAL CHINESE MEDICINE (TCM)

Treating patterns of Eczema may be seen as wind-heat Skin level or heat in the blood. Some forms of TCM may be chosen singly or together for the best treatment plan and holistic response.

(See skin chart under Dermatitis)

EDEMA

Edema is not a disease, however, it is a symptom of what could be a serious health issue. Edema means swelling caused by fluid in your body's tissues. It usually occurs in the feet, ankles and legs, but it can involve your entire body.

CAUSES

- Sunburn
- Heart failure
- Kidney disease
- Liver problems from cirrhosis
- Pregnancy
- Problems with lymph nodes, especially after mastectomy
- Pharmaceutical Drugs
- Standing or walking a lot when the weather is warm

To keep swelling down, your health care provider may recommend keeping your legs elevated when sitting, wearing support stockings, limiting how much salt you eat, or taking a medicine called a diuretic, also called a water pill.

CONVENTIONAL TREATMENT

Edema should not be treated until the doctor has a specific diagnosis of the origin. If it is related to kidney function you may be prescribed a diuretic, but be aware that they strip the body of much needed calcium and magnesium. If the cause is due to an infection in the bowel tract (IBS) you will probably be prescribed anti-biotics.

NATURAL TREATMENT

Again, a competent practitioner must diagnose the cause of the edema. If it is from decreased kidney function it is important to know if there are kidney stones and the size. If they are small you can try a kidney cleanse or stone buster formula. If there is scar tissue in the kidney, this can be improved by natural remedies.

Most medical doctors will tell you to cut down on your consumption of salt. This can be counterproductive, since the body is nearly 70% salt water. Use a good brand of sea salt instead that contains all the natural minerals from the sea.

It has a grayish tone and much healthier than the sexy pink Himalayan salt that is the rage. Himalayan is ROCK salt and does not have an ionic charge (negative charge), which the body needs to function efficiently. It also does not have the proper composition of minerals, as sea salt does.

Try natural diuretics. Natural diuretics stimulate the kidney to produce more urine by reducing the amount of water and salts that the kidney reabsorbs into the bloodstream.

This improves the functioning of tissues and organs, and prevents fluids from pooling in tissue matrices.

Bringing the pH levels of the blood is an efficient means of avoiding edema. pH levels can be monitored by measuring saliva and urine with pH strips or a pH meter. Normal saliva levels are 7.3-7.5 and urine is 6.8-7.0. When they are balanced there will be no edema. Normal pH protects kidneys, contributes to urinary alkalization and treats chronic metabolic acidosis, An efficient means of accomplishing this is with the use of sodium bicarbonate (baking soda).

Dissolve ¼-1/2 tsp. in 4-8 ounces of water. Drink twice daily on an empty stomach. Your doctor may have told you to stay away from salt, but the bicarbonate is the part the body utilizes. The body uses the bicarbonate ion to destroy free radicals, thereby relieving oxidative stress. Continue to monitor pH levels and consult your doctor for assistance.

ADDITIONAL SUGGESTIONS FOR RELIEF

- Elevating the affected area for 30-40 minute intervals will help to drain fluid
- Gently moving around
- Massaging the area gets fluids moving
- Compressing the area with wraps, swabs or stockings (can soak dressing in baking soda solution)

SUPPLEMENTS AND TREATMENTS

- Apple Cider Vinegar
- Cornsilk
- Coriander
- Cucumber
- Comfrey
- Flaxseed
- Tea Tree oil
- Green Tea
- Parsley
- Stinging Nettle
- Artichoke
- Celery
- Dandelion

HOMEOPATHIC REMEDIES

A qualified homeopathic practitioner can prescribe a Constitutional remedy to improve overall health and wellbeing and reduce the causes of edema. The following remedies are symptom specific.

- **APIS-** below the eyes, ankles and feet, better from cold applications.
- **CALCARIA CARBONICUM-** worse from sitting, unless the legs are supported; weight problems, easily fatigued, worse from exertion; hands and feet are often cold and clammy (although the feet may heat up at night).
- **FERRUM METALLICUM-** comes on after fluid loss; better from walking; may be anemic, flushes easily.
- **GRAPHITES-** swelling of the lower extremities and develops in stout persons with a tendency toward skin problems (cracks behind the ears, on the fingertips, etc.). Pain in the lower back and trouble becoming alert after waking in the morning.
- **KALI CARBONICUM-** swelling above the eyes; sensitive soles of feet; swelling in lower extremities, improved by slow movement.
- **LEDUM-** for tender swollen ankles and feet; better from cold packs; for swelling after injury or puncture wound.
- **PULSATILLA-** swelling related to premenstrual symptoms or from over indulging in rich foods, worse from warmth, better from gentle motion.

GEMMOTHERAPY is an effective method of reducing fluids in the body. Choose the tinctures appropriate for your issues. Can customize combinations for your particular needs.

- BLACK CURRANT- blood
- BLACK POPLAR- overall drainage
- CEDAR OF LEBANON- skin
- COWBERRY- intestines
- GIANT REDWOOD- prostate (if there is no cancer)
- JUNIPER- liver & kidney drainage
- ROSEMARY- liver & kidney drainage
- SWEET CHESTNUT- Lymph

ACUPUNCTURE & TRADITIONAL CHINESE MEDICINE (TCM)

Treating patterns of Edema may be seen as water accumulation; Spleen deficiency with damp/cold; Kidney yang deficiency or yin deficiency with damp. Some forms of TCM may be chosen singly or together for the best treatment plan and holistic response.

ENURISIS (SEE BEDWETTING)

FEVER

A fever is a body temperature that is higher than normal. It is not an illness. It is part of your body's defense against infection. Most bacteria and viruses that cause infections do well at the body's normal temperature (98.6 F). A slight fever can make it harder for them to survive. Fever also activates your body's immune system.

Infections cause most fevers. There can be many other causes, including:
- Medicines
- Heat exhaustion
- Cancer
- Autoimmune diseases

CONVENTIONAL TREATMENT

Treatment depends on the cause of your fever. Your health care provider may recommend using over-the-counter medicines such as acetaminophen or ibuprofen to lower a very high fever. Adults can also take aspirin, but children with fevers should not take aspirin. It is also important to drink enough liquids to prevent dehydration.

NATURAL TREATMENT

Fever is a positive thing and it is important to allow a fever to run its course. As mentioned above, fever is the body's means of fighting infection. Its presence indicates an ongoing battle with bacteria, virus or parasites. The fever helps to eliminate the intruder, or at least prevent it from spreading. Drugs such as acetaminophen or ibuprofen are not necessary in the initial stages and interrupt the healing process.

HOMEOPATHIC REMEDIES

Homeopathy has a number of remedies that resolve fever without interference. The fever is not driven inward; instead the immune system is stimulated by the instructions presented by the remedy. The following are some commonly used Homeopathic remedies for fever:

- **ACONITUM-** fever during cold, dry weather, exposure to cold during hot, dry weather, worry, restlessness, fear of death, dizzy and pale on sitting up.
- **BELLADONNA-** fever with sweating, red, hot cheeks, dilated pupils, sleep-walking, convulsions, muttering, irritable.
- **BRYONIA-** not wanting to move, gastric complications, dry hacking cough, must sit up, worse after eating and drinking, chill with hot head and red face.

- **CHINA-** fevers that come and go, worse from light, noise, odors; throbbing headache, rattle in chest.
- **FERRUM PHOSPHORICUM-** flushed cheeks, nosebleeds, early stage of ear infection, cough with sore chest predisposition to colds and sore throats.
- **GELSEMIUM-** achy, tired, chilled, heaviness, muscular weakness, influenza.
- **IPECACUANHA-** nausea, not better from vomiting; aversion to food, heavy cough, irritable, stomach pain worse around navel.
- **NUX VOMICA-** a feeling of heaviness or lethargy, stomach complaints, irritable.
- **RHUS TOXICONDENDRON-** following a cold bath, patient has the need to move around.

ACUPUNCTURE & TRADITIONAL CHINESE MEDICINE (TCM)

Treating patterns of Fever may be seen as heat in all 3 jiaos (upper/mid/ lower body); wind-heat; Lung heat; damp heat in Lun or; yin deficiency with false heat. Some forms of TCM may be chosen singly or together for the best treatment plan and holistic response.

FEVER REMEDY CHART:

CAUSE:
Fever is the body's defense against infection. It activates the body's immune system.

Heat exhaustion and teething can also cause fever.

SYMPTOM:
Body temperature that is higher than normal (98.6°F, 37°C)

ACONITUM:
exposure to cold, dry weather
great anxiety thirst
shortness of breath
hot hands, cold feet

GELSEMIUM:
fever with influenza
great muscular soreness
chills mixed with heat
dizziness

BRYONIA:
gastric complications
dry hacking cough, must sit up,
worse after eating or drinking,
chill with hot head and red face

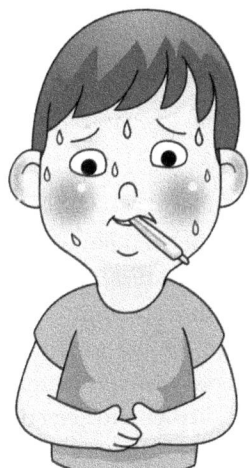

FERRUM PHOS:
alternates pale face with redness
early stages of ear infection
cough with sore chest
predisposition to colds and sore throat

CHINA:
fevers that come and go
worse from light, noise, odors, pai
throbbing headache
ratting in chest

BELLADONNA:
red, hot skin, flushed face
throbbing pain, earache
worse from light or noise
sleepwalking or muttering

Copyright © 2018 Elena Upton, PhD

FROZEN SHOULDER

Your shoulder joint is composed of three bones: the clavicle (collarbone), the scapula (shoulder blade), and the humerus (upper arm bone). Your shoulders are the most movable joints in your body. They can also be unstable because the ball of the upper arm is larger than the shoulder socket that holds it. To remain in a stable or normal position the shoulder must be anchored by muscles, tendons and ligaments. Because the shoulder can be unstable, it is the site of many common problems. They include sprains, strains, dislocations, separations, tendonitis, bursitis, torn rotator cuffs, frozen shoulder, fractures and arthritis.

Usually shoulder problems are treated with RICE. This stands for Rest, Ice, Compression and Elevation. Other treatments include exercise, medicines to reduce pain and swelling, and surgery if other treatments don't work.

This sounds really painful, and it is, but hanging (stretching the arm up as high as possible) and letting the arm carry as much body weight as you can stand. If you do it for a few minutes, multiple times per day, each time you will be able to raise the arm a little more until it releases completely.

This is a very common condition for menopausal women…yes there is a connection. If you fall in this category be sure to pay attention to the changes in your body. (see the section on Menopause)

CONVENTIONAL TREATMENT

Pain medication, intra-articulate steroid injections, physical therapy, and/or surgery

NATURAL TREATMENT

A frozen shoulder can almost always be rectified by one or more natural therapies. Find a practitioner in any of the following therapies; Acupuncture, Chiropractic, Osteopathic, Cranial Sacral Therapy treatments and combine with Homeopathic remedies. I was able to relieve a frozen shoulder with the use of Homeopathic remedies and 'hanging.' (Ouch!) Yes, it did hurt, but I suffered through hanging daily from a bar attached to a door jam. Each day I stretched a bit further and stayed longer. Within a few weeks it was gone. (Beats surgery)

HOMEOPATHIC REMEDIES

- **ARNICA-** helps to relieve pain, bring down swelling and any bruising.
- **CALCAREA FLUORICA-** a powerful tissue remedy and should be combined with others to promote healing of any torn tissues.
- **FERRUM PHOSPHORICUM-** first stages of all inflammatory conditions; increases circulation.
- **RHUS TOX-** when pain is improved by movement.
- **RUTA GRAV-** can help to relieve joint pain when worse from movement.

- **SEPIA-** in menopausal women.
- **SILICEA-** encourages repair of cartilage when taken daily with Vitamin C and a multi-mineral.

THE BANERJI PROTOCOL™ REMEDIES

Solving the issue of a frozen shoulder takes a minimum of two to three months. Be patient and you will be completely satisfied with the results of natural therapy. The following medicines must be taken for a minimum of 13 weeks. If there is not enough improvement with the first line move on to the second, after this time frame. If still not completely resolved, move on to the third line. THE POTENCIES SPECIFIED MUST BE FOLLOWED.

FIRST LINE MEDICINES

- **RIGHT SHOULDER-** CUPRUM METALLICUM 200C, 2 X'S daily
- **LEFT SHOULDER-** SYPHILICUM 200C, 2 doses daily and HYPERICUM 200C, 2 doses daily

SECOND LINE MEDICINES

- **SYMPHYTUM 200C**, two x's daily
- **HYPERICUM 200C,** two x's daily

THIRD LINE MEDICINES

- **SYMPHYTUM 200C**, two x's daily
- **RHUS TOXICODENDRON 30C,** two x's daily
- **TRACE MINERAL THERAPY-** connective tissue weakness, *Fluoride*

ACUPUNCTURE & TRADITIONAL CHINESE MEDICINE (TCM)

Acupuncture treatments are very effective in working with soft tissue injuries. Understanding how patterns may manifest differently in each individual who have the same symptoms or allopathic diagnosis (i.e. type II adult onset diabetes) allows this medical system to be unique. With the expertise of the licensed provider of Chinese Medicine a correct pattern/s for your symptom/s may be chosen from one of several that fall under a certain disease or condition category.

Treating patterns of Frozen shoulder may be seen as qi and blood stagnation. Some forms of TCM may be chosen singly or together for the best treatment plan and holistic response.

FUNGAL INFECTIONS (SEE CANDIDA ALSO)

If you have ever had athlete's foot or a yeast infection, you can blame it on a fungus. A fungus is a primitive organism. Mushrooms, mold and mildew are examples. Fungi live in air, in soil, on plants and in water. Some live in the human body. Only about half of all types of fungi are harmful.

Some fungi reproduce through tiny spores in the air. You can inhale the spores or they can land on you. As a result, fungal infections often start in the lungs or on the skin. You are more likely to get a fungal infection if you have a weakened immune system or most likely have taken antibiotics.

Whenever there is a fungal infection, you can be sure there is acidosis. This means your pH levels are too low and the body cannot operate properly protecting you from infection. One way to correct this is with sodium bicarbonate (baking soda.) Start with ¼-½ tsp. in 4-8 ounces of water twice daily on an empty stomach. Monitor your pH level with pH strips or a pH meter. Optimum level for saliva is 7.3-7.5 and urine is 6.8-7.0. (Do not exceed 2 tsp. of baking soda in a 24-hour period.)

You can also drink fresh lemon water or apple cider vinegar to raise pH levels.

For skin and nail infections, you can apply medicine directly to the infected area, but the infection must be treated at the source, which is the gut. See Candida for further treatment options. You can also apply a baking soda solution topically directly to the affected area.

- **GENERAL FUNGAL INFECTIONS-** Hepar Sulph Calcarea
- **FUNGAL PATCHES ON SKIN-** Mercurius Viv or Mercurius sol
- **NAIL FUNGUS-** Graphites
- **RINGWORM-** Tellurium 200C or Rhus Tox
- **FUNGUS WORSE FROM SUGAR-** Arsenicum album + Sulphur, or Helonias
- **FREQUENT VAGINAL/KIDNEY DISORDERS-** Helonias

GERD/ACID REFLUX/ HEARTBURN

This digestive disturbance is categorized under 'Conditions', since it is not a 'disease.' Instead what is referred to as GERD is an imbalance of acids in the gut with inappropriate pH (potential of hydrogen). When acid reflux is present it is food and acid rising up into the esophagus from the stomach. Heartburn can cause burning behind the sternum, in the chest and throat, as well as in the stomach.

SYMPTOMS

- Gas
- Bloating
- Belching
- Sour eruptions
- Lack of appetite
- Shortness of breath
- A bad taste in the mouth
- Regurgitation of fluid into the mouth

The causes are varied and may be from infection from various pathogens (bacterial, fungal or parasitic); stress; eating too fast with improper chewing over a long period of time; prescription drugs; ulcers and also elevated estrogen and/or progesterone levels.

Disease is always a possibility so consult a physician in the event of hypothyroidism, anemia and malabsorption. Esophageal Cancer can also create acid reflux symptoms so be sure to seek the advice of a qualified doctor.

Bill Thompson, co-author with Parhatsathid Napatalung in their book **pH- Balanced for Life**, writes:

> "Millions of people suffer from digestive problems that are caused by a lack of stomach acid."

> They state their protocols benefit adults or children who eat a normal amount of food but remain either underweight or overweight because of a digestive problem.

Their protocol is recommended to those who have the following problems:

- GERD or Reflux problems
- Poor Digestion (This problem can also be caused by parasites or candida)
- Lack of Bicarbonates in the Pancreatic Juices

"Stomach digestion must occur in an acid environment. Proper pH levels of stomach acidity trigger pepsin, a protease enzyme. Stomach muscles mash the food. Proper pH levels from stomach acid kill all pathogens incoming with food (most important!!).

"The correct and proper pH acid level in the stomach crucially triggers the secretin hormone. This hormone makes the pancreas secrete important digestive enzymes and alkaline bicarbonates into the duodenum (upper intestines) for Main Stage digestion to successfully occur. The duodenum should be at an alkaline to neutral pH, not acidic, or proper digestion cannot take place."

Before attempting any protocol using HCL, it is imperative to first do an acid test to determine if you lack hydrochloric acid. Try this method…the next time you have heartburn take a tablespoon of apple cider vinegar (ACV). If it alleviates the heartburn, then you are in need of HCL. If it however aggravates, this means you are too acidic and should avoid HCL, as well as vinegars.

(Drink a large glass of water to neutralize the vinegar if it did cause aggravation.)

If the test reveals that you are low acid, drinking apple cider vinegar in a glass of water with meals as one alternative to the above protocol. If this relieves your symptoms and you stop the ACV and the heartburn returns, then you know you have again eaten foods that create an acid gut.

Read about **HIATAL HERNIA** under **ACID-REFLUX** to see if this condition might be a missed diagnosis. It has an easy fix and can clear up many digestive issues, both acute and chronic.

You should also seek proper testing for parasites, H-Pylori, Candida and/or any other infections, as well as food allergies that may be the underlying cause of the stomach distress. If the situation is not cleared properly (rather than covered up with ant-acid medicines) it can lead to much more serious conditions in the future.

HOMEOPATHIC REMEDIES

There are a number of Homeopathic remedies that relieve the symptoms of GERD. The following remedies are specific to digestion issues with their common indications. It is best to find the underlying cause, especially if it is a result of prescription drugs or poor diet.

- **ABIES NIGRA-** burning in the stomach and abdomen with heart palpitations; sensation of a rock in upper portion of stomach; acid belches; chronic indigestion in the elderly; worse after a large meal, smoking or drinking tea.
- **ANTIMONIUM CRUDUM-** burning in the pit of stomach; stomach feels heavy; heartburn, nausea, vomiting; irritability, does not want to be touched; craves pickles, wine and other vinegar foods; belching tastes like food eaten; distress from overeating; thick (white) coating on tongue; worse from fats, acids, alcohol and sweets.
- **ARGENTUM NITRICUM-** sugar cravings, but aggravated by; stomach pain after eating; worse from heat and relief from warm drinks and alcohol; flatulence and belching; food gets caught in pharynx; worse from heights or anticipation of upcoming events; regularity of heartbeat may also be affected.

- **ARSENICUM ALBUM-** heartburn exhibits lots of burning like fire; desires small sips of hot liquids even though heat aggravates; better from milk; worse from cold drinks; nausea, diarrhea; nervous type personality with fears about health, restless and worse after midnight.
- **BRYONIA-** bitter taste; watery burps (water brash), better after burping; dry mouth with great thirst for cold drinks; dryness of mucous membranes; may have rheumatism alternating with digestive issues; stomach sensitive to touch, feels like a stone; coated tongue; better from less movement; heartburn from cold drinks when overheated; irritable wanting to be left alone; craves coffee and wine, worse from acid foods and warm drinks.
- **CALCAREA CARBONICA-** heavy people who gain weight easily; craves eggs; loud belching; stomach acid with burning, worse during and after eating; bloated abdomen; acid rises and food will not go down from stricture of the esophagus; throat feels like it contracts after swallowing food; can have sour perspiration and profuse sweating from scalp; anxiety over health with stubbornness; many foods aggravate such as dairy, beans, sugar, fats, vegetables and cold drinks.
- **CARBO VEGETABILIS-** constipation, diarrhea, dyspepsia, belching, flatulence, bad breath & taste, nausea, distension of stomach, heartburn, sore stomach.
- **CHELIDONIUM-** if there is stomach pain and incomplete bowel movements.
- **LYCOPODIUM-** suited to those with low self-esteem, fear of public speaking and/or anger from contradiction; distended and full after the slightest amount of food; heavy sensation in stomach; flatulence; pressure from clothing aggravates; worse from 4:00-8:00 P.M.; craves sweets, alcohol and warm drinks; aggravated by cold drinks, milk, gluten, onions, beans, wine, beer and cabbage.
- **NATRUM PHOSPHORICUM-** heartburn with trouble swallowing; sour acid reflux; belching with stomach pains; coated tongue (yellow); sour fluid is regurgitated; solid food tolerated better than liquids; distended stomach after little food; high uric acid levels; worse 2 hours after eating, especially from sugar, dairy and fatty foods; craves eggs, beer, spicy food and fried fish. Taken before meals aids digestion.
- **NUX VOMICA-** similar symptoms to Chelidonium but with over indulgence from food, alcohol, sweets, etc.
- **SULPHUR-** burning in throat; heartburn from overeating; sour watery eruptions; feels as though there is a lump in the throat; worse in the a.m. after eating eggs and dairy; hunger at 11:00 a.m.; worse before menses; skin issues that may alternate with gastric distress; rotten egg taste in the mouth; shortly after meal there is regurgitation with acid taste; eats too quickly not chewing food well.

WINNING COMBINATIONS (REPEAT FOR 2-3 MONTHS)
- **BLOATING-** Lycopodium 200c + Arsenicum album 6c
- **OVERINDULGENCE-** Chelidonium 30 c + Nux Vomica 200c
- **FOOD SENSITIVITIES-** Bovista 200c + Lycopodium 200c
- **DAIRY SENSITIVITY-** Aethusa 200c + Lycopodium 200c
- **SUGAR SENSITIVITY-** Helonias 200c + Nux Vomica 200c

SUPPLEMENTS
- **ALOE VERA JUICE-** helps to stimulate bile and heals the stomach.
- **DEGLYCYRRHIZINATED LICORICE-** an anti-inflammatory and anti-microbial; can heal ulcers of the gastrointestinal tract (Avoid if you are taking diuretics or steroids, also if you have high blood pressure, low potassium, liver disease, heart failure, kidney disease or are pregnant.)
- **PAPAYA-** contains beneficial enzymes and works to reduce heartburn and indigestion.
- **PINEAPPLE-** also contains beneficial enzymes.
- **PROBIOTICS-** beneficial bacteria, especially if you have taken antibiotics previously.

ACUPUNCTURE & TRADITIONAL CHINESE MEDICINE (TCM)

Treating patterns of Gerd may be seen as Stomach fire with rising Stomach qi or Liver qi stagnation. Some forms of TCM may be chosen singly or together for the best treatment plan and holistic response.

DIGESTION CHEAT SHEET

Serious digestive issues should be treated by a trained professional. Many of the following homeopathic remedies can be taken to improve symptoms. Remedies can be combined.

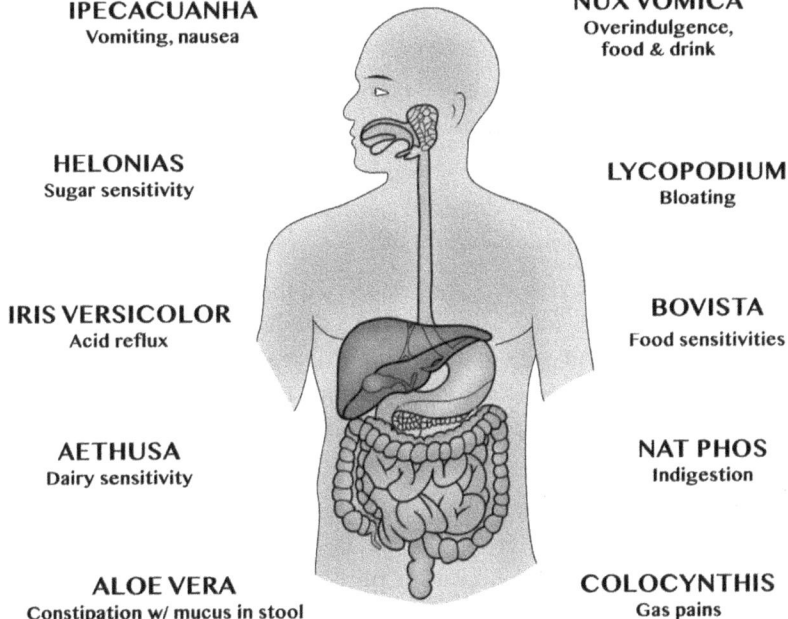

CALC PHOS — Poor appetite, teething

ARSNICUM ALBUM — Food poisoning, diarrhea, vomitting

IPECACUANHA — Vomiting, nausea

NUX VOMICA — Overindulgence, food & drink

HELONIAS — Sugar sensitivity

LYCOPODIUM — Bloating

IRIS VERSICOLOR — Acid reflux

BOVISTA — Food sensitivities

AETHUSA — Dairy sensitivity

NAT PHOS — Indigestion

ALOE VERA — Constipation w/ mucus in stool

COLOCYNTHIS — Gas pains

PLUMBUM — Constipation

Copyright © 2018 Elena Upton, PhD

GINGIVITIS

Gingivitis is inflamed gum tissue and can lead to periodontal disease. I have included Gingivitis under Common Ailments, rather than Disease because it is not a condition one needs to suffer from. Most cases of gingivitis, if the person has proper hygiene, are a result of spirochetes. Spirochetes (also spelled Spirochaetes) are spiral-shaped bacterial/parasitic critters that live in the mouth, specifically in and around the gums. There are different species such as Treponema, Leptospira and Borrelia. They are free living and do not require oxygen (anaerobic). Each species of spirochetes is disease causing, including Lyme disease and intestinal disease. They tend to be overlooked by dentists and therefore not diagnosed as the cause of the gingivitis. As they progress oral health declines further from gingivitis into a diagnosis of periodontal disease (Pyorrhea).

Spirochetes can be contracted from kissing another person who is infected.

If you were able to locate a 'biological' dentist with a dark field microscope, he would examine a sample of your gum tissue and tarter under the microscope and would project the image on a computer for you to observe them swimming in all their glory.

A deep cleaning that brings the colony numbers down considerably, followed by Homeopathic treatment brings the gingivitis under control.

Another place to look for the cause of gingivitis is the gut. If there are severe digestive issues it will be reflected in the condition of your teeth and gums. In other words, the infection stretches from your gut to your mouth.

There are a number of home remedies for detoxifying the mouth such as lemon rubbed over gums, mustard oil with salt; castor oil with camphor and honey; and oil pulling. Oil pulling is an ancient Ayurvedic remedy that uses sesame oil, coconut oil, olive or sunflower oil to pull harmful bacteria, fungus and other organisms from the mouth and gums. About a tablespoon of cold pressed, organic oil is placed in the mouth and swished around for about 10-15 minutes and then spit out.

You can also balance the pH of saliva by drinking a dissolved solution of sodium bicarbonate (baking soda) twice daily. Even swishing it in your mouth will help to pull bacteria and fungus that causes gingivitis. Check your pH levels with pH strips or a pH meter. Optimal saliva range is 7.3-7.5.

HOMEOPATHIC REMEDIES

Homeopathic remedies can be very effective in clearing gingivitis with the most efficient ones being:

- **CALC-FLUOR-** deficient enamel, boils, swelling
- **HEPAR SULPH CALCAREA-** helps to drain infection
- **KREOSOTUM-** helps to clear inflammation
- **MERCURIUS VIVUS-** drains infection
- **PHOSPHORUS-** helps with sore, bleeding gums
- **SILICEA-** removes old tissue

HAY FEVER

Each spring, summer, and fall, trees, weeds, and grasses release tiny pollen grains into the air. Some of the pollen ends up in your nose and throat. This can trigger a type of allergy called hay fever.

SYMPTOMS

- Sneezing, often with a runny or clogged nose
- Coughing and post-nasal drip
- Itching eyes, nose and throat
- Red and watery eyes
- Dark circles under the eyes

CONVENTIONAL TREATMENT

Your health care provider may diagnose hay fever based on a physical exam and your symptoms. Sometimes skin or blood tests are used. Taking medicines and using nasal sprays can relieve symptoms. You can also rinse out your nose, but be sure to use distilled or sterilized water with saline.

- Allergy shots

NATURAL TREATMENT

There are many very effective natural remedies for the treatment of hay fever and also the desensitization to resolve the issue. Monitor your pH levels. If you stay in an alkaline state you will be bothered by hay fever far less.

HOMEOPATHIC REMEDIES

- **ALLIUM CEPA-** singers' cold with acrid discharge; better open air, burning nasal discharge, teary eyes (non-burning).
- **AMBROSIA-** watery nasal discharge, tearing and itchy, burning of the eyes, some throat irritation.
- **DULCAMARA-** Sudden change of weather with watery mucus discharges.
- **EUPHRASIA-** burning tears from the eyes, bland nasal discharge that is worse at night; eyes and cheeks become red with irritation.
- **GALPHIMIA-** sensitive to weather changes; runny nose and eyes; skin sensitivity and/or herpetic eruptions; gastric complaints.
- **KALI BICHROMICUM-** thick, gooey, stringy yellow nasal discharge, post-nasal drip, pain at root of nose; sneezing; can have sore throat; all symptoms worse from exposure to cold.

- **SABADILLA-** Chilly, thirstless patients with sore throat, better by warm food, sneezing.
- **SKOOKUM CHUCK-** Hay fever with dry skin and profuse discharge and constant sneezing.
- **SULPHER-** summer hay fever, aggravated by heat and sun, nose runs outside, stuffed up when indoors; red nose and eyes, nasal discharge burns; can develop into asthma.
- **WYETHIA-** Itching of posterior of throat that feels swollen and creates hacking cough, constant clearing and swallowing saliva constantly with difficulty; worse in the afternoon; itching behind the nose.

Ease hay fever symptoms by alternating three pellets of each, three times per day on a regular basis during pollen season:
- **ARSENICUM ALBUM, HISTAMINUM, SABADILLA**
- **CALCAREA CARBONICA 200C**, can be taken once per week for those who get sick often and for over-all immunity; after time allergies will subside.

ACUPUNCTURE & TRADITIONAL CHINESE MEDICINE (TCM)

Treating patterns of Hay fever may be seen as wind-cold with fluid congestion and/or damp-heat with fluid congestion. Some forms of TCM may be chosen singly or together for the best treatment plan and holistic response.

PHENOLIC THERAPY

One of the main uses of phenolic remedies is to desensitize the body against allergens. Different practitioners have different methods to determine which substances are the offending causes of your symptoms. You can also refer to the chart of symptoms listed in Chapter III. It is an inexpensive, efficient method of relieving the body of allergic reactions.

OSTEOPATHIC TREATMENT

Osteopathy works to unblock trapped energy in the body. When energy flows in a balanced manner everything works better, including having more tolerance to the environment.

(SEE REMEDY CHART UNDER ALLERGIES)

HEADACHES

Almost everyone has had a headache. Headache is the most common form of pain. It's a major reason people miss work or school or visit the doctor.

The most common type of headache is a tension headache. Tension headaches are due to tight muscles in your shoulders, neck, scalp and jaw. They are often related to stress, depression or anxiety. You are more likely to get tension headaches if you work too much, don't get enough sleep, miss meals, or use alcohol.

Other common types of headaches include migraines, cluster headaches, and sinus headaches. Most people can feel much better by making lifestyle changes, learning ways to relax and taking remedies to relieve the root cause.

Not all headaches require a doctor's attention. But sometimes headaches warn of a more serious disorder. Let your health care provider know if you have sudden, severe headaches. Get medical help right away if you have a headache after a blow to your head, or if you have a headache along with a stiff neck, fever, confusion, loss of consciousness, or pain in the eye or ear.

Many women experience headaches as a result of their monthly cycle. Many times natural balancing of hormones can relieve chronic headaches.

HEADACHES, MIGRAINES

If you suffer from migraine headaches, you're not alone. About 12 percent of the U.S. population gets them. Migraines are recurring attacks of moderate to severe pain. The pain is throbbing or pulsing, and is often on one side of the head. During migraines, people are very sensitive to light and sound. They may also become nauseated and vomit.

Migraine is three times more common in women than in men. Some people can tell when they are about to have a migraine because they see flashing lights or zigzag lines or they temporarily lose their vision.

Many things can trigger a migraine. These include:

- Anxiety
- Stress
- Lack of food or sleep
- Exposure to light
- Hormonal changes (in women)

CONVENTIONAL TREATMENT

Doctors used to believe migraines were linked to the opening and narrowing of blood vessels in the head. Now they believe the cause is related to genes that control the activity of some brain cells. Medical doctors prescribe medicines to help suppress the causes of migraine attacks or help relieve symptoms of attacks when they happen. For many people, treatments to relieve stress can also help.

NATURAL TREATMENT

Headaches are a symptom of a variety of issues within the body. Having a headache can be miserable and it is easy to reach for pain medication. Looking into the cause of chronic headaches will reveal the underlying issues that need to be resolved.

ACUPUNCTURE & TRADITIONAL CHINESE MEDICINE (TCM)

Diagnostics are made beginning with subjective intake of the patient's chief complaint and accompanying symptoms. A Lic. Ac. will incorporate observation, palpation, pulse and tongue diagnosis. Each individual organ and pattern is mapped in the tongue as well as the pulse. Gathering this information allows the practitioner to formulate a holistic individual diagnosis within Traditional Chinese Medicine. Treatment plan based on this diagnosis may utilize some of the more commonly known branches of TCM and may include acupuncture, herbs, nutrition, exercise and tuina (Chinese medical massage/manipulation).

OSTEOPATHIC OR CRANIAL SACRAL THERAPY

Unblocking trapped energy can help blood flow more efficiently and resolve issues related to headaches. Also, the movement of trapped energy makes information in the body flow more efficiently.

HOMEOPATHIC REMEDIES

Often a Homeopath can dispense a constitutional remedy that will reach the cause of the offending headaches. The following are some remedies based on symptom picture. Repeat two times daily, or as needed.

- **ANTIMONIUM CRUDUM-** exposure to too much heat, from a cold bath.
- **AURUM METALLICUM 200c-** depression, exhaustion, esp. in men.
- **ARGENTUM NITRICUM-** feels like a band around the head.
- **BELLADONNA-** onset of a cold, from a haircut, being angry; worse from noise and light, throbbing, temples or right side of head (migraines) Combines well with **LEDUM 200c**.
- **BRYONIA-** from constipation; the onset of a cold; coughing; moving or blinking eyes, thirsty.
- **CALCAREA PHOS-** from too much over-thinking, children's headaches.
- **GLONOINUM 30c-** too much exposure to the sun, throbbing migraine.
- **KALI BICHROMICUM-** headache from sinus pain, worse barometric change.
- **LYCOPODIUM-** over eating (greasy food) or from missing a meal.
- **NATRUM SULPH-** mild head trauma, even old trauma can be treated.

- **NUX VOMICA-** overeating, indigestion, irritable, drinking coffee.
- **RHUS TOX 30C-** from muscle fatigue; getting wet.
- **ACONITUM 200C** for neck stiffness.
- **SEPIA-** female headaches, left sided.
- **SPIGELIA-** behind left eye.

THE BANERJI PROTOCOL™

- **SANGUINARIA 200C mixed with BELLADONNA 3X,** headaches with nausea; can repeat every 15-30 minutes initially, then every 3 hours until resolved
- **TRACE MINERAL THERAPY-** Cobalt, Molybdenum, Manganese, (Frontal) Bismuth

HEARTBURN (SEE ACID-REFLUX & GERD ALSO)

Heartburn is a painful burning feeling in your chest or throat. It happens when stomach acid backs up into your esophagus, the tube that carries food from your mouth to your stomach. If you have heartburn more than twice a week, you may have what has been labeled as Gerd. But you can have Gerd without having heartburn.

Pregnancy, spicy foods, alcohol, and some medications can bring on heartburn. Treating heartburn is important because over time reflux can damage the esophagus.

It is important to find the underlying cause of heartburn and resolve the issue, since digestion is one of the most important functions in the body. If heartburn is continually suppressed with anti-acids or other medicines that only cover the pain, it can lead to much more serious issues in the future.

If you have symptoms such as crushing chest pain, it could be a heart attack. Seek help immediately.

CONVENTIONAL TREATMENT

There are many pharmaceutical drugs that suppress the symptoms of heartburn, however they do not resolve the cause.

NATURAL TREATMENT

Heartburn is far more prevalent today than in years past and occurring at a younger age. This is due to the contaminated food supply of modern times, the manner in which they are prepared and damage from pharmaceutical drugs. Cleaning up your diet and eating as much organic as possible is the first place to look in resolving heartburn. Removing unnecessary chemical drugs is the second.

Over-looked issues are pH balance and HIATAL HERNIA. Most who suffer from stomach disorders also suffer from acidosis and/or a stomach out of its proper position. Refer to Acid-Reflux and GERD for further information and under the heading Hiatal Hernia.

ACUPUNCTURE & TRADITIONAL CHINESE MEDICINE (TCM)

Treating patterns of Heartburn may be seen as Stomach fire. Some forms of TCM may be chosen singly or together for the best treatment plan and holistic response.

HOMEOPATHY

Homeopathy is very efficient at resolving the issues associated with heartburn. It is also prudent to pay attention to dietary intake to isolate the foods that trigger the discomfort.

- **ARSENICUM ALBUM-** when heartburn is accompanied by diarrhea or nausea.
- **CARBO VEGETABILIS-** slow digestion, the simplest foods distress, belching, heaviness, fullness and sleepiness.
- **NUX VOMICA-** repeat often for heartburn due to over eating or drinking (great for hangovers).

THE BANERJI PROTOCOL™

- **LYCOPODIUM 200C mixed with ARSENICUM ALBUM 3C**, 2 times daily for gastro related pain (may also have palpitations).
- **IPECACUANHA 30C** combined with **MERCURIUS SULPH 6C**, two times daily when related to food intolerance.
- **BOVISTA 200C**, two times daily for a minimum of 3 months for gluten intolerance

HEAVY METAL TOXICITY

Heavy metals are chemical elements that have a specific gravity (a measure of density) at least five times that of water. There are many causes for metal toxicity, beginning with mercury amalgam fillings to cooking with aluminum cookware, to vaccines laced with mercury. Lead poisoning can also be traced to the use of lead-based glazes on pottery that is used for food. Another huge area of contamination is cosmetics and dyes. Most women never think to look at the ingredients on the box of hair dye they purchase, or ask their hairdresser for an ingredient list. Paying attention to labels usually becomes a concern only after health issues arise, especially allergies.

Arsenic is also a major contaminate in modern times. Most exposure comes about through environmental pollution when arsenic is released from the smelting process of copper, lead and zinc and through manufacturing chemicals and glass. It is also contained in insect poisons and some linseed oil. This in turn has contaminated our water supply, which then contaminates our fish. An arsenic-based additive is also used in chicken feed to promote growth, kill parasites and improve pigmentation of chicken meat. Another reason to only eat organic chicken.

If your level of health has shifted and you are experiencing any of the following symptoms with no clear diagnosis, consider heavy metal testing.

SYMPTOMS

- Chronic malaise; fatigue and general discomfort
- Brain fog; forgetfulness and confusion
- Depression
- Allergies; new ones that keep developing
- Anemia
- Edema in the lungs
- Loss of words; the brain can't seem to grasp the correct words
- Chronic pain; muscles, tendons and soft tissue
- Digestive issues; bloating, gas, diarrhea, constipation, heartburn, cramping
- Chronic Candida infections
- Kidney problems
- Headaches, dizziness, sweating
- Mood swings
- Numbness and tingling in isolated spots, or throughout the body
- Visual disturbances

TESTING

Your Medical doctor may suggest blood tests, but be aware that they may not be accurate. Many metals quickly pass from your blood to your tissues, where they lodge, and are not detected. As a result, serious long-term health problems can go unchecked or misdiagnosed.

Heavy metals do not stay present in the urine for extended periods of time either. Lead, for instance, migrates from the blood into the body's organs and over time is incorporated into the bones. If someone was chronically exposed to lead, then he might have lead in his blood, urine, organs and bones.

Fecal testing can be done during 'chelation' therapy, since the chelating agent provokes excretion of the heavy metals. It is a good measure of what is being extracted.

The testing used by most holistic practitioners is hair analysis. Hair is collected from the nape of the neck and analyzed for its mineral content. Hair holds a history of the past 3 months. There is controversy concerning the effectiveness of this type of testing, but it has been scientifically validated. Forensic specialists use this type of testing because of its accuracy.

NATURAL TREATMENT

Heavy metal detoxification is crucial to your health because metals negate the electrical charge in the body. Heavy metal poisoning creates the same environment as a battery that has lost its charge.

Detoxification of heavy metals should always be done under the guidance of a qualified practitioner. The following list are tools used for this purpose, but which method, in which order depends solely on the health of the patient. The body requires a lot of energy to remove unwanted toxins and only a trained professional can monitor your health through the process.

Chelation Therapy is a mainstream treatment used to treat heavy metal poisoning. However, the term is also used to promote an alternative therapy used to treat heart disease, cancer, and other conditions. It most often involves the injection of ethylene diamine tetra-acetic acid (EDTA), a chemical that binds, or chelates, heavy metals, including iron, lead, mercury, cadmium, and zinc. The term "chelation" comes from the Greek word chele, which means, "claw," referring to the way the chemical grabs onto metals.

For more than 40 years the U.S. Food and Drug Administration (FDA) as a treatment for lead poisoning, have approved Chelation Therapy using EDTA. The human body cannot break down heavy metals, which can build up to toxic levels in the body and interfere with normal functioning. EDTA and other chelating drugs lower the blood levels of metals such as lead, mercury, aluminum, cadmium, and zinc by attaching to the heavy metal molecules, which helps the body remove them through urination.

Because EDTA can reduce the amount of calcium in the bloodstream, some practitioners suggest chelation therapy may help reopen arteries blocked by mineral deposits, a condition called atherosclerosis or hardening of the arteries. It has shown to be an effective and less expensive alternative to coronary bypass surgery, angioplasty, and other techniques designed to unclog blocked arteries.

Chelation Therapy has also been promoted as an alternative treatment for many unrelated conditions, such as gangrene, thyroid disorders, multiple sclerosis, muscular dystrophy, psoriasis, diabetes, arthritis, Alzheimer's disease, and the improvement of memory, sight, hearing, and smell.

Some alternative practitioners utilize Chelation Therapy as a cancer treatment. It is said to remove "environmental toxins" from the body and block the production of harmful molecules called 'free radicals' that cause cell damage.

CHLORELLA is a tiny green single-celled fresh water algae. It is a nutrient- dense superfood that contains 60% protein, 18 amino acids (including all the essential amino acids), and various vitamins and minerals. Studies have shown that chlorella is a natural chelating agent that helps to remove many heavy metals. It is an efficient supplement to detoxify heavy metals.

CILANTRO- this popular herb mobilizes mercury and other toxic metals from the brain and central nervous system into other tissue by changing the charge on the intracellular mercury to a neutral state. The reason for the powerful binding ability is chlorophyll. Any green plant high in chlorophyll has the ability to cross the blood/brain barrier.

Once the chlorophyll has done its job of binding to the metals, it is then imperative to pull them out of the body with the use of fulvic acid minerals. The charged minerals will complete the process of chelation by attaching to the heavy metals and excrete them out of the body through the urinary tract and bowels.

The use of an infrared sauna can assist in the process by sweating out toxins through the skin, once they are mobilized.

Distilled water- drink ONLY *distilled water* while detoxifying. The body will have an easier time removing the metal through the kidneys if there are no dissolved minerals in your water. It is important to also have a negative charge to the water, to help collect the metals. Positively charged minerals have been removed from distilled water. It is important to *drink a lot of water when detoxifying*. Your health care practitioner will suggest an amount based on your weight.

ACUPUNCTURE & CHINESE HERBS

Acupuncture can assist with Kidney, Lymph and other organ detoxification. When heavy metals are being pulled through the body they need to flush quickly and not pool in other organs. Chinese herbs can also assist in mobilizing the process of removing heavy metals from the body.

GEMMOTHERAPY

Gemmotherapy is very successful in chelating heavy metals from the body. It is a process that happens over time and with diligence you will see a considerable shift in health. Whichever Gemmos are chosen from the following list should be combined with **Juniper** and **Rosemary** to be certain there is proper drainage through the liver and kidneys.

- **Black Poplar-** all toxic metals; chlorinated solvents and nitrates; petroleum.
- **Grape Vine-** removes lead.
- **Mountain Pine-** all toxic metals.
- **Silver Birch-** removes waste matter from the body.
- **White Willow-** mercury and other metals (do not give to children).
- **European Alder-** removes toxic metals including aluminum; pesticides.
- **Bilberry-** aluminum, cadmium and lead.
- **Judas Tree-** affects cadmium.

SUPPLEMENTS

- **Milk Thistle** protects the liver while detoxifying.
- **SAMe** - a methyl donor and will help to bind arsenic.
- **Magnesium, B-Vitamins, Vitamin E and Alpha Lipoic Acid.**
- **L-Cysteine, and L-Glutamine** will help to naturally increase glutathione, while binding toxins to the cholesterol for removal through the bodies detoxification pathways.
- **Liposomal Vitamin C,** to be effective, Vitamin C needs to be coated to pass through the acid in the gut (Or Sufficient C™ is another efficient Vitamin C product.)
- **Turmeric** (Curcumin) keeps in check any inflammation and continues to naturally build glutathione.

Foods important to metal detoxification:

- Butter, which has a high content of Selenium
- Seaweed
- Garlic
- Eggs
- Beans
- Onions

Combine *Apple Cider Vinegar* and *honey* in distilled water to taste daily to hasten the detoxification process. Monitor your pH levels regularly. Use pH strips or a pH meter. Fungal infections tend to increase as heavy metals are released. An alkaline environment will help to destroy excess fungus.

Drinking 1/4-1/2 tsp. of sodium bicarbonate (baking soda) in 4-8 ounces of water twice daily is another efficient means of balancing pH.

HEMORRHOIDS

Hemorrhoids are swollen, inflamed veins around the anus or lower rectum. They are either inside the anus or under the skin around the anus. They often result from straining to have a bowel movement. Other factors include pregnancy, aging and chronic constipation or diarrhea.

Hemorrhoids are very common in both men and women. About half of all people have hemorrhoids by age 50. The most common symptom of hemorrhoids inside the anus is bright red blood covering the stool, on toilet paper or in the toilet bowl. Symptoms usually go away within a few days.

CONVENTIONAL TREATMENT

If you have rectal-bleeding, you should see a doctor. You need to make sure bleeding is not from a more serious condition such as colorectal or anal cancer. Treatment may include warm baths and a cream or other medicine. If you have large hemorrhoids, a doctor may recommend surgery and other treatments.

NATURAL TREATMENT

Removing the cause, which is almost always constipation, will immediately improve this condition. Constipation can be caused by an upset in bowel flora from antibiotic use, or poor diet, or food allergies. Sugar, dairy and wheat allergies are the biggest offenders. High doses of probiotics for an extended period of time can help. Monitor pH levels also. Acidosis contributes greatly to constipation.

ACUPUNCTURE & TRADITIONAL CHINESE MEDICINE (TCM)

Treating patterns of Hemorrhoids may be seen heat in large Intestines. Some forms of TCM may be chosen singly or together for the best treatment plan and holistic response.

HOMEOPATHIC REMEDIES

THE BANERJI PROTOCOL™

In external or internal piles, when there is no outside swelling, the following protocols can be very effective.

FIRST LINE MEDICINES

- **SULPHUR 200C**, one dose every other day
- **NUX VOMICA 30C**, one dose daily
- **SULPHUR 200C + RATANIA 200C**, two doses per day when there is acute pain. Can also repeat dosage every 3 hours when there is severe pain and burning, until it subsides

SECOND LINE MEDICINES
- **SULPHUR 200C + HAMAMELIS VIRGINICA 200C**, two x's per day
- **NUX VOMICA 30C,** one dose per day

If these fail, **COLLINSONIA CANADENSIS 30C,** one dose per day

GEMMOTHERAPY
- **HORSE CHESTNUT** and **SERVICE TREE** work well together
- **RASPBERRY-** In females only, to arrest bleeding
- **BILBERRY-** When associated with diarrhea
- **BOXWOOD-** when associated with diarrhea and person is immune compromised
- **HORSETAIL-** when associated with other skin ailments that do not heal rapidly
- **GRAPEVINE-** when associated with leukopenia and autoimmune conditions as well as diarrhea
- **TAMARISK-** when associated with anemia

HIATAL HERNIA

A hiatal hernia is a condition in which the upper part of the stomach bulges through an opening in the diaphragm. The diaphragm is the muscle wall that separates the stomach from the chest. The diaphragm helps keep acid from coming up into the esophagus. When you have a hiatal hernia, it's easier for the acid to come up. The leaking of acid from the stomach into the esophagus has been named gastroesophageal reflux disease (GERD). If the cause of the disturbance, the hernia is fixed the GERD symptoms clear up. For this reason, I have categorized this as a condition, rather than a disease.

The GERD condition may cause symptoms such as:

- Heartburn
- Problems swallowing
- Dry cough
- Bad Breath

Hiatal hernias are common, especially in people over age 50. If you have symptoms, eating small meals, avoiding certain foods, not smoking or drinking alcohol, and losing weight may help.

CONVENTIONAL TREATMENT

Antacids or other medicines; if these don't help surgery may be suggested. (There are much more efficient methods, continue reading)

NATURAL TREATMENT

Dr. Phil Selinsky has written extensively on the topic of Hiatal Hernia. He brilliantly describes the condition as, "A tear or stretching of connective tissue." A hiatus is a port or opening. There is an opening or hiatus in the diaphragm that allows the esophagus (food tube from your mouth to your stomach) to go through. The diaphragm is a parachute shaped muscle that separates the thoracic (chest) cavity from the abdominal (tummy) cavity.

The diaphragm is used as a bellows in the breathing process. Sometimes the hole or hiatus tears or stretches and when you breathe or put pressure on your abdomen, a part of the stomach gets literally sucked up into your chest cavity. This can put pressure on the heart, giving you symptoms of a heart attack. Or it can displace the lung capacity, giving you shortness of breath or a feeling like someone is sitting on your chest.

Sometimes instead of the diaphragm tearing, the esophagus stretches just as it attaches to the stomach. Or the valve between the esophagus and the stomach becomes weak or damaged, and acid leaks into the esophagus and burns the esophagus and we have what western medicine calls "reflux esophagitis", or Gastro-Esophageal-Reflux-Disease or GERD. In either case, the stomach is physically "injured". If you've ever had a sliver in your finger and could not get it out, after a week or so your whole arm becomes achy and sore. The pain "creeps". The same thing happens to your food tube. Eventually your entire digestive tract becomes enflamed and irritated. Then you experience "colitis", "enteritis", "gastroenteritis", all the itises you can think of.

In his book, **THE HUMAN MACHINE; A Trouble Shooter's Manual**, Selinsky describes an easy fix for the hiatal hernia that plagues millions without their knowledge. His book describes the human body as an electrochemical machine and is a must read for those looking for a clear understanding of the workings of the body.

CHIROPRACTIC TREATMENT

A Chiropractor trained in working on Hiatal Hernia can easily work with rectifying the problem.

ACUPUNCTURE & TRADITIONAL CHINESE MEDICINE (TCM)

Treating patterns of Hiatal hernia may be seen as Spleen qi deficiency/ sinking qi or Liver heat effecting Stomach. Some forms of TCM may be chosen singly or together for the best treatment plan and holistic response.

HIVES (URTICARIA)

Hives are red and sometimes itchy bumps on your skin. An allergic reaction to a drug, a chemical, environmental or food usually causes them. Allergic reactions cause your body to release the chemical histamine, among others, that can make your skin swell up in hives. People who have other allergies are more likely to get hives than other people. Other causes include infections and stress.

CONVENTIONAL TREATMENT

Conventional medicine believes hives are very common and will go away on their own, but if you have a serious case, they may administer pharmaceutical drugs or a shot. In rare cases, hives can cause a dangerous swelling in your airways, making it hard to breathe, which is a medical emergency.

NATURAL TREATMENT

Hives are a symptom of the body's reaction, or over-reaction to a substance or condition it cannot deal with properly. It is important to find out what the reaction is from in order to treat properly.

When my granddaughter was a baby she was breaking out in hives on her exposed skin areas only. This meant the aggravating factor was something that her skin was coming in direct contact with. With my daughter-in-law's keen observation, she noticed that the baby would break out within minutes of being put on the carpet. Since it was spring and the windows were open, she assumed it must be allergy to pollens. I told her to give the baby the Homeopathic remedy APIS. She called me amazed that the hives cleared in about 30 minutes. She gave her 2 doses per day for the next 3 days and the hives have never returned.

That was an easy case, but an example of how attentive observation and finding a specific cause solved the problem. When my son was a young teen he would come in with large hives that looked like welts on his legs after playing soccer. He also had joint pain. At first I thought it was exposure to the cold, but when the first remedy I tried did not work I looked at the circumstances again. I changed the remedy to Urtica Urens and the hives cleared.

HOMEOPATHIC REMEDIES

There are many Homeopathic remedies that address hives. Success comes when you are able to match not only the cause, but also the symptoms. The following are a few of the most commonly used remedies for Urticaria.

- **ANTIMONIUM CRUDUM-** from eating meat, gastric discomfort.
- **APIS MELLIFICA-** pinkish looking, itchy, flushed face, swollen lips, rash on uncovered areas of skin.

- **ARSENICUM ALBUM-** irritability, restlessness and maybe accompanied by upset stomach.
- **CALCAREA CARBONICA-** milk white spots, cold to the touch, boils, psoriasis.
- **CALCAREA SULPHURICA-** bumps with yellow secretions.
- **DULCAMARA-** from drinking milk.
- **FRAGARIA VESCA-** eating strawberries.
- **NATRUM MURIATICUM-** exposure to the sun.
- **RHUS TOXICONENDRON-** red, swollen, intense itch, dry, hot.
- **SULPHUR-** unhealthy skin, dry, scaly, itchy, worse at night, worse from heat, irritated by scratching and washing.
- **URTICA URENS-** strenuous exercise, joint pain, after taking a bath or eating seafood.

PHENOLIC THERAPY

If the exciting factor behind the hives is discovered and reduced to environmental pollens or foods, they can then be treated with the specific phenol prepared homeopathically. Being treated with the drops over time can desensitize the person, alleviating the allergic reaction. See the chart of phenolics in Chapter III.

ACUPUNCTURE & TRADITIONAL CHINESE MEDICINE (TCM)

Treating patterns of Hives may be seen as wind-heat at Skin level; blood heat; damp-heat or toxic heat. Some forms of TCM may be chosen singly or together for the best treatment plan and holistic response.

HYPERTENSION (HIGH BLOOD PRESSURE)

High Blood Pressure is not a disease it is a symptom of a disturbance in the body. Blood pressure is the force of your blood pushing against the walls of your arteries. Each time your heart beats it pumps blood into the arteries. Your blood pressure is highest when your heart beats, pumping the blood. This is called systolic pressure. When your heart is at rest, between beats, your blood pressure falls. This is called diastolic pressure.

Your blood pressure reading consists of these two numbers. Usually the systolic number comes before or above the diastolic number. Recently, the American Medical Association changed what they believe to be 'normal' range to lower numbers vs. pre-HBP or HBP. It does not seem other countries are following the change at this time? For that reason, I am not listing ranges for *ideal, pre-high blood pressure* and *high blood pressure*.

As mentioned previously, hypertension is a *symptom*, not a pathology. Many times you can control this issue through healthy lifestyle habits.

CONVENTIONAL TREATMENT
- Pharmaceutical drugs

NATURAL TREATMENT

HBP can be controlled through diet, exercise, lessening of stress and natural supplementation. HBP can be related to slowed kidney function, since blood pressure is related to the osmotic pressure regulated by the kidneys. The top Homeopathic remedies to drain kidneys and revitalize function are:

- **BERBERIS**
- **CANTHARIS**
- **SOLIDAGO**

SUPPLEMENTS

NATTOKINESE- an enzyme extracted from the traditional Japanese soy food Natto. Natto is soybeans that have been boiled and fermented with a specific bacterium called Bacillus natto. Nattokinase decreases the ability of the blood to clot. It reinforces the actions of the enzyme plasmin to break down the natural clotting agent in blood called fibrin. By inhibiting the actions of fibrin, Nattokinase is able to reduce the chances of abnormal blood thickening and subsequent clotting.

Nattokinase also helps the interior walls of your blood vessels stay smooth and flexible.

ACUPUNCTURE & TRADITIONAL CHINESE MEDICINE (TCM)

Treating patterns of Hypertension may be seen as damp-heat Liver; Liver yang rising with Liver and Kidney yin deficiency; qi and blood stagnation; excess heat in all 3 jiaos; damp and phlegm accumulation. Some forms of TCM may be chosen singly or together for the best treatment plan and holistic response.

HOMEOPATHIC REMEDIES

A Constitutional remedy dispensed by a professional Homeopath may work best for this issue. The following are some remedies common to the onset of hypertension.

- **ACONITUM NAPELLUS 200C-** brought on my shock, trauma or sudden stress; 2 doses per day for 8-10 weeks
- **IGNATIA AMARA 200C-** brought on my grief or loss; 2 doses per day for 8-10 weeks

GEMMOTHERAPY- TINCTURES CAN BE COMBINED

- **HAWTHORN-** a natural beta-blocker
- **MISTLETOE-** diuretic
- **OLIVE-** bladder infections
- **HAZEL-** edema of lower extremities
- **MAIDENHAIR-** hypotensive
- **LINDEN TREE-** hypertension caused by stress
- **BRAMBLE-** arterial hypertension
- **LEMON TREE-** aspirin alternative without the risk of ulcers

TRACE MINERAL THERAPY

- **Iodine-** Fluctuating blood pressure
- **Molybdenum-** Blood flow, Cerebral
- **Cobalt-** Blood flow, peripheral

HYPOGLYCEMIA (ALSO SEE INSULIN SHOCK)

Hypoglycemia means low blood glucose, or blood sugar. Your body needs glucose to have enough energy. After you eat, your blood absorbs glucose. If you eat more sugar than your body needs, your muscles, and liver store the extra. When your blood sugar begins to fall, a hormone tells your liver to release glucose.

In most people, this raises blood sugar. If it doesn't, you have hypoglycemia, and your blood sugar can be dangerously low.

SYMPTOMS

- Hunger
- Headache
- Shakiness
- Dizziness
- Confusion
- Irritability
- Difficulty speaking
- Feeling anxious or weak

CAUSES include certain medicines or diseases, hormone or enzyme deficiencies, and tumors. In people with diabetes, hypoglycemia is often a side effect of diabetes medicines.

CONVENTIONAL TREATMENT

Eating or drinking something with carbohydrates can help. If it happens often, your health care provider may need to change your treatment plan.

You can also have low blood sugar without having diabetes. Laboratory tests can help find the cause. The treatment depends on why you have low blood sugar.

NATURAL TREATMENT

Adults and children alike suffer from hypoglycemia and it is often missed in small children. Sometimes that tantrum and outrageous behavior is because the child has gone too long between meals and their blood sugar level has dropped. It is a condition that is often misdiagnosed and underdiagnosed. It is not a disease and can be rectified with proper eating habits and if necessary, supplementation to rebalance the pancreas.

If an adult suddenly is catapulted into hypoglycemia, it usually means there is a systemic infection in the body. It can be caused by food poisoning or candida. If you have had this experience, look deeper into possible infections.

HOMEOPATHY

The following are remedies suggested by the Banerji Clinic to help balance hypoglycemia.

- **CHELIDONIUM-** 6C, two times daily (Liver/ GB issue)
- **HELONIAS-** 200C, two times daily (sugar sensitivity)
- **SYZYGIUM-** mother tincture, 5 drops, two times daily (pre-diabetic)

ACUPUNCTURE & TRADITIONAL CHINESE MEDICINE (TCM)

Treating patterns of Hypoglycemia may be seen as Spleen and Heart blood deficiencies and qi, blood, yin, yang deficiency. Some forms of TCM may be chosen singly or together for the best treatment plan and holistic response.

GEMMOTHERAPY- can combine tinctures as needed

- **SWEET CHESTNUT-** improves venous congestion
- **BLACK CURRANT-** blood detoxifier (do not use with elevated cortisol)
- **JUNIPER-** supports the liver and kidneys
- **LINDEN TREE-** relaxes the nervous system
- **OAK-** helps liver to stimulate hormones
- **FIG-** balances Hypo disturbances

SUPPLEMENTS

- **FENUGREEK-** very effective as a tea, in seeds, or as a supplement to balance blood sugar levels.
- **CHROMIUM-** an essential trace mineral that can help to cut cravings for carbohydrates, fight body fat and control blood sugar levels.
- **CINNAMON-** not only a spice for food, but can reduce fasting blood glucose, total cholesterol, triglycerides, and "bad" LDL cholesterol, while raising "good" HDL cholesterol.
- **VANADIUM-** a trace mineral that has the ability to lower blood sugar levels and improve sensitivity to insulin in people with type 2 diabetes.

IMMUNE SUPPORT

This topic can fill a book in and of it itself so I have touched on the main issues.

There are many ways to be proactive to ward off acute and chronic illnesses. Diet is always the first place to start, followed by nutritional supplementation for any deficiencies you may be aware of. Disease is caused by an immune imbalance and paying attention to the basics like drinking fresh, clean water, balancing stress and taking care of emotional situations will help to transcend issues that might otherwise plague your health.

CONVENTIONAL TREATMENT

None known at this time, since it is not an area medical doctors are trained to work with. A small percentage of doctors are now suggesting probiotics after anti-biotic use. (Do not take during, anti-biotics will negate)

NATURAL TREATMENT

Natural medicine is all about prevention, which translates into supporting, and if necessary, rebuilding the immune system. There are many choices and directions to follow based on your health needs. Are you concerned with heavy metal poisoning, or herpes, or digestive issues and are now getting sick often? A qualified holistic doctor can help with finding the correct program to fit your health needs. The following are a few suggestions.

ACUPUNCTURE & TRADITIONAL CHINESE MEDICINE (TCM)

Treating patterns of Immune Support may be seen as tonifying wei qi; qi/blood/yin/yang deficiency; Lung and Kidney deficiencies and yuan qi deficiency. Some forms of TCM may be chosen singly or together for the best treatment plan and holistic response.

GEMMOTHERAPY

The most efficient means of supporting the immune system is with the use of drainage remedies to cleanse and detoxify the major organs. This can be done twice yearly, Spring and Fall to keep the body 'tuned.' The following are the major immune building tinctures:

- **BEECH-** stimulates immunity, especially in immune suppressed states
- **BLACK CURRANT-** stimulates endocrine system
- **BLACK ELDER-** wards off cold and flu
- **BOXWOOD-** acts as an anti-biotic
- **DOG ROSE-** stops chronic runny nose
- **GRAPE VINE-** fights inflammation
- **HAWTHORN-** detoxifies heart and arteries
- **JUNIPER-** liver/kidney detoxification
- **MISTLETOE-** balances blood pressure
- **ROSEMARY-** increases white blood count to fight infection

- **SILVER BIRCH-** induces apoptosis
- **SILVER FIR-** multi-mineral for children

HOMEOPATHY

Visiting a Classical Homeopath and receiving a constitutional remedy is a pro-active way to maintain balance in your life. Whenever there is an illness or trauma you will have the remedy to fall back on to re-dose and rebalance.

Homeopathic remedies that work to help stimulate the immune system:

- **THYMULINE-** A remedy made from potentized thymus gland, which can help to encourage a strong immune system, especially during changes of seasons. Best to source in low potencies, such as 9c and repeat for a short period of time, as needed.
- **CALCARIA CARBONICA-** Works on impaired nutrition through proper assimilation of calcium affecting the glands, bones and skin. Helpful to those who get sick often (especially children). Take once per week for an extended period of time to rebalance these functions of the body.
- **SULPHUR-** This remedy is especially useful for clearing colds, flu and other illnesses that linger. Take a 30c or 200c potency for a few days, as needed, to finish up after other remedies have failed to clear symptoms completely.

CELL SALTS

Taking cell salts regularly is a powerful tool. This is a much more efficient means of assisting the immune system than stocking up daily on multiple vitamins and other supplements. Children, in particular, do well with cell salts daily for teething, growing pains and other childhood structural issues. (SEE CHAPTER III)

NATUROPATHIC MEDICINE

A Naturopathic doctor will take your case, usually administer some type of testing and put together a custom protocol using herbs, supplements, homeopathy and other forms of therapy to help to maintain optimum health.

SUPPLEMENTS

I am not a huge proponent of supplements for the sake of taking supplements. Over the years I have had hundreds of clients come in with bags of supplements they are taking for one reason or another. Most of them are of questionable quality, not combined correctly, their purpose is overlapping, dosages are inappropriate and most of all, they don't suit their particular health needs.

There are many supplements advertised for immune support and anti-aging. The biggest issue with supplements is that many contain "fillers", may be chemically based and may contain too many ingredients for your body to metabolize. If you are looking for a multi-vitamin be sure it is derived from food sources, not synthetics. (80% of vitamins sold today are synthetic) Fillers are the 'also contains' that you read on the label. It is a way to fill the rest of the capsule beyond the main ingredient.

Keep it simple. Do not take numerous combinations of supplements because you heard it was good for this or that. Seek the advice of a professional. In the long run you will save money and be healthier by taking only what is appropriate for your body as determined by a professional. If you do seek the advice of a professional and they dispense numerous supplements, walk away. This is not the most efficient means of building your immune system.

Here are a few suggestions that are beneficial to add to most health regimes as needed.

- **BOSWELLIA-** 400 mg three times daily can help to balance the immune system; an anti-inflammatory been used for thousands of years.
- **ECHINACEA + GOLDENSEAL-** two powerful herbs that support the immune system. They should not be taken year long, but rather spring and fall for support during the change of seasons.
- **ELDERBERRY** (SAMBUCUS)- a powerful anti-oxidant. Especially helpful to children to ward off colds and flu in winter.
- **VITAMIN C-** taking high doses of Vitamin C goes a long way to supporting the immune system. It is especially helpful if you are harboring a virus, such as Herpes. Be sure to source a liposomal Vitamin C (coated) so that it survives your stomach acids. (Or a brand like Sufficient C™)
- **UMCKA-** a remedy that shortens the duration, speeds recovery and reduces the severity of the common cold, nasal, throat and bronchial irritations. It is made from the African Geranium and works with the immune system to help support the body's own natural defense mechanisms.
- **OMEGA 3 Fish Oil…** be sure it is pharmaceutical grade, or DON'T buy it.
- **TURMERIC (CURCUMIN)-** a powerful antioxidant and anti- inflammatory that slows down oxidative stress.
- **COLLOIDAL MINERALS-** natural combination minerals are actually more important than vitamins. If you are eating organic fruits and vegetables, you are already getting the vitamins needed. However, minerals are another story, since most have been farmed out of the soil in this day and age of 'modern' farming.
- **MUSHROOMS-** There are many mushrooms that support immune health. The top 3 are: *Shiitake, Reishi and Maitake.*

TRACE MINERAL THERAPY

- **Selenium-** anti-oxidative protection
- **Zinc-** memory, concentration
- **Copper-Gold-Silver-** antimicrobial
- **Manganese-Copper-** Susceptible to infections (Respiratory)

Above all, monitor your pH levels regularly. It is impossible for the immune system to function properly if your body is too acidic.

INDIGESTION (DYSPEPSIA) (SEE ACID REFLUX ALSO)

Nearly everyone has had indigestion at one time. It's a feeling of discomfort or a burning feeling in your upper abdomen. You may have heartburn or belch and feel bloated. You may also feel nauseated, or even throw up.

You might get indigestion from eating too much or too fast, eating high-fat foods, or eating when you're stressed. Smoking, drinking too much alcohol, using medicines, being tired, and having ongoing stress can all cause indigestion or make it worse. Sometimes the cause is a problem with the digestive tract, like an ulcer or GERD. This section addresses less severe acute indigestion.

CONVENTIONAL TREATMENT

Avoiding foods and situations that seem to cause the problem will help. Because indigestion can be a sign of a more serious problem, see your health care provider if it lasts for more than two weeks or if you have severe pain or other symptoms. Your health care provider may use x-rays, lab tests, and an upper endoscopy to diagnose the cause. They would prescribe medicines to treat the symptoms.

NATURAL TREATMENT

Indigestion is a symptom of a disturbance in the gut. You may have been given multiple antibiotic treatments that accumulatively can change the natural balance of chemistry in the gut and bowel tract. Another cause of symptoms could be unresolved food poisoning, Giardia (from drinking water in foreign lands) or even H-Pylori (the bacteria that causes ulcers). Natural health practitioners will look for the underlying cause of the symptoms to establish a correct protocol to resolve the situation.

Be sure to monitor saliva and urine pH levels. Acidosis will surely cause problems with digestion.

ACUPUNCTURE & TRADITIONAL CHINESE MEDICINE (TCM)

Treating patterns of Indigestion may be seen as spleen qi deficiency; damp-heat Intestines; food stagnation and/or Liver qi stagnation. Some forms of TCM may be chosen singly or together for the best treatment plan and holistic response.

HOMEOPATHIC REMEDIES

The following are the more common remedies used for indigestion. There are others and are symptom specific. You do not need to have ALL the symptoms to use the remedy.

- **ARSENICUM ALBUM-** bloating, stomach pain, diarrhea, vomiting, irritability, anxiety about health, food poisoning.
- **CARBO VEGETABILIS-** slow to digest, heaviness, belching.

- **LYCOPODIUM-** food takes several hours to digest; bloated after meals; need a long nap after meals.
- **NUX VOMICA-** need a short nap after meals, overeating aggravates, stomach feels too full, back of the tongue can be coated, over drinking (great 'hangover' remedy).
- **PULSATILLA-** intolerance to fats, ice cream, pastries, pork.

SUPPLEMENTS

The following supplements can be sourced in many ways. *Ginger* is best used fresh in your food, or steeped as a tea. Fresh *papaya*, as well as papaya tablets, is effective for acute indigestion. Fresh *peppermint* makes a great tea or added to your water, as well as purchased in a concentrate as an oil.

- **GINGER**
- **PAPAYA**
- **PEPPERMINT**

INSOMNIA

Insomnia is a common sleep disorder. If you suffer from it, you may have trouble falling asleep, staying asleep, or both. As a result, you may get too little sleep or have poor-quality sleep. You may not feel refreshed when you wake up.

Symptoms of insomnia include:

- Lying awake for a long time before you fall asleep
- Sleeping for only short periods
- Being awake for much of the night
- Feeling as if you haven't slept at all
- Waking up too early

CONVENTIONAL TREATMENT

Your doctor will diagnose insomnia based on your medical and sleep histories and a physical exam. He or she also may recommend a sleep study. A sleep study measures how well you sleep and how your body responds to sleep problems. Treatments include lifestyle changes, counseling, and pharmaceutical prescriptions. Sleeping pills can be addictive and difficult to wean off of over time.

NATURAL TREATMENT

There are many natural remedies and therapies to improve sleep. Most with sleep issues have difficulty turning off their brain. They are over stressed, over worked, and/or unhappy in some area of their lives. This is the record that plays over and over preventing sleep. Making changes in your life is the first obstacle to overcome. Most will say this is not possible, but even changing your attitude about the situation, if you are unable to change the situation itself can help.

ACUPUNCTURE & TRADITIONAL CHINESE MEDICINE (TCM)

Treating patterns of Insomnia may be seen as Liver qi stagnation; Liver and Kidney yin deficiencies; Spleen and Heart blood deficiencies and/or blood stagnation. Some forms of TCM may be chosen singly or together for the best treatment plan and holistic response.

HOMEOPATHIC REMEDIES

Seeing a Classical Homeopath for a Constitutional remedy can help to resolve underlying issues that cause sleep issues. Here are some "go to" remedies for acute situations. Take 4 pellets ½ hour before bed and repeat if necessary on waking during the night.

- **ACONITUM NAPELLUS-** from being frightened.
- **ARSENICUM ALBUM-** due to worry, busy mind, digestive issues.

- **AMBRA GRISEA-** retires tired, wakes from worry, anxious dreams, helpful to the elderly.
- **AVENA SATIVA-** chronic insomnia from mental exertion.
- **AURUM METALLICUM-** depression.
- **BELLADONNA-** unpleasant images when closing eyes.
- **COCCULUS-** from staying up too late.
- **COFFEA CRUDA-** after hearing bad news, too much thinking, waking due to nerve pain, drinking too much coffee.
- **GELSEMIUM-** from fear, afraid you can't sleep, after bad news.
- **IGNATIA-** upsetting emotional disturbance, grief.
- **KALI PHOS-** night terrors of children, sleepwalking, sleeplessness, from work troubles, restlessness with heat, amorous dreams.
- **LITHIUM BROMATUM-** prolonged mental exertion.
- **NUX VOMICA-** hung over, muscle cramps, indigestion.
- **PASSIFLORA-** calms the nervous system, insomnia of infants and the elderly.
- **PHOSPHORIC ACID-** sleepy by day, hot and wakeful at night.
- **ZINCUM METALLICUM-** constant desire to move legs.

SLEEP DISORDERS IN CHILDREN

- **BELLADONNA-** children who moan and toss about; frightful dreams; sees frightful visions on closing eyes.
- **STRAMONIUM-** children who are afraid of dark and need light on.
- **SULPHUR-** their feet are hot and need to be uncovered to cool off.
- **THERIDION-** wakes from the slightest noise.

GEMMOTHERAPY

A combination of **LINDEN TREE** and **FIG** work well together to relax the nervous system, as well as the brain to affect a more restful sleep. Take before retiring and can be repeated if sleep is disturbed during the night.

PHENOLIC THERAPY

Phenolic therapy can help to balance brain chemistry, allowing for a deeper, more relaxed sleep. (See Chapter III)

SUPPLEMENTS

- **AVENA SATIVA-** tincture- chronic insomnia, worse during convalescence. Sleeplessness from mental exertion.
- **B VITAMINS-** (6 & 12 specifically).

- **MAGNESIUM-** relaxes the nervous system.
- **MELATONIN-** this supplement will either work like a charm or make you wired, it depends on your brain chemistry.
- **VALERIAN-** act like a sedative on the brain and nervous system.
- **ST JOHN'S WORT-** affects the nervous system.
- **SAMe-** affects brain chemistry.

JET LAG

The term 'Jet Lag' refers to the body's negative reaction to flying long distances in an airplane. There is less oxygen in the cabin of a plane than under normal circumstances. You are crossing time zones, sitting in close proximity to a large number of people with little filtration, as well as breathing in chemical disinfectant sprays used by many airlines. The food may be foreign to you, as well as the water, if not bottled.

Symptoms of Jet Lag can include:

- Confusion/ Disorientation
- Dehydration
- Diarrhea
- Fatigue
- Irritability
- Insomnia
- Swelling of legs and/or feet

Jet Lag can be avoided, or at the very least kept to a minimum by following a few easy steps.

- Start out your flight being rested
- Exercise the day before
- Bring as little emotional stress as possible
- Drink lots of bottled water during flight
- Do not drink alcohol (it dehydrates)
- Do not drink caffeine (too harsh on the liver)
- Do not drink orange juice (too acidic for stomach)
- Get up and move around as much as possible
- Do simple in-seat exercises to keep circulation optimum
- Bring comfort items; ear plugs, blindfold, blow-up pillow
- Take remedies before, during and after the flight
- Immediately shift your mindset to the time zone where you land

IONIZER

Wear a mini ionizer. You can find them advertised on the Internet. They are battery operated and about the size of a matchbox. They emit negative ions that kill pathogens you might be breathing from your neighbors or the cabin air.

NASAL SPRAYS

Since the sinus passages are one of the main entries for pathogens, it is wise to carry a nasal spray. Repeat every couple of hours, before, during and even after the flight. You'll be pleasantly surprised how seldom you get sick using this method. Look for a Colloidal Silver Spray, or a homeopathic combination formula called REBOOST™.

HOMEOPATHIC REMEDIES

Combine any of the following remedies as needed. Be sure to start taking remedies a few hours before you fly, during flight if crossing time zones, and continue to take at least another 12 hours after landing.

- **ACONITUM-** for emotional trauma.
- **ARNICA MONTANA-** overall first aid, including pain.
- **ARSENICUM ALBUM-** diarrhea, nausea, stomach distress.
- **BELLIS-** venous congestion.
- **CHAMOMILLA-** irritability, anxiety.
- **GELSEMIUM-** fear of flying or anticipatory fear.
- **IPECACUANHA-** dehydration.
- **LYCOPODIUM-** stimulates liver function, curbs anxiety.
- **NUX VOMICA-** stomach distress.
- **RADIUM BROMATUM-** exposure to radiation.

SUPPLEMENTS

- **CLOVE OIL**
- **OREGANO OIL**
- **PEPPERMINT OIL**

Put a dab of any of the oils just below the nose. This will discourage pathogens from entering the sinus passages.

LARYNGITIS

Voice is the sound made by air passing from your lungs through your larynx, or voice box. In your larynx are your vocal cords, two bands of muscle that vibrate to make sound. For most of us, our voices play a big part in who we are, what we do, and how we communicate. Like fingerprints, each person's voice is unique.

Many things we do can injure our vocal cords. Talking too much, screaming, constantly clearing your throat, or smoking can make you hoarse. They can also lead to problems such as nodules, polyps, and sores on the vocal cords. Other causes of voice disorders include infections, upward movement of stomach acids into the throat, growths due to a virus, cancer, and diseases that paralyze the vocal cords.

Signs that your voice isn't healthy include:

- Your voice has become hoarse or raspy
- You've lost the ability to hit some high notes when singing
- Your voice suddenly sounds deeper
- Your throat often feels raw, achy, or strained
- It's become an effort to speak

Treatment for voice disorders varies depending on the cause. Most voice problems can be successfully treated when diagnosed early.

NATURAL TREATMENT

- Gargle with warm water and salt
- Make a tea with honey and lemon to sooth

HOMEOPATHIC REMEDIES

- **ACONITUM-** after exposure to dry cold.
- **ARGENTUM METALLICUM-** a feeling of having a thorn in the throat when swallowing.
- **ARUM TRIPHYLLUM-** partial or total loss of voice after straining vocal cords.
- **CAUSTICUM-** sharp pains with voice loss.
- **IGNATIA AMARA-** voice loss from anxiety or nervousness.
- **PHOSPHORUS-** pain worse in the evening accompanied by hoarseness.
- **RHUS TOXICODENDRON-** when voice loss relieved by speaking.

SUPPLEMENTS

- **COUCH GRASS** and **SLIPPERY ELM** have a high mucilage content that helps to coat the tissues of the throat and this protective layer helps to prevent dry throat.
- **LICORICE ROOT** contains glycyrrhizin, an anti-inflammatory agent.
- **GINGER ROOT and MARSHMALLOW** herb are excellent laryngitis remedies to brew into a tea.
- **ZINC** lozenges.
- **SINGER'S® Soothing Throat Spray**.

ACUPUNCTURE & TRADITIONAL CHINESE MEDICINE (TCM)

Treating patterns of LARYNGITIS may be seen as plum pit qi; wind-heat invasion and Lung dryness with phlegm. Some forms of TCM may be chosen singly or together for the best treatment plan and holistic response.

LARYNGITIS REMEDY REFERENCE CHART

Laryngitis is the loss of sound from the voice box

CAUSES:
- Infections
- Smoking
- Talking or singing too much
- Stomach acids
- Screaming

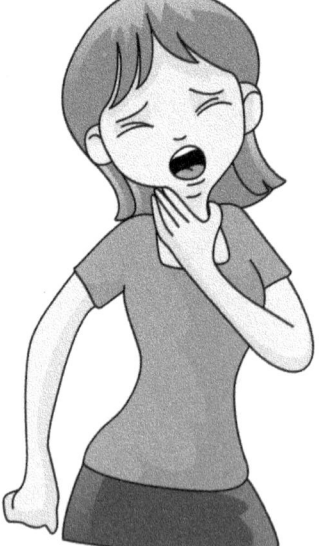

BROMIUM
Swollen tonsils
< Swallowing liquids
< Evening

ALLIUM CEPA
Hoarseness & Tickling
Pain in ears

CAUSTICUM
From voice strain
Sticky discharge
Cries easily

ARNICA
First sign of hoarseness
From screaming
health

PHOSPHORUS
Fears about
< Evening

ARG MET
Raw, < yawning
Singer's laryngitis

RUMEX
Heavy mucus
Lump in throat
Throat is raw

SULPHUR
Burning redness and dryness
Dry cough, neck is red

< worse

Copyright © 2018 Elena Upton, PhD

LEAKY GUT SYNDROME

I did not find a definition for leaky gut syndrome in conventional medical references which is probably why it is not a widely recognized condition among the medical establishment.

Dr. Andrew Weil, an Integrative Medical doctor describes Leaky Gut as the following:

> "Conventional physicians do not recognize leaky gut syndrome, but evidence is accumulating that it is a real condition that affects the lining of the intestines. The theory is that leaky gut syndrome (also called increased intestinal permeability), is the result of damage to the intestinal lining, making it less able to protect the internal environment as well as to filter needed nutrients and other biological substances. As a consequence, some bacteria, and their toxins; incompletely digested proteins and fats; and waste not normally absorbed may "leak" out of the intestines into the blood stream. This triggers an autoimmune reaction, which can lead to gastrointestinal problems such as abdominal bloating, excessive gas and cramps, fatigue, food sensitivities, joint pain, skin rashes, and autoimmunity. The cause of this syndrome may be chronic inflammation, food sensitivity, damage from taking large amounts of non-steroidal anti-inflammatory drugs (NSAIDS), cyto-toxic drugs and radiation or certain antibiotics, excessive alcohol consumption, or compromised immunity."

Leaky gut syndrome may trigger or worsen such disorders as Crohn's disease, Celiac disease, Rheumatoid arthritis, and Asthma.

Some alternative medical practitioners also relate the cause of migraines, bad breath and insomnia to leaky gut syndrome. They may recommend a home kit that measures intestinal permeability. This test measures the ability of two non-metabolized sugar molecules, mannitol and lactulose to get through the digestive lining.

If you feel you have symptoms of leaky gut it is recommended to avoid alcohol, NSAIDS, refined sugars, artificial sweeteners and any foods you might be allergic to, especially wheat and dairy products. Choose a diet rich in fibers and lots of essential fatty acids, like fish.

SYMPTOMS

- Gas, bloating, diarrhea or Irritable Bowel Syndrome (IBS)
- Seasonal allergies or asthma
- Hormonal imbalances such as PMS
- Diagnosis of an auto-immune disease such as Rheumatoid arthritis, Hashimoto's Thyroiditis, Lupus, Psoriasis, or Celiac disease
- Diagnosis of Chronic Fatigue or Fibromyalgia
- Depression, anxiety, ADD or ADHD
- Skin issues such as acne, rosacea, or eczema

- Candida overgrowth (fungal infection)
- Food allergies or food intolerances

NATURAL TREATMENT

There is much that can be done to repair Leaky Gut Syndrome. It is a very real disturbance and without proper treatment can lead to many serious illnesses. The digestive tract is the brains of the body and when it does not function properly nothing else can function properly.

Be sure to monitor pH levels in the saliva and urine. With the use of pH strips, or a pH meter you can regularly check to see if saliva is in the normal range of 7.3-7.5 and urine, 6.8-7.0. Drinking a solution of sodium bicarbonate (Baking Soda) daily will help to keep pH in check. Also fresh lemon water or apple cider vinegar.

As a side note; It is very difficult for baking soda to escape stomach acids. An efficient means of ingesting sodium bicarbonate is to coat it with a fat, so that it's benefits will not be destroyed before reaching the intestines. A method of accomplishing this is to melt some butter (not margarine), dissolve baking soda into the butter and refrigerate. (Spoon out the desired quantity as needed. An ice-cube tray works well.)

ACUPUNCTURE & TRADITIONAL CHINESE MEDICINE (TCM)

With the expertise of the licensed provider of Chinese Medicine a correct pattern/s for your symptom/s may be chosen from one of several that fall under a certain disease or condition category. Some forms of TCM may be chosen singly or together for the best treatment plan and holistic response.

GEMMOTHERAPY

Gemmotherapy is a very efficient means of healing the gut. The tinctures work slowly over time and can resolve the necessary healing. Gemmos can be combined as needed.

- **BLACK CURRANT-** anti-inflammatory without the tendency to create ulcers (as steroids and NSAIDS can).
- **EUROPEAN ALDER-** gastric drainer acting as an anti-inflammatory.
- **FIG-** gastric drainer, heals the mucosa, regulates gastric secretions and esophageal motility (also indicated in GURD).
- **HOLLY-** gastritis.
- **LINDEN TREE-** antispasmodic, acts on the chronic inflammation of the digestive mucosa.
- **JUNIPER-** gentle liver drainage.
- **ROSEMARY-** anti-microbial, analgesic, astringent.
- A powerful combination for the treatment of Leaky Gut is **FIG, ASH** and **COWBERRY.**

HOMEOPATHY

In Homeopathy there is no remedy specifically for 'leaky gut' since Homeopathy is designed to treat issues that exhibit the cause of the disturbance. Remedies are based on an individuals' description of symptoms, such as the type of stomach distress and related discomfort. However, a Constitutional remedy dispensed by a professional Homeopath can help to begin the process of healing. The following are remedies for specific symptoms related to or a result of 'leaky gut syndrome.'

DIARRHEA

- **ARSENICUM ALBUM-** as soon as symptom begins and repeated often as needed.
- **ALOE-** loose stool, gas and acidity.
- **VERATRUM ALBUM + CUPRUM METALLICUM,** one dose every two hours after the passing of stool.

BLOATING

- **ARSENICUM ALBUM-** food sensitivities, diarrhea, nausea.
- **LYCOPODIUM-** worse after meat, takes a long time to digest food, rumbling.
- **BRYONIA-** sensation there is a stone in the stomach.
- **NUX VOMICA-** feels too full, needs a nap after eating, over-indulgence.

FOOD ALLERGIES

- **PULSATILLA-** worse from fats, ice cream, sweets.
- **BOVISTA-** worse from gluten.
- **FERRUM METALLICUM-** issue with eggs.
- **HELONIAS-** sensitive to sugar.
- **IPECACUANHA + MERCURIUS SULPH-** general food intolerances, taken 2 times daily for an extended time.

GASTRO WITH PALPITATIONS

- **LYCOPODIUM** combined with **ARSENICUM ALBUM,** two times daily for at least 10 weeks.

SUPPLEMENTS

- **ACIDOPHILUS-** initially double the dose recommended on the bottle.
- **DIGESTIVE ENZYMES-** with each meal; sauerkraut and other fermented vegetables can also assist in more efficient digestion.
- **GLUTAMINE-** especially if you have had chemotherapy or radiation.
- **OMEGA3 Fatty Acids** (pharmaceutical grade).

SEE REMEDY CHART UNDER DIGESTION ALSO

MASTITIS (BREAST INFECTION)

A breast infection is an infection in the tissue of the breast. Breast infections are usually caused by a common bacterium, (Staphylococcus aureus) found on normal skin. The bacteria enter through a break or crack in the skin, usually on the nipple.

The infection takes place in the fatty tissue of the breast and causes swelling. This swelling pushes on the milk ducts. The result is pain and lumps in the infected breast. Breast infections usually occur in women who are breastfeeding.

CONVENTIONAL TREATMENT
- Anti-biotics

NATURAL TREATMENT
If nursing, consider that the baby will also receive the drug therapy. There are many anti-bacterial remedies and herbs. If the infection is caught early natural therapy can help to efficiently resolve infection.

ACUPUNCTURE & TRADITIONAL CHINESE MEDICINE (TCM)
Treating patterns of Mastitis may be seen as Liver qi stagnation with phlegm and heat. Some forms of TCM may be chosen singly or together for the best treatment plan and holistic response.

HOMEOPATHIC REMEDIES
Treating the presenting symptoms works amazingly well to resolve mastitis. In acute prescribing repeat remedies as often as every 15 minutes. Remedies can be combined or changed as symptoms change.
- **ACONITUM-** cracked nipples, breasts hard and tense, possible milk fever and toothache, FEAR, worse at night and to the touch, better from fresh air.
- **APIS-** inverted nipples, swollen, hard, threatening to ulcerate, jealous and weepy, worse from touch, and from 3-5 pm, better from open air.
- **ARNICA-** nipples cracked, violent stitching, pain in middle of left breast, ulcerated, feels bruised, says they are fine, worse from touch.
- **ARSENICUM-** cracked nipples, retracted, burning, itching, lump in breast, sensitive to touch, and fear of being alone, demanding.
- **BELLADONNA-** sudden onset, acute swelling burning plane, worse in right breast, red streaked from center to circumference, inflamed, engorged, tender, hot, throbbing, bright red and shiny, swollen, high fever, flushed face, dilated pupils, toothache, headache after breast feeding, excitable, possible delirium, worse jarring, better lying down.

- **BRYONIA-** electric-like shocks, pale, inflamed, engorged, tender, hot, stony hardness, pain on slightest movement, left breast worse, high fever, nausea, extreme thirst, bursting headache after breastfeeding, lips cracking, irritable when disturbed, worse from cold and slightest movement, better being alone and supporting breasts.
- **CALCAREA CARBONICA-** hot, swollen, hard, distended swollen glands, pains as of excoriation and ulceration of nipples, great debility, fever, head perspires at night, watery milk refused by baby, toothache, headache after breast feeding, FEAR that something might happen, chilly and worse from cold air.
- **CHAMOMILLA-** cracked, tender, inflamed nipples, hard glands, can hardly bear the pain of breastfeeding, fever, pain in uterus during breast feeding, milk is cheesy with blood and pus, headache after nursing, irritable, worse from touch, better from uncovering.
- **GRAPHITES-** nipples cracked, blistered, swollen; very sensitive lymph, inflamed weeps without cause, worse in the night.
- **HEPAR SUPLH CALCAREA-** great for draining abscess; chilly and intolerant of becoming cold; stitching or splinter-like pains; complains intensely from pain; abscess with skin healing slowly; cracking skin (*anti-biotic alternative*).
- **MERCURIUS SOL OR VIVUS-** offensive eruptions; worse from heat (*anti-biotic alternative*)
- **PHOSPHORUS-** cracked, inflamed, hot, bluish nipples; swollen, anxious feeling below left breast, burning in right breast with heat extending to the head, cramping pains, bitter tasting burps, increased sexual desire, stitching pains, toothache, headache after breastfeeding, wants sympathy, massage and is easily reassured, worse from slightest touch.
- **PHYTOLACCA-** nipples crack, swollen, inflamed, sensitive and tender; breast inflamed and hard like a stone, lumpy, unbearable pain when breastfeeding starting from the nipple, radiating over the entire body and streaking up and down the spine; elevated temperature, abscesses and pus, milk with blood, bad breath; unbearable pain, irritable, indifferent and restless; better supporting breasts.
- **PULSATILLA-** cracked, burning, itchy nipples; breasts swollen, feel stretched and intensely sore; pains extended to chest, neck and down the back, pain changes location; thin, watery milk; pain in uterus while breastfeeding, white discharge, headache after breastfeeding; weeps while breastfeeding; better from sympathetic company; can be used to restore adequate milk supply following breast infection.
- **SILICEA-** nipples cracked, bleeding, inverted like a funnel, burning, itchy, cutting pain; breasts inflamed, lumpy, deep red in center with rose colored periphery, burning pains worse in left breast, pain extends from breast to shoulder; cutting pains in uterus, head sweat at night, constipation, back pain, fever, milk with blood, refused by baby, headache after breastfeeding; chilly, anxious, excited, yielding; better from warmth.

THE BANERJI PROTOCOL™ FOR BREAST ABSCESS

- **HEPAR SULPH CALCAREA 6C and BELLADONNA 3C,** alternate every 3 hours. With acute pain repeat every hour.
- If abscess is draining, **HEPAR SULPH CALCAREA 6C** and **HYPERICUM PERF 200C + ARSENICUM ALBUM 200c,** alternating every 3 hours.
- **COLLOIDAL SILVER** is antibacterial and can be added to any treatment.

MENOPAUSE

Menopause is the time in a woman's life when her period stops. It usually occurs naturally, most often after age 45. Menopause happens because the woman's ovaries stop producing the hormones estrogen and progesterone.

Conventional medical text will state that women reach menopause when they have not had a period for one year. Changes and symptoms actually begin several years earlier and continue for up to a decade and beyond.

SYMPTOMS

- A change in periods – shorter or longer, lighter or heavier, with more or less time in between
- Hot flashes and/or night sweats
- Trouble sleeping
- Vaginal dryness
- Mood swings
- Weight gain
- Trouble focusing
- Hair loss, possible increase on face

Some symptoms require treatment. Talk to your doctor about how to best manage menopause. Make sure the doctor knows your medical history and your family medical history. This includes whether you are at risk for heart disease, osteoporosis, or breast cancer.

CONVENTIONAL TREATMENT

- Hormone replacement therapy (HRT)
- Anti-depressants

NATURAL TREATMENT

Some holistic practitioners will tell you they use 'bio-identical hormones'. They claim it is a 'natural' method of hormone replacement therapy. This is not correct, since all hormone therapies are chemically based. There are many other means of relieving the symptoms of menopause without introducing hormones into the body at a time when women are meant to *naturally lower* hormone levels. Female cancers have more than tripled since HRT was introduced into the marketplace.

Always request a full blood panel including thyroid, cortisol levels, testosterone as well as estrogens, progesterone and pregnenolone. Also a good opportunity to test ferritin levels (iron). Review test results for yourself. Most conventional doctors only take note of results 'Out of Range', however, being at the *bottom* of any range is not optimal for your wellbeing.

Many women notice they begin to put on weight more easily during menopause. You may be eating the same amount and exercising just as much, to no avail. One of the many changes during this time is a lowering of body temperature (even though you feel like you are heating up). As a result, metabolism begins to slow, meaning the thyroid may need support. If your practitioner is using *Organotherapy*, they would dispense a natural thyroid glandular. A Homeopath may dispense the remedy *Thyroidinum 4C*, that can naturally stimulate thyroid activity. An alternative thyroid treatment is *Thyroidinum 200c + Bromium 6c* for a minimum of three months. Often it is necessary to support the adrenals when stimulating the thyroid. Re-test blood work to monitor results.

You may also be low in *IODINE*, important food for the proper functioning of the thyroid. As we age our iodine levels drop. An easy test to determine if you are low in iodine is to purchase a bottle of Lugol's Iodine. Rub one drop into the bend of your left elbow and note how long it takes for the body to absorb the iodine stain. If it is gone in a few hours you are in need of iodine. If it takes overnight, then you do not. (Seek the help of a professional in regulating iodine and thyroid levels.)

Gaining some weight as we age is normal. The body stores estrogen in fat cells, staying stick thin and/or completely muscular does not help to feel better during this time of transition. It might help your ego, but not your physical body. Digestion also slows as we age. See below for remedy suggestions for digestive issues.

HOMEOPATHY

A qualified Homeopath can take your case and dispense a 'Constitutional' remedy that suits your symptoms and particular health profile. Having said that, the following are a number of commonly used remedies for issues of menopause. Remedy selection does not depend on having all the symptoms. Also, do not be afraid to mix remedies and re-dose as needed. **AMMONIUM CARBONICUM 200C** taken twice daily is an excellent over-all remedy to help balance changes during menopause. It can improve circulation, which in turn improves many symptoms.

HOT FLASHES

- **CALCAREA CARBONICA-** profuse sweating at the slightest activity (mostly head & neck); skin can feel cold and clammy.
- **LACHESIS-** intense hot flashes (head & neck); but can feel overheated all the time; can have cold extremities; intolerant of anything tight around neck, wrists or waist.
- **PHOSPHORUS-** hot flashes with heart palpitations, lightheadedness, dizziness and anxiety.
- **PULSATILLA-** hot flashes brought on by anxiety; may have irregular heartbeat; craves fresh air; worse in a congested room.
- **SEPIA-** tends to be chilly but changes to overheated when in bed at night; can have drenching sweats followed by chills. Does not sleep well and as a result

is tired during the day. Women who are stressed and overworked and agitated with partner.

- **SANGUINARIA-** intense heat; flushed face; pulsating sensation all over body; headaches; humming in ears.
- **SULPHUR-** feels overheated all the time; sweats from head, feet, under arms and has an odor; heat rashes; uncovers feet at night.

INSOMNIA

- **ACONITUM-** sleeplessness after bad news, shock or trauma.
- **ARSENICUM-** restlessness; anxiety; wakes after midnight with worries of work, money, health, failure, etc.
- **AVENA SATIVA-** nervous exhaustion.
- **AURUM METALLICUM-** depression.
- **COFFEA CRUDA-** due to anticipation or overexcitement; can't turn off brain from work and/or ideas.
- **IGNATIA-** intense grief or loss; cries, even in sleep.
- **NUX VOMICA-** difficulty falling asleep; tense people; wake between 2:00 and 4:00 with difficulty going back to sleep; chronic insomnia related to work; desires alcohol and stimulants.
- **PHOSPHORUS-** awaken from anxious dreams; difficulty going back to sleep; fear of being alone, from dark and of loud noises.

DIGESTION ISSUES

- **CALCARIA CARBONICA-** increase in upper body weight, flabby; intolerant of exercise; hard worker, conscientious; constipation and/or diarrhea (especially if there is a craving for milk and dairy products).
- **CARBO VEGETABILIS-** bloating, gas; low vitality; may have bad breath or body odor; constipation and/or diarrhea.
- **LYCOPODIUM-** gas and bloating, especially after sugar or carbohydrates; liver issues; low blood sugar that can cause fatigue mid-day. Combines well with **ARSENICUM ALBUM.**
- **LACHESIS-** constipated for days at a time, will then pass large stools; hemorrhoids.
- **MAGNESIA PHOSPHORICA-** gas pains and constipation; cramping (leg cramps).
- **NATRUM MURIATICUM-** can have emotional eating disorders; reluctant to use public restrooms; craves salt; fluid retention.
- **NUX VOMICA-** nausea and heartburn after meals; craves rich foods, alcohol and stimulants; irritability; headache; constipation with small hard stools; difficulty relaxing.

HAIR LOSS

The Banerji Protocol™

- **PHOSPHORIC ACID-** for falling out of hair from grief, also for graying, and/or loss of eyelashes or eyebrows.
- **PHOSPHORUS-** hair falls out in handfuls, or in spots.
- **NATRUM MURIATICUM-** hair loss in temples (or in general), can be greasy.

FIRST LINE MEDICINES

- **HEPAR SULPH CALCAREA 1M-** once per week in water.
- **USTILAGO 200c-** two times daily.

SECOND LINE MEDICINES

- **PHOSPHORUS 1M-** in liquid once every 10 days for 3 months.

THIRD LINE MEDICINE

- **FLUORICUM ACIDUM 200C-** every third day if due to radiation or chemotherapy.

TRACE MINERAL THERAPY FOR HAIR LOSS- Copper.

HEADACHES

If you experienced headaches before or during your regular cycle you are more at risk for headaches during menopause. However, you may have the opposite reaction and be finally rid of the monthly discomfort. If you already have a prescription medicine for headaches, remedies can still be used at the first sign of a headache according to your particular symptoms.

- **BELLADONNA-** for acute pain if there is throbbing, right-sided, worse bending or stooping. Can be combined with **Picric Acid 200c** and repeated every 3 hours.
- **IRIS VERSICOLOR-** pain comes on with relaxing after strain or tension; many times vision is affected (tunnel vision or spots).
- **LACHESIS-** headache worse with sleep, wakes with headache; sinus congestion.
- **LYCOPODIUM-** headache appears in the afternoon with a drop in energy, stomach distress.
- **MAGNESIA PHOSPHORICA-** tension headache with tightness of muscles in neck and around forehead; better with warm compresses or massage.
- **NUX VOMICA-** headache symptoms are like that of a hangover; nausea; irritability; stomach distress; sensitive to noise, light and smells.
- **SANGUINARIA-** worse from being overheated; throbbing pain; flushed face; red eyes; better from cold compresses.

- **SEPIA-** chronic left-sided headache; depleted; depressed; chilliness; insomnia. Repeat remedy every seven days.

INCONTINENCE

Urinary incontinence is a common problem during and after menopause due to vaginal tissue losing moisture in the tissues. This is a common result of lower estrogen and a thinning of the mucus membranes. Along with the use of remedies you can also do what is called the *Kegel* exercise. This exercise can help to restore tone to the pelvic muscles. For best results the exercise must be done *daily*, not sporadically. However, it can be done anywhere at any time. When you first begin to do the exercise you may not be able to do it for more than a couple of minutes, but it is easy to build up to longer periods of time. Some who write about this exercise claim 5 minutes twice a day is enough…***it is not***. If you want results you need to build up to longer periods of time, even if you have to break it up throughout the day.

Put your attention to the vagina and imagine urinating, then cutting off the flow. That's it, that squeezing motion is the exercise. You'll find that if you count, even in blocks of 10 it will be easier to reach 50, then 100, then 500. This helps not only the tone of the pelvic area, but also bladder and rectal function.

Often times incontinence is due to a fungal infection (from anti-biotics or passed on by your partner) in the bladder, urethra, kidneys or vagina. No one needs to wear diapers! See CANDIDA for suggestions to clear this and/or do KEGELS!

- **NATRUM MURIATICUM-** urine escapes in spurts during laugh or cough.
- **PULSATILLA-** urine escapes from anxiety, being overheated or coughing; urinates frequently.
- **SEPIA-** sense of weakness and weight in pelvis and bladder; constipation; loss of urine with exertion.

ACUPUNCTURE & TRADITIONAL CHINESE MEDICINE (TCM)

Treating patterns of Menopause may be seen as yin deficiency with deficient heat. Some forms of TCM may be chosen singly or together for the best treatment plan and holistic response.

GEMMOTHERAPY

Gemmotherapy can be a very efficient therapy for menopause. It works gently and naturally over time to assist the endocrine system in adjusting to the changes. A doctor who practices Integrative Medicine will use your blood work to match the correct Gemmos needed as symptoms change.

- **BLACK CURRANT-** hormonal deficiency.
- **CHASTE TREE-** insomnia, hot flashes.
- **COWBERRY-** anti-aging*, hot flashes, constipation or diarrhea.
- **CRAB APPLE-** anti-aging**, hot flashes, constipation.
- **DOGWOOD-** resentful of changes, nervousness, hot flashes.

- **FIG-** depression and insomnia.
- **GREY ALDER-** *vaginal dryness* accompanied by resentment of menopause.
- **LINDEN TREE-** insomnia and anxiety (mixes well with **FIG**).
- **MAIZE-** hot flashes, *vaginal atrophy*.
- **MISTLETOE-** hypertension.
- **RASPBERRY-** regulates balance between estrogen and progesterone.
- **SERVICE TREE-** circulation issues and tinnitus.

SUPPLEMENTS

- **ALPHA LIPOIC ACID-** this powerful antioxidant is an amino acid that turns on the brain, improving memory and assists B Vitamins in producing energy from the proteins, fats and carbohydrates in your food.
- **OMEGA 3 FATTY ACIDS-** (Pharmaceutical grade) helps with the production of hormones.
- **MULTI-B VITAMINS-** important for brain and nervous system function (raw, not synthetic).
- **RED CLOVER-** the isoflavone compounds (lignan & phyoestrogens) attach to estrogen-like receptors to stimulate a response in the body similar to estrogen.
- **BLACK COHASH-** contains phytochemicals that have an effect on the endocrine system.

FEMALE REMEDY REFERENCE CHART

UTIs- Cantharis

Cramps- Colocynthis or Mag Phos 6x

PMS- Sepia

Breast tenderness- Bryonia

Edema under eyes- Lycopodium

Low libido- Sepia

Anemia- Ferrum Phos 6x + Kali Mur 6x

Exhausted/ overwhelmed- Sepia

Weepy/Depressed- Ignatia or Aurum metallicum

Regulate hormones after BC- Sepia

Spotting between menses- Sabina

Vaginal Itching- Ars alb + Kreosotum

Hot flashes- Lachesis or Sulphur

Insomnia- Arnica, Ignatia or Coffea cruda

Vaginal dryness- Sepia

Edema during pregnancy- Lycopodium

Morning sickness- Tabacum or Ars alb + Ipecac

Post-partum depression- Sepia

MENSTRUAL ISSUES

Menstruation, or period, is normal vaginal bleeding that occurs as part of a woman's monthly cycle. Every month, your body prepares for pregnancy. If no pregnancy occurs, the uterus, or womb, sheds its lining. The menstrual blood is partly blood and partly tissue from inside the uterus. It passes out of the body through the vagina.

Periods usually start between age 11 and 14 and continue until menopause at about age 50. They usually last from three to five days. Besides bleeding from the vagina, you may have:

- Abdominal or pelvic cramping
- Lower back pain
- Bloating
- Sore breasts
- Food cravings
- Mood swings and irritability
- Headache
- Fatigue

Premenstrual Syndrome, or PMS, is a group of symptoms that start before the period. It can include emotional and physical symptoms.

Consult your health care provider if you have big changes in your cycle. They may be signs of other problems that should be treated.

CONVENTIONAL TREATMENT

Many doctors will put their patients on the birth control pill (BCP) as soon as there is a sign of menstrual discomfort. Ultimately, this is NOT the adjustment the body is looking for. Taking chemical hormones and putting the body into an artificial state of pregnancy is suppressive, especially at a young age. Statistics show that female cancers have risen tremendously since the advent of the BCP.

NATURAL TREATMENT

There are a number of natural therapies, including supplements that adjust moods, pain, flow and other issues successfully. A proper diagnosis may be necessary to know where the imbalance is coming from. The following types of practitioners and their therapies all have something to offer in this area.

HOMEOPATHY

Homeopathy can be very powerful in adjusting the discomforts of menses. A Classical Homeopath can dispense a 'Constitutional' remedy that can re-balance the body based on your particular symptoms and sensations. When seeking a remedy prioritize your symptoms and measure the severity. Notice if they are acute or chronic. The following are some commonly used remedies for specific issues.

PMS- (Premenstrual Syndrome) The severity of symptoms before periods can range from mildly troubling to almost debilitating. They may also change in severity from month to month according to stress. If symptoms last longer than 3 months, see a health care practitioner. Remedies are recommended for at least two cycles before changing remedies.

- **SEPIA-** (may have some or all of the symptoms) emotional distress preceding period, fatigue, weight gain, headaches, abdominal bloating, breast tenderness, constipation, loss of sex drive and/or depression. (*Two times weekly*)
- **COCCULUS-** painful pressure in uterine region, weakness, fearful. (*Two times daily*)
- **CIMICIFUGA-** backache, revousness, pain across pelvis, better with flow. (Two times daily)
- **PLATINUM METALLICUM (PLATINA)-** arrogance, haughty, disdain, increased sexual desire.(*Two times weekly*)
- **STRAMONIUM** (mother tincture)- anger, rage, irritability. (*5 drops in water two times daily*)

BALANCING PERIODS IN YOUNG GIRLS

- **CHAMAMILLA-** repeat 2x daily when there is irritability, moodiness and they are over-emotional. Dose when symptoms arise, repeat until improvement.
- **CALCAREA CARBONICA-** headache, chilliness or pain before period, may have burning and itching before and after period. Repeat once daily until improvement.
- **COLOCYNTHIS-** cramping, repeat often, stop when symptoms are gone.
- **IGNATIA-** too early, heavy, suppressed from grief, great fatigue with spasmodic pains (history of passing out). Repeat 2x daily
- **PULSATILLA-** painful, irregular, breakthrough bleeding, (repeat *twice weekly*) to regulate periods. May take up to 6 cycles.
- **MAG PHOS 6X-** if there is a history of bed wetting, repeat 2 x's daily for 6-8 weeks.

MISSED PERIODS (AMENORRHEA)

- **ACONITUM-** after being frightened or catching cold.
- **COLOCYNTHIS-** after being angry.
- **NATRUM MUR-** after mental strain (stress).
- **PULSATILLA-** after getting wet.

LIGHT PERIODS
- **PULSATILLA-** light flow that stops and starts again.
- **SEPIA-** fewer days of flow than normal.

PAINFUL PERIODS (DYSMENORRHEA)
- **BELLADONNA-** sensation of heaviness in lower pelvic region, worse moving around, pain in right ovary.
- **CAULOPHYLLUM-** pain radiates in all directions.
- **CHAMOMILLA-** intolerable pain.
- **COLOCYNTHIS-** cramping, worse eating or drinking, boring pain in ovary (repeat as needed).
- **MAG-PHOS-** pain usually before flow; better from heat and bending over (repeat or alternate with **COLOCYNTHIS**).
- **PULSATILLA-** painful cramps with nausea.
- **SABINA-** pain in thighs, sacrum or pubic bone, spotting between periods.
- **VERATRUM ALBUM-** pain with cold sweating, worse from least exertion.

HEAVY PERIODS (MENORRHAGIA)
- **ACONITUM+ RHUS TOX-** if accompanied by headache.
- **AMMONIUM CARB 200C-** every 10 days if occurance is every month.
- **ARNICA or SABINA-** every 3 hours to slow heavy bleeding.
- **CINCHONA-** heavy periods with fatigue, alternate with **HELONIAS**.
- **CROCUS SATIVUS-** heavy period with black or dark blood.

ANEMIA
- **KALI MURIATICUM 6X+FERRUM PHOSPHORICUM 6X-** two times daily.

APLASTIC ANEMIA
- **HAMAMELIS + ARNICA-** two times daily.

If there is *flooding* add the supplement **Dessicated Liver to cleanse and strengthen liver function.

LEUCORRHEA- ABNORNAL DISCHARGE (COLOR, ODOR)
- **KREOSOTUM-** violent itching, burning soreness, yellow or green discharge, worse between periods. (*every other day*)
- **PSORINUM-** if there are skin issues or depression, much backache and debility, pain in sacrum. (*two times weekly*)

VOMITING
- **ARSENICUM ALBUM-** every 3 hours until improvement.
- **IPECACUANHA-** persistent nausea and vomiting, bright red bleeding (possible hemorrhaging).
- **PULSATILLA-** timid, emotional, tearful, changeable moods.
- **VERATRUM ALBUM-** extreme chilliness and weakness, vomiting with cramps in limbs.

SUPPRESSED OR ABSENT PERIODS
- Athletes many times experience the loss of, or infrequency of periods. Eating disorders in young girls can also affect an otherwise normal flow. The remedy **Calcarea Carbonicum** taken weekly can help to correct.
- If eating disorders is the cause look to **IGNATIA Amara** *(two times daily)*, especially if there is grief or sadness. **AURUM Metallicum** if the picture of depression is more like hopelessness. *(Two times per week)* If OCD tendencies are present, **Natrum Muriaticum Aurum** *(twice daily.)*

BALANCING AFTER BIRTH CONTROL
- **SEPIA 200c-** A valuable remedy for rebalancing hormones after birth control *(every 7 days for a few months)*.
- **AMMONIUM CARBONICUM 200C-** for synthetic hormone use *(every other day for 6-8 weeks or as needed)*.

FREQUENT URINARY TRACT INFECTIONS
- **CANTHARIS*-** as soon as symptoms arise, repeat every 2-3 hours.
- **BORAX-** white discharge, nausea and pain in stomach extended to small of back. *(Twice daily)*
- **MEDORRHINUM-** thick fishy discharge, intense itching. *(repeat twice daily)*
- **MERCURIUS SOL(or VIV)-** thick white discharge with itching, worse urinating. *(repeat 2-3 times daily)*
- **PYROGEN-** sepsis-like conditions, fever, offensive odor, acute throbbing pain. *(repeat every 3 hours)*
- **STAPHYSAGRIA-** infections after sex, if not enough resolve add **Medorrhinum**. *(repeat twice daily)*
- **TEREBINTHINA-** intense burning in uterine region, especially with heavy periods.

TOXIC SHOCK SYNDROME- when a tampon has been left in and infection arises
- **PYROGEN (PYROGENIUM)-** repeat 3-4 times daily until improvement.

ACUPUNCTURE & TRADITIONAL CHINESE MEDICINE (TCM)

With the expertise of the licensed provider of Chinese Medicine a correct pattern/s for your symptom/s may be chosen from one of several that fall under a certain disease or condition category. TCM is very effective for female issues.

GEMMOTHERAPY

The following are the Gemmos most used for female issues:

- **ASH-** can increase adrenal production of cortisol.
- **BLACK CURRANT-** can stimulate endocrine system.
- **COWBERRY-** post menopausal, anti-aging.
- **CRABAPPLE-** anti-aging, hot flashes.
- **DOG ROSE-** can rejuvenate adrenals, supports thyroid.
- **DOG WOOD-** affects thyroid (do not use in hypothyroidism).
- **HAWTHORN-** palpitations in hyperthyroidism.
- **OAK-** helps liver to stimulate hormones.
- **RASPBERRY-** regulates menstrual cycles, can induce labor.

MEMORY ISSUES

Memory issues used to occur mostly in women during menopause and severe cases that extended into later years was labeled *Dementia*. In recent times it has become an epidemic labeled as *Alzheimer's*. It has also struck men almost as often as women.

There is usually a lack of memory of recent events, confusion, mood swings and sometimes irritability. In this section I will not address the more severe symptoms of further deterioration, such as loss of language skills and bodily functions. For the purposes of this discussion we are addressing mild memory loss. When there is intervention early on through diet, exercise, natural therapies and supplements the decline can be arrested.

The change in farming methods in the 1950s that introduced fungicides into our food supply is said to be one reason for the epidemic. Another reason is aluminum, which is very toxic to the brain. Aluminum cooking pans, aluminum cans for food packaging and a rise in aluminum in the soil from chemtrails contributes to the increased exposure. We also come in contact with over 300,000 chemicals in our daily lives.

The brain is still not completely understood by the medical community and as discoveries continue, so will new methods of treatment. Those methods however, will be pharmaceutical drugs and adding more chemicals may not be the answer.

There are a number of natural therapies and supplements for brain function. The following is a small sampling. The topic warrants a book in and of itself, so I will keep it brief for the context of this book.

THE IMPORTANCE OF pH

The first place to start is by measuring pH levels in the body. Optimal ranges are 7.3-7.5 for saliva and 6.8-7.0 for urine. You can monitor levels regularly with the use of pH strips or a pH meter. If you are too acidic (below normal range), start with ¼ -1/2 tsp. of sodium bicarbonate (baking soda), two times daily. Adjust intake as your levels rise. Fresh lemon water or apple cider vinegar can accomplish the same end goal.

DIET

Diet is the most important place to start. Technically speaking, your gut is the first brain, since the brain cannot function without proper nutrition or uptake of hormones.

Eat as much fresh, locally grown organic foods as possible. The importance of feeding your brain with good, clean food cannot be stressed enough. Stay away from GMO foods (Genetically Modified Organisms). Interestingly enough the issue of *memory loss in mass numbers did not exist before the advent of GMO foods*.

If you are interested in researching a clean, substantial diet for optimal brain function research the 'Weston Price Foundation'. Their website is jam packed with information about proper eating habits and how food can be your medicine.

If the onset of depression coincided with your memory issues you may not be receiving the correct balance of neurotransmitters to the brain. This would mean improper uptake of serotonin, dopamine or the pre-cursor to dopamine, L-dopa, to name a few. You can ask your doctor to test your levels of neurotransmitters. Also make sure your thyroid levels and ferritin levels (iron) are well in normal range.

HOMEOPATHY

There are many Homeopathic remedies that address memory. The most efficient means of finding the correct one for you is by visiting a qualified Homeopath to take your case and dispense a 'Constitutional' remedy.

ACUPUNCTURE & TRADITIONAL CHINESE MEDICINE (TCM)

Treating patterns of Memory may be seen as Heart and Kidney deficiencies; Spleen and Heart deficiencies and/or Liver wind with 'shen' disturbance. Some forms of TCM may be chosen singly or together for the best treatment plan and holistic response.

PHENOLIC THERAPY

Memory loss can sometimes be related to allergic reactions and/or sensitivities that slow brain function. Chapter III has a brief explanation of phenolic therapy. If you can isolate your particular issue, phenolic therapy can be a means of desensitization to allergens to bring about balance.

As an example, if you have food sensitivities such as wheat or gluten that are interfering with digestion, you may not have the proper uptake of Dopamine or Serotonin to the brain. Specific phenolic tinctures can help to reduce the symptoms brought on by the disturbance. Chapter III includes charts of phenols and their symptoms for a clearer idea of the possibilities for this type of therapy.

SUPPLEMENTS

- **OMEGA 3 FATTY ACIDS-** pharmaceutical grade helps the transport of nutrients to the brain.
- **ALPHA LIPOIC ACID-** an amino acid that crosses the blood/brain barrier combined with Acetyl L-Carnitine has been shown to improve memory.
- **B VITAMINS-** Folic Acid, B6 and B12 can lower blood levels of homocysteine, which is associated with brain shrinkage.
- **LECITHIN-** an important phospholipid needed in all cells and can improve brain memory function.
- **COCONUT OIL-** supplies the brain with energy and prevent neuro-degenerative disease states.
- **GINKGO-** according to new research encourages the development of neural stem cells.

MORNING SICKNESS

Nausea and vomiting that happen during pregnancy, especially during the first trimester, is often called "morning sickness." Despite its name, morning sickness can occur at any time of the day.

In some instances, morning sickness is considered severe if you cannot keep any food or fluids down and begin to lose weight. This condition is called hyperemesis gravidarum.

Although it is not known for certain what causes morning sickness, it is most likely due to increasing levels of hormones during pregnancy. Sometimes the multi-vitamin with iron you are taking may be the culprit. If the iron is not from an herbal or food source (such as Floridex™) it may exacerbate your symptoms. Your pre-natal vitamin should be organic and list ingredients from food sources, rather than generic chemical based vitamins.

CONVENTIONAL TREATMENT

Your health care provider will first investigate whether your nausea and vomiting are due to morning sickness or if there is another medical cause. If other causes are ruled out, certain medications may be prescribed. Diclegis®, a combination antihistamine and chemical form of Vitamin B6 (along with numerous other chemicals) may be suggested. If you are dehydrated from loss of fluids, replenishment through an IV may be administered.

NATURAL TREATMENT

Taking in any drugs during pregnancy may pose a risk, since they can affect the fetus. There are a number of natural solutions to "morning sickness." You can start with paying attention to diet and eating a number of small meals throughout the day. Do not go to bed hungry. Even having a high protein snack on the bedside table, if you wake during the night and feel hungry can be helpful. Try having a snack before getting out of bed in the morning. Avoid spicy foods, strong smells that may be bothersome, get plenty of rest and drink lots of clean water.

- Increase Vitamin B-complex intake (especially B6)
- Try adding 25 mg of Zinc per day
- Drink fresh ginger steeped in hot water
- Other teas that may help- Peppermint, Anise or Raspberry
- Add Brewer's yeast to your food
- Fennel and cinnamon help to keep blood sugars normalized
- Suck on lozenges, natural lemon flavor, etc

ACUPUNCTURE & TRADITIONAL CHINESE MEDICINE (TCM)

With the expertise of the licensed provider of Chinese Medicine a correct pattern/s for your symptom/s may be chosen from one of several that fall under this condition.

HOMEOPATHIC REMEDIES

The homeopathic remedy that will work best for you must be symptom specific. Here are the most common remedies for morning sickness.

- **ANTIMONIUM TARTARICUM-** extreme nausea that comes in waves, anxiety, frequent vomiting followed by exhaustion, worse after vomiting, better lying on right side, inclined to want to sleep.
- **ARSENICUM ALBUM-** anxious and restless; extreme nausea and retching; can have vomiting without nausea, worse after vomiting, perspiration during vomiting; after drinking cold drinks, worse in the afternoon and from the smell of food, diarrhea, burning in the stomach, desire for sour things and coffee, better from heat and warm drinks.
- **IPECACUANHA-** constant nausea not relieved by vomiting, belching, feels like stomach is hanging down, cold perspiration, shortness of breath, thirstless, worse after vomiting, after eating, from smell of food or tobacco, worse being warm or from movement, better in open air and from cold drinks.
- **NUX VOMICA-** irritable, angry, sensitive to smells and noise; constant nausea, relieved after vomiting, eating or dry heaves; feels like heavy weight in stomach after eating; vomits bile, mucus, that is bitter; heartburn, faintness, copious saliva, craving for stimulants; worse immediately after eating, smell of tobacco smoke, from pressure of clothes, better after vomiting.
- **PHOSPHORUS-** fearful, requires sympathy when ill, easily comforted, gregarious personality; nausea after food and drink becomes warm in the stomach, sour burps; heat between shoulder blades; vomits bile, mucus that is yellow and bitter; craves ice cold drinks and salt; aversion to tea, coffee meat; feels weak and has burning pains, worse from hot drinks, and warm water brings on nausea.
- **PULSATILLA-** easily hurt, mild mannered, yielding, easily moved to tears not relieved from vomiting; bad taste in the morning; desire for sour refreshing things; worse after eating or drinking coughing, hot drinks, rich or fatty foods, stuffy room, fruit; better from fresh air and cold drinks.
- **SEPIA-** nausea intermittently, gnawing pains; feels like dragging down in abdomen, empty feeling; vomits bile; backache; desire for sour things, sweets, wine, aversion to bread, fatty foods, milk; worse from minimal effort, company, not eating, worse in the morning and again from 3-5, smell of food; temporarily better after eating, snappy and indifferent due to exhaustion.

OTITIS MEDIA (SEE EAR INFECTION)

PAIN

Pain is a feeling triggered in the nervous system. Pain may be sharp or dull. It may come and go, or it may be constant. You may feel pain in one area of your body, such as your abdomen, back or chest or you may feel pain all over, such as when your muscles ache from the flu. There are just as many causes of pain as there are treatments.

Pain can be helpful in diagnosing a problem. Without pain, you might seriously hurt yourself without knowing it, or you might not realize you have a medical problem that needs treatment. Once you take care of the problem, pain usually goes away. However, sometimes pain goes on for weeks, months or even years. This is called chronic pain. Sometimes chronic pain is due to an ongoing cause, such as cancer or arthritis. Sometimes the cause is unknown.

CONVENTIONAL TREATMENT

Treatment varies depending on the cause of the pain. Traditional medical doctors try various prescription pharmaceutical drugs to help mask pain. It is important to be aware that pharmaceutical pain meds can lead to addiction. In some cases, your doctor may recommend surgery when the diagnosis is specific and fits a particular injury or medical condition

NATURAL TREATMENT

There are numerous avenues of successful pain treatment offered within natural therapies. The avenue you choose depends on the circumstances. Body pain can be greatly improved and even cured by a Chiropractor, Acupuncturist, Osteopath, Cranial Sacral Therapist and Naturopath who is trained in any of these areas.

ACUPUNCTURE & TRADITIONAL CHINESE MEDICINE (TCM)

Treating patterns of Pain may be seen as qi and blood stagnation. Some forms of TCM may be chosen singly or together for the best treatment plan and holistic response. TCM can be very effective in the treatment of pain.

HOMEOPATHIC REMEDIES

There are a number of Homeopathic remedies that assist with pain and are symptom specific. The following are a few of the most commonly used. Remedies can be combined and repeated often in acute situations.

- **ACONITUM-** if there is great anxiety from the pain.
- **ARNICA MONTANA-** pain from sprains, bruising, swelling, contusions, painful healing of fractures, muscular aches, sports training, any over exertion, pre and post-op. The most commonly used remedy for overall symptoms of pain.
- **ARSENICUM ALBUM-** anxiety, depression, fear of health, body ache during influenza.
- **BELLADONNA-** headaches, throbbing pain during fever, sensitive to light, noise and being moved.
- **BELLIS PERENNIS-** excitable, feels bruised, pain from varicose veins, uterus sore during pregnancy.
- **GELSEMIUM-** can have sudden emotions of grief; pain from influenza; chills; pain in temple extended to ear, apathy toward illness.
- **HYPERICUM-** painful wound after an injection or from damaged nerves, combines well with Arnica.
- **LEDUM-** relief from puncture wounds.
- **NUX VOMICA-** stomach pain from over eating or drinking; too much mental strain; can be sensitive to noise, odors or light; irritable and impatient.
- **PHOSPHORUS-** sensitive to pain, overly fearful, sympathetic pain.
- **RHUS TOXICODENDRON-** joint pain, pain that is better from motion, but continued motion may aggravate; back strain or injury, better lying on something hard; worse with exposure to wet or cold; worse at night.
- **RUTA GRAVIOLA-** joint pain, pain that is worse from motion; back- vertebrae slip in and out easily; backache from injury or strain; sprains with weakness in joint.
- **TOPICAL REMEDIES- Arnica** creams, some include **Hypericum** also for relief from nerve damage.

SUPPLEMENTS CANCER PAIN

***Salvestrol** is made from natural plant compounds found in fruits, vegetables and herbs. Dr. Danny Burke (Professor Emeritus of Pharmaceutical Metabolism) while on the staff of Aberdeen University Medical School, Scotland discovered a protein in 1995 that exists only in cancer cells. That protein, named CYP1B1 is the very reason cancer cells do not die, (apoptosis) but instead continue to replicate. In fact, CYP1B1 is the only difference between a cancer cell and a normal cell.

Dr. Burke looked to nature to find a means of turning off the CYP1B1 protein. He found that Salvestrols are found throughout the plant kingdom and form a part of a plants defense mechanism. For example, when a ripe fruit comes under attack by fungus the synthesis of a pathogen-specific Salvestrol is induced. In other words, the Salvestrol phyto-nutrient comes to the rescue. Salvestrol is a natural anticancer prodrug. It is harmless and inactive until it is inside a cancer cell its structure is then changed by the CYP1B1 enzyme and goes to work to correct the defect in the cell inducing apoptosis.

STEROL 117- a plant sterol with antioxidants and a polypeptide/essential fatty acid blend that supports immune function, blood lipid levels. It reduces pain by being an anti-inflammatory. This supplement made from plant sterols is an important supplement and worth taking a look at. It has been shown to reduce oxidative damage to proteins and DNA in the body. It is the highest tier of antioxidants available in supplement form. It is a proprietary blend of proteins, amino acids and essential fatty acids.

CLOVE OIL- very effective for any type of pain topically and even taken internally if using pharmaceutical grade.

DMSO (Dimethyl sulfoxide)- initially used as a commercial solvent, DMSO is FDA approved at this time for interstitial cystitis and preserving organs for transplant. Laboratory studies suggest that DMSO cuts pain by blocking peripheral nerve C fibers. Several clinical trials have demonstrated its effectiveness. Burns, cuts, and sprains have been treated with DMSO. Relief is reported to be almost immediate, lasting up to 6 hours. A number of sports teams and Olympic athletes have used DMSO. It has the ability to quickly lessens pain and change the "quality" of the pain. There is much written about percentage of dilution in regards to its effectiveness.

PAIN REMEDY REFERENCE CHART

Pain can be improved or relieved with Homeopathic remedies. The cause, sensations, and symptoms of what affects pain for better or worse are important in selecting the best remedy. For many types and locations of pain, Arnica is the "Go-To" remedy. For more specific choices refer to individual conditions. The following are some of the remedies that help to relieve pain. Arnica can be combined with any of the other remedies. Clove oil is also an efficient topical pain reliever.

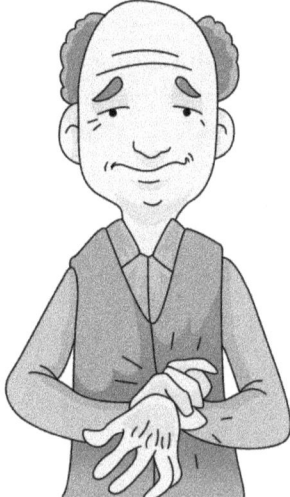

JOINT PAIN
Rhus Tox or Rhuta Grav

FIBROMYALGHIA
Rhus Tox + Symphytum

MENSTRUAL PAIN
Colocynthus or Mag Phos

GOUT
Colchicum + Benzoic Acid

NERVE PAIN
Hypericum

HEADACHES
Belladonna, Sepia

SINUS PAIN
Kali Bic or Hepar Sulph

HEMORRHOIDS
Hamamelis

SINUS HEADACHE
Sanguinaria or Sabadilla

TOOTHACHE
Hypericum + Hepar Sulph

Copyright © 2018 Elena Upton, PhD

PARASITES

Parasites are organisms that derive nourishment and protection from other living organisms known as hosts. They may be transmitted from animals to humans, from humans to humans, or from humans to animals. Several parasites have emerged as significant causes of food borne and waterborne illness. These organisms live and reproduce within the intestinal tract, tissues and organs of infected human and animal hosts, and are often excreted in feces.

Parasites are transmitted from host to host through consumption of contaminated food and water, skin contact, insect bites, air, pets, and soil contact.

Parasites are of different types and range in size from tiny, single-celled, microscopic organisms (protozoa) to larger, multi-cellular worms (helminths) that may be seen without a microscope. The size ranges from 1 to 2 µm (micrometers) to 10 meters long.

Some common parasites are Ancylostoma duodenale/Necator americanus (hookworms), Blastocystis hominis, Giardia lamblia, Cryptosporidium parvum, Cyclospora cayetanensis, Entamoeba bhistolytica, Enterobius vermicularis (pinworm), Helminths (macroscopic multi-cellular worms), Toxoplasma gondii, Trichinella spiralis, Taenia saginata (beef tapeworm), and Taenia solium (pork tapeworm), Trichuris trichiura (whipworm).

Parasites are under-diagnosed in America, especially in cases of IBS, Crohn's and other abdominal/bowel disturbances, as well as some skin conditions. A number of years ago I experienced this very situation first hand. After returning from a trip to the south of France I had a bout of diarrhea and cramps, then began losing weight. I saw a doctor who suggested it was possibly food poisoning and/or stress. Anti-biotics were prescribed. After more than a month of continued symptoms, I did some research and called a friend, Dr. Omar Amin. Dr. Amin had been a Professor of Parasitology at Arizona State University. He sent a stool collection kit and when I received my results it included a picture of the creepy Cryptosporidium that was found in my stool.

Dr. Amin explained that if this condition had gone unchecked it would have led to a number of chronic illnesses. The other valuable information I learned from Dr. Amin is that it is vitally important to collect specimens the first and third day of the full moon for best results. He further explained, "Because of the lack of uniform in structure and/or composition and the cyclic nature of some of the most common human parasites, infections may not be detected in a fecal sample if collected when parasites are not running in the main fecal flow. For instance, intervals of many days may intervene between amebic "runs" which may make the microscopic examination of multiple stool specimens necessary to confirm a positive Entamoeba histolytica infection. The same kind of periodicity and/or adherence to the intestinal lining is also known to occur in Giardia lamblia and Cyclospora cayetanensis. This explains the intermittent shedding and cyclic recovery of these parasites in fecal samples collected for testing. It is important to test for cyclic parasites when they are "running." (In other words, to detect certain specimens, collection is imperative during runs.)

The stool collection kit at PCI Lab, which was developed by Dr. Amin, collects 2 separate fecal samples on 2 different days to maximize parasite recovery rate. On some occasions, however, testing may need to be repeated.

PARASITES AND DAMAGE TO THE BODY

Amin states, "Parasites will compromise the host immune system as well as the person's state of physical, mental, and emotional well-being to various degrees. The tapeworm Diphyllobothrium latum will deplete the body of half its vitamin B12 resources, which are essential for proper central nervous system function, propagation of nerve impulse, muscle coordination, and recall. When this 30-foot long worm is expelled after proper treatment, above functions will be restored to normalcy. Host-parasite relationships causing physical or psychological trauma, may go undetected from early childhood years. Progressive or sudden overt disease outcome may then occur later in life. This reactivation of infection is usually related to depressed immune status, age, hormonal changes, and physical or psychological pressures."

Parasitic infection can also be very damaging by direct injury to the tissue of the digestive tract or liver, among other organ systems. In addition, the most destructive effects may not be caused by the parasite itself, but by its toxic by-products, which are produced unintentionally as part of its living process. Parasites can disrupt digestive activity, can cause malabsorption and can interfere with the action of digestive enzymes and nutrients. In addition, parasites can compromise the human immune system in order to promote and ensure their own survival.

Amin has documented numerous cases of Irritable Bowel Syndrome (IBS), Crohn's, and many other 'diseases' that cleared after the patient was treated for parasitic infection and its subsequent damage.

HOW WE GET INFECTED:

- Drinking water or juice: Giardia, Cryptosporidium.
- Skin contact with contaminated water: Schistosomiasis, swimmers itch.
- Food (fecal or oral infections): most protozoans, Blastocystis, Entamoeba spp and worms: Ascaris.
- Arthropods: Lyme disease, plague, typhus, etc.
- Air: Upper respiratory tract infections (viruses, bacteria), flu, Valley fever, Hanta virus.
- Pets: Hydatid cyst disease, heartworm; larva migrans (dogs).
- Toxoplasma (cats); Taenia spp. (beef, swine tapeworms).
- People (contagious diseases): AIDS, herpes.
- Soil: hookworms, thread worms.

GET TESTED IF YOU HAVE ONE OR MORE OF THESE SYMPTOMS:
GI SYMPTOMS

- Diarrhea/constipation
- Irritable bowel
- Cramps
- Gas & Bloating
- Bleeding
- Appetite changes
- Malabsorption
- Mucus
- Rectal itching
- Gut leakage
- Poor digestion

SYSTEMIC/ OTHER SYMPTOMS

- Fatigue
- Skin rash
- Dry cough
- Brain fog/ memory loss
- Lymph blockage
- Allergies
- Nausea
- Muscle or joint pain
- Dermatitis
- Headaches
- Insomnia

DIFFICULTIES IN DIAGNOSIS

Parasitic infections have long been considered diseases of the tropics, so physicians often do not consider them when diagnosing common illnesses. Parasitology is seldom discussed in mainstream medical journals, and traditionally there has been little reporting of parasite incidence. For example, Giardia has been widely tracked by the Centers for Disease Control (CDC) only since 1987. When physicians receive their training, very little information is provided on parasitology in medical school and in professional medical journals in the US. Given the lack of information and minimal clinical exposure, doctors don't usually consider parasites as a possible cause of illness, especially when the symptoms aren't confined to the digestive tract.

This was exactly the experience I had and it was fortunate I could call on a Parasitologist like Dr. Amin for accurate testing.

CONVENTIONAL TREATMENT

Pharmaceutical drugs- many are irritating to the gut and may cause toxic shock syndrome and not clear the condition completely. It is important to retest after treatment has been completed. If improper dose is given for improper duration, drug resistant parasite strains will develop creating pockets of residual infections that are harder to treat.

NATURAL TREATMENT

Accurate testing is first and foremost. Most labs do parasite analysis along with many other types of microbiology and blood work. They lack specialized training and are not as accurate as a lab that concentrates on parasite analysis only.

While RX anti-parasitics can be useful, Amin, developer of PCI Labs, formulated a 3-part product called Freedom, Cleanse, and Restore to help rid the body of parasites and other organisms based on his many years of research and experience. All-natural products represent one of the best options for the treatment of parasites. The formulas are based on Amin's research and experience that covers known remedies from the Ancient Egyptians and Ancient Chinese.

A good botanical remedy for the restoration of optimal digestive health is one that accomplishes 3 things:

- Defends the body from parasitic infections causing intestinal imbalance
- Cleanses the colon from toxins and promotes regularity
- Supports the integrity of damaged tissues

The 3 PCI formulas accomplish these three functions.

Amin is a nationally and internationally recognized authority in his field. He has over 220 major articles and books published in American and foreign professional journals worldwide on human and animal parasites. Amin is a Fulbright Scholar and has received many other honors, awards and Parasitology research grants.

MYSTERIOUS SKIN DISORDER

- Do you feel pinpricks on your skin?
- Have lesions that have broken out on your body?
- Do you feel like a bug is crawling all over your face?

A patient by the name of Stacy went to seek the advice of Dr. Amin after visiting numerous doctors about the symptoms listed above. The common name for the symptoms is Morgellon's syndrome, which the CDC doesn't recognize as legitimate. Critics say it's a mental issue and patients are called delusional.

"I'm a hard-core, old-fashioned scientist," said Amin.

Amin believes the problem actually comes down in most cases to dental materials that are not compatible with the body's immune system. The exposure to those toxins causes nerve damage, which makes it feel like the skin is crawling.

Amin says, "The nerve cells will misfire. You have no normal nerve impulse anymore, and that misfiring will cause the sensations of movement and pinpricking. The lymphatic system tries to eliminate those toxins through the skin, which breaks out in sores and invites other biological organisms to nest, like spores that grow long-stemmed fungus."

"Everybody who has dental work, and that's just about everybody who lives in this culture of ours, is an open game," he said.

Amin calls the disorder, NCS, for Neurocutaneous Syndrome. Stacy took homeopathic remedies and her dentist started replacing her fillings with more compatible material based on her individual blood tests. You would need to find a biological dentist who works in this way.

The concept is new to science and easy to dismiss, but Amin warns thousands are at risk. The same symptoms can be caused by exposures such as toxic fumes in the work place, insecticides or allergenic sprays, household chemicals, mold, implants, recreational drugs, e.g., crystal methamphetamine and/or cocaine, medications, creams, hot sulfur/mineral springs, and any other environmental exposures to which the patient is allergic.

WHERE TO GET TESTED

Parasitology Center, Inc. (PCI) in Scottsdale, Arizona has state of the art testing equipment and highly trained technicians. They use the new Protofix (fixative) & the CONSED (stain) system. The fixative & stain qualities are superior to those of other tests required by US Government testing agencies. They detect & identify 50-80% more species and individuals of intestinal parasites in fecal specimens than found using other standard tests. You or your doctor can call PCI or go on line to order a stool collection kit. Only your physician or clinic is authorized to receive and discuss your results.

HOMEOPATHY

Parasites are a serious condition and must be monitored by a doctor. There are a number of Homeopathic remedies that address parasites and worms. The remedies must be continued until all worms are eliminated and symptoms resolve completely. Remedies should be prescribed by a professional who can match symptoms with the correct medicine. The following are some of the major remedies that address parasitic infestation.

- **CINA 6C-** most common parasite remedy, especially for children
- **BARYTA CARBONICUM**
- **CALCAREA CARBONICUM**
- **NATRUM PHOSPHORICUM**
- **SILICEA**
- **SPIGELLIA**
- **SULPHUR**

pH BALANCE (POTENTIAL OF HYDROGEN)

pH is a measure of acidity in aqueous solutions (liquids). Solutions less than 7 are considered acid and greater than 7 is considered alkaline. The body needs both measurements to function properly. In fact, the body has a natural circadian rhythm that enables acid levels to fluctuate regularly in a healthy person. If you were to test your first urine of the day you would see it is much more acidic than later in the day (or at least it should be.) This is because the body eliminates toxins during the night by bringing them through the kidneys and bladder into the urine. As the day goes on, pH level rises. If it does not, it means the body is too acid (acidosis) and leads to numerous disorders.

A more in-depth explanation of the importance of pH would fill a book in and of itself. Simply stated, the relationship to positive and negatively charged ions is the key to good health. Just as a battery cannot operate unless there is a proper electrical charge, the human body cannot operate properly without this same balance.

Cations are positively (+) charged particles and anions (-) are negatively charged particles. Junk food, cigarettes, all chemicals and polluted air contain cations. On the other hand, a walk at the beach and fresh organic foods contain anions. Everything you come in contact with affects your health by affecting your pH values. This is why you feel awful after binging on chicken wings and beer, and feel great after a walk at the ocean (salt water emits negatively charged ions) and/or eating a healthy, clean, balanced meal.

Medical doctors are not trained to put attention to a patient's pH values. It is an overlooked marker that signals illness. A number of years ago the topic of pH was very controversial within the medical community and the legal system when a doctor was brought up on charges for healing his patients simply by balancing their saliva and urine pH. The following is a brief overview of the brilliant breakthrough of Dr. Carey Reams.

DR. CAREY REAMS

Dr. Carey Reams (1903-1985) was both a physician and an agronomist. His medical degree, completed in England, included an undergraduate degree in chemistry. Upon returning to the US to practice medicine, Reams chose to retain his independence by avoiding membership in the AMA (American Medical Association).

Dr. Carey Reams was a mathematical genius, chemical engineer for the department of US agriculture, and close friends with Albert Einstein. He lived a controversial life, healing people with "irreversible" conditions and involved in a number of court battles with the AMA and the FDA. It is written that he was mysteriously poisoned in Prison.

While practicing medicine in Orlando, Florida, Reams opened a health retreat in Georgia and used his accumulated practical experience and research to develop what he termed the Reams Human Health Equation. This is a diagnostic and analytical tool based on the testing of urine and saliva. The body fluids were tested with the identical LaMotte soil testing approach that Reams favored when evaluating soil health. The test measured energy loss in his patients, and Reams accurately diagnosed specific diseases based upon small reductions in energy loss, without actually seeing his clients.

Using math alone he determined which "diseases" a person had had, what parts of their body were chronically aching, intimate details concerning function of their body and its superficial appearance; even what single point on the body might be highly sensitive to the touch. He determined these things by inserting their numbers in a series of complex algorithms. Ream's was often quoted as saying, "Why guess, when you can be sure."

Reams was a master at bringing people back from the brink of death by adjusting and balancing the pH in their urine and saliva, along with diet. There is much written on his techniques and his testing kits are also available online for purchase.

(If you are interested in researching his methods, it is advised that his lemon water fast and other protocols be followed under the guidance of a trained professional.)

NATURAL TREATMENT

There is much controversy that exists within the holistic health community also, in regards to pH balancing. There are high pH water products (9.5 to as high as 11) that have come to the marketplace in recent years to address the rampant issue of acidity. Attempting to balance pH through water intake is not solving the issue of acidity at a deeper level. In fact, if the pH level in the body is artificially elevated for long periods of time it interferes with the natural detoxification process mentioned above.

Many people have discussed feeling great once they started drinking high pH water. This is understandable for some. For those people it is a quick fix to a very acid gut, which then helps to kill off pathogens. Various viral, bacterial, fungal and parasitic infestations can only survive in an acid environment. The die-off would surely improve their immediate condition. Long term, however, a pH of over 7.5 is not natural, or necessary, to the normal functions of the human body.

A clean, balanced diet along with drainage therapy can quickly shift the body into a healthy, negatively charged state. There are many supplements on the market that claim to balance pH. It is not an easy proposition for supplementation, since the substance has to survive the strong stomach acids and make its way intact into the intestines. A successful means of accomplishing this is with plain old baking soda (sodium bicarbonate). There is a trick to it though. Even baking soda will not survive the power of stomach acids and needs to be in a liposomal base. This means it needs to be coated with fat. The fat will help to successfully carry the baking soda to its final destination where it will chemically adjust the pH level to a normal range.

How do you do this? With butter (never use margarine). Melt some organic butter in a pan just until it becomes liquid. Remove from heat immediately. Pour in enough baking soda until it dissolves in the butter. "Fill" the butter up with the baking soda. Pour into a container (even an ice cube tray) and refrigerate. Once it is solidified it is ready to use.

Two to three times daily ingest ¼ - ½ a teaspoon or more of the preparation. Your level of health will determine how much is necessary for you to take each day. You will be amazed at how quickly your body responds. Arthritis, chronic pain, allergies will improve with this method.

I broke a finger about twenty years ago. In recent years, arthritis was beginning to develop. I began the baking soda method and 24-hours later the swelling and pain was already down. Continuing the protocol, I noticed an improvement in digestion also.

Another easy method of improving pH is with boric acid. It can be purchased in a pharmacy, along with empty capsules. Fill seven capsules with the boric acid and insert one filled capsule rectally every night at bedtime for one week. Test your pH using pH strips to see if you need to extend the protocol beyond one week.

DR. HAZEL PARCELL'S FORMULA TO ALKALIZE & HYDRATE

Dr. Parcells was a leading researcher in the field of detoxification and energy healing. Her work has changed the lives of many who credit her with their renewed health. This amazing teacher and practitioner continued her research to the age of 106. The following is the formula she shared:

- ½ tsp Cream of Tartar Spice
- ¼ tsp Sea Salt
- ¼ tsp Baking Soda
- 8-10 oz. of spring or filtered water

Drink whenever you feel brain fog, or need a lift.

PRE-MENSTRUAL SYNDROME (PMS) (SEE MENSTRUAL ISSUES)

RESTLESS LEG SYNDROME

The National Institutes of Health (NIH) describes restless legs syndrome (RLS) as a disorder that causes a strong urge to move your legs. This urge to move often occurs with strange and unpleasant feelings in your legs. Moving your legs relieves the urge and the unpleasant feelings.

People who have RLS describe the unpleasant feelings as creeping, crawling, pulling, itching, tingling, burning, aching, or electric shocks. Sometimes, these feelings also occur in the arms.

The urge to move and unpleasant feelings happen when you're resting and inactive. Thus, they tend to be worse in the evening and at night.

RLS can make it hard to fall asleep and stay asleep. It may make you feel tired and sleepy during the day. This can make it hard to learn, work, and do other daily activities. Not getting enough sleep also can cause depression, mood swings, or other health problems.

Research suggests that the main cause of restless legs syndrome (RLS) is a faulty use of iron or a lack of iron in the brain. The brain uses iron to make the neuro-transmitter dopamine and to control other brain activities. Dopamine works in the parts of the brain that control movement.

Many conditions can affect how much iron is in the brain or how it is used. These conditions include kidney failure, Parkinson's disease, diabetes, rheumatoid arthritis, pregnancy, and iron deficiency anemia. All of these conditions increase your risk of RLS.

CONVENTIONAL TREATMENT

If a medical condition or medicine triggers RLS, the disorder may go away if the trigger is relieved or stopped. For example, RLS that occurs due to pregnancy tends to go away after giving birth. Kidney transplants (but not dialysis) relieve RLS linked to kidney failure.

Treatments for RLS include lifestyle changes and medicines. Some simple lifestyle changes often help relieve mild cases of RLS. Medicines often can relieve or prevent the symptoms of more severe RLS.

Certain medicines are known to trigger RLS. These include:
- Anti-nausea medicines (used to treat upset stomach)
- Antidepressants (used to treat depression)
- Antipsychotics (used to treat certain mental health disorders)
- Cold and allergy medicines that contain antihistamines
- Calcium channel blockers (used to treat heart problems and HBP)

RLS symptoms usually get better or may even go away if the medicine is stopped.

NATURAL TREATMENT

RLS is a secondary problem brought on by other imbalances in the body. As with all disorders the place to start is with proper diet and the balancing of stress. The next place to look is pathology. A leading cause of RLS is **bacterial infection** in the gut. Just as food allergies and digestive maladies can cause pain in the feet, *a bacterial infection in the colon can cause RLS*. The following are natural treatments that can reach the main cause.

HOMEOPATHIC REMEDIES

Treatment by a Classical Homeopath to find a Constitutional remedy that suits your health profile can be very beneficial. Listening to your symptoms, beyond the RLS, are clues to the underlying issue.

- **HOMEOPATHIC PENICILLIN-** well tolerated by even those with intolerance to pharmaceutical antibiotics.
- **PYROGENIUM-** especially if you have a history of food poisoning.
- **NUX VOMICA+ARSENICUM ALBUM-** if there is diarrhea and/or food intolerances.
- **HEPAR SULPH CALCAREA-** if you experience any discharges with color or odor.
- **MERCURIUS SOL OR VIV-** if you experience bad breath and any sensitivity to temperature changes.

ACUPUNCTURE & TRADITIONAL CHINESE MEDICINE (TCM)

Treating patterns of RLS may be seen as Liver wind rising with lack of nourishment tendons/sinews; qi/blood stagnation and blocked dai mai vessel. Some forms of TCM may be chosen singly or together for the best treatment plan and holistic response.

OSTEOPATHIC TREATMENT

Osteopathic treatment can be another effective means of getting to the root cause of your symptoms. If, for example, your RLS is a result of improper utilization of iron this type of treatment can help the body to function more efficiently once again.

RINGWORM

Ringworm in humans, also known as dermatophytosis, is one of the most common superficial fungal infections. *Tinea* is the name of a group of diseases caused by a fungus. Types of tinea include ringworm, athlete's foot and jock itch. These infections are usually not serious, but they can be uncomfortable. You can get them by touching an infected person, from damp surfaces such as shower floors, or even from a pet.

Symptoms depend on the affected area of the body:

- Ringworm is a red skin rash that forms a ring around normal-looking skin. A worm does not cause it.
- Scalp ringworm causes itchy, red patches on your head. It can leave bald spots. It usually affects children.
- Athlete's foot causes itching, burning and cracked skin between your toes.
- Jock itch causes an itchy, burning rash in your groin area.

CONVENTIONAL TREATMENT

Over-the-counter creams and powders can help with many tinea infections, particularly athlete's foot and jock itch. Other cases can require prescription medicine. Chemical treatments can be suppressive.

NATURAL TREATMENT

There are a number of natural remedies that quickly clear ringworm. Since it is not a worm at all, but a fungus, most anti-fungal solutions will efficiently resolve the infection.

It is not enough to eradicate only the affected area. If you were capable of manifesting a fungal infection, it indicates an overall acid environment in the blood. If the issue is not rectified, pathogenic infections will continue to proliferate. A simplistic method of reversing acidosis is with the use of sodium bicarbonate (baking soda). Refer to pH Balance previously in this chapter.

- **TEA TREE OIL** is a very efficient anti-fungal. Spread over affected area 2-3 times daily.
- **CLOVE OIL** is a wonderful ancient anti-fungal. Use multiple times per day and it will clear quickly.
- **COLLOIDAL SILVER** internally and topically.

HOMEOPATHY

Although tea tree oil and clove are a very efficient means of clearing ringworm, there are Homeopathic remedies that can go deeper into the causation. For this reason, both methods of treatment work well together. Some homeopathic scholars are of the belief that Tea Tree Oil can antidote remedies, but this has not been my experience.

- **CALCAREA CARBONICUM-** if you have perspiration from the head, get sick frequently, bone issues, cold damp feet, skin feels cold.
- **CALC SULPH-** ringworm of scalp or beard.
- **GRAPHITES-** eruptions worse from heat, moist & crusty, oozing, rawness.
- **NATRUM MURIATICUM-** raw, red, inflamed, dry eruptions itch and burn.
- **PHYTOLACCA-** dry, itchy, best used in early stages.
- **SEPIA-** ringworm in isolated spots, blotchy, cracked, itchy, relieved by scratching.
- **TELLURIUM-** ring-shape lesions, circular patches of eczema, small red pimples, very bright red with minute vesicles, itching or pricking, worse in cool air.
- **THUJA-** itching and burn violently, worse from cold bathing, worse scratching.

SCABIES

Scabies is an itchy skin condition caused by the microscopic mite Sarcoptes scabei. It is common all over the world, and can affect anyone. Scabies spreads quickly in crowded conditions where there is frequent skin-to-skin contact between people. Hospitals, child-care centers, and nursing homes are examples. Scabies can easily infect sex partners and other household members. Sharing clothes, towels, and bedding can also spread scabies. You cannot get scabies from a pet. Pets get a different mite infection called mange.

SYMPTOMS

- Pimple-like irritations or a rash
- Intense itching, especially at night
- Sores caused by scratching

Your health care provider diagnoses scabies by looking at the skin rash and finding burrows in the skin.

The infected person's clothes, bedding and towels should be washed in hot water and dried in a hot dryer. Treatment is also recommended for household members and sexual partners.

CONVENTIONAL TREATMENT

Over the counter chemical based lotions are available to treat scabies.

NATURAL TREATMENT

Refer to the segment 'pH BALANCE' earlier in this chapter to learn how to balance the acid condition that enables bugs to survive in the body and on the skin.

There are a number of effective anti-parasitic remedies in nature. The following are a few topical treatments:

- **NEEM OIL-** (Azadirachta indica) an anti-parasitic plant.
- **STICKY SNAKEROOT-** (Eupatoriume Adenophorum) from the daisy family, can kill scabies mites.
- **TEA TREE OIL-** (Melaleuca alternifolia) can effectively treat scabies. It has anti-parasitic constituents to help kill the mites.

HOMEOPATHY

The following remedies are symptom specific, except for Sulphur. Sulphur is the number one skin remedy that works for most. Repeat remedy often and consult with a professional as needed.

- **ARSENICUM ALBUM-** skin symptoms can alternate with asthma or internal disorders; dry rough, scaly skin, worse from the cold.
- **CARBO VEGETABLIS-** skin burning and itching.
- **CAUSTICUM-** soreness in folds of skin and behind ears, between thighs.
- **KALI SULPH-** dry skin, burning, yellow, jaundice ulcers, oozes thin yellow water.
- **SELENIUM-** dry, scaly, itchy eruptions, palms and ankles, between fingers, tingling, great desire to scratch.
- **SEPIA-** rough, raw, hard, cracked skin, thick crusts on elbows, thick crusts form on joints.
- **SULPHUR-** skin eruptions can alternate with other illnesses; dry, scaly unhealthy skin itchy, worse at night, heat of bed, scratching, and washing.

SCIATICA

Sciatica is a symptom of a problem with the sciatic nerve, the largest nerve in the body. It controls muscles in the back of your knee and lower leg and provides feeling to the back of your thigh, part of your lower leg, and the sole of your foot. When you have sciatica, you have pain, weakness, numbness, or tingling. It can start in the lower back and extend down your leg to your calf, foot, or even your toes. It usually occurs on only one side of your body.

CAUSES

- A ruptured inter-vertebral disk
- An injury such as a pelvic fracture
- A herniated disk (may require surgery)
- Sleeping on a new mattress
- Emotional stress
- Narrowing of the spinal canal that puts pressure on the nerve, called spinal stenosis

In many cases no cause can be found.

Piriformis Syndrome can contribute to the symptoms of sciatica. The symptoms include tenderness or pain in the buttock muscle that can radiate down the back of the leg into the hamstring muscles, or even the calf muscles. It is a soft tissue impingement that comes from the buttocks when nerve bundles get compressed, or if there is not enough tissue to properly bundle the nerves. Sometimes there is too much muscle or it is too tight. The sciatic nerve runs very close to this muscle and in some people even runs through the muscle fibers. If the piriformis muscle becomes tight it can compress the sciatic nerve and cause pain that can radiate down the leg.

CONVENTIONAL TREATMENT

Sometimes sciatica goes away on its own. Treatment, if needed, depends on the cause of the problem. It may include exercises, medicines, and some doctors might recommend surgery.

NATURAL TREATMENT

There are many natural therapies that can help to resolve Sciatica. For Piriformis Syndrome *Acupuncture* is a much better choice of treatment than *Chiropractic* adjustment. Since there is nothing really to "adjust" a properly trained Acupuncturist can work with the soft tissue of the muscle to increase circulation and remove the advancement of the histamine response. Histamine is the swelling agent causing inflammation.

OSTEOPATHY

An Osteopath who works with hands on therapy can help to restore proper energy flow through the tissues relieve the source of pain.

CRANIAL SACRAL THERAPY

Cranial Sacral Therapy is similar to Osteopathy. Refer to previous chapters for specific descriptions of each therapy.

MASSAGE

Body work that manipulates tissue can go a long way to helping to release the underlying cause of the condition.

ACUPUNCTURE & TRADITIONAL CHINESE MEDICINE (TCM)

Treating patterns of Sciatica may be seen as qi/blood stagnation; coldness and deficiency of low back/ Kidney. Some forms of TCM may be chosen singly or together for the best treatment plan and holistic response.

HOMEOPATHY

Homeopathy can assist with pain and discomfort while seeking any of the treatments mentioned. Sciatica, as with many back issues, can have an emotional component. For this reason, a Constitutional remedy given by a classically trained Homeopath can address the emotional burden, along with the physical symptoms. The following are some commonly used remedies for sciatica.

DEPENDING ON CIRCUMSTANCES:
AGGRAVATED FROM:

- **AMMONIUM MURIATICUM-** when sitting.
- **BRYONIA-** on the slightest movement.
- **KALI IODATUM-** at night.
- **RHUS TOXICODENDRON-** when resting in bed; by exposure to humidity.
- **SULPHUR-** when standing.
- **TELLURIUM-** from cough, sneezing or passing stools.

BETTER FROM:

- **BRYONIA-** lying on the painful side.
- **COLOCYNTHIS-** by bending leg upward.
- **MAGNESIUM PHOSPHORICA-** by pressing on the leg, by applying heat.
- **RHUS TOXICODENDRON-** by moving around or walking.

DEPENDING ON SENSATIONS
- **ARSENICUM ALBUM-** a burning sensation that is relieved by heat.
- **BRYONIA-** prickly pains.
- **KALI BICHROMICUM-** pain seems to move along the leg.
- **MAGNESIUM PHOSPHORICA-** shooting pains.
- **NUX VOMICA-** a sensation of cramps.
- **CAUSTICUM-** If the sciatica is paralyzing.

SINUSITIS

Sinusitis means your sinuses are inflamed. The cause can be an infection or another problem. Your sinuses are hollow air spaces within the bones surrounding the nose. They produce mucus, which drains into the nose. If your nose is swollen, this can block the sinuses and cause pain. The mucus can also drain down the back of your throat and this is called post-nasal drip. Post-nasal drip can cause sore throats or hoarseness.

Sinus drainage can also continue down into the chest. You might think your chest symptoms are a separate issue, but the cause may be coming from the sinus.

There are several types of sinusitis, including:

- Acute, which lasts up to 4 weeks
- Sub-acute, which lasts 4 to 12 weeks
- Chronic, which lasts more than 12 weeks and can continue for months or even years
- Recurrent, with several attacks within a year

Acute sinusitis often starts as a cold, which then turns into a bacterial infection or a fungal infection, or both. *Allergies*, nasal obstructions and certain diseases can also cause acute and chronic sinusitis.

SYMPTOMS

- Fever and chilliness
- Headache
- Weakness/fatigue
- Chronic sinus drainage
- Ear pain
- Cough
- Congestion

There may be mucus drainage in the back of the throat, called post-nasal drip. Your health care professional diagnoses sinusitis based on your symptoms and an examination of your nose and face. You may also need imaging tests.

CONVENTIONAL TREATMENT

Treatments include anti-biotics, decongestants, and pain relievers. Using heat pads on the inflamed area, saline nasal sprays, and vaporizers can also help. Many times sinusitis will return after the use of anti-biotics. This is usually because the underlying infection is fungal. People who have systemic Candida infections will have reoccurring sinus infections. An overall Candida cleanse will go a long way to removing the chronic sinus issue.

NATURAL TREATMENT

To get things moving in the right direction your first line of defense is to use steam inhalation. It helps to begin draining the sinuses. An acidic environment supports sinusitis. For that reason, it is important to balance the pH of the body. Refer to 'pH BALANCE' previously in this chapter for further information.

There are many choices within holistic medicine to treat sinusitis. Chinese herbs can very efficiently bring down inflammation of the sinus passages. Homeopathy has many symptom-driven remedies for sinus infection. Spagyric tinctures have also shown to help boost the immune system and clear pathogens.

HOMEOPATHY

If the chosen remedies fit your situation and the issue is not completely resolved, add **Arsenicum album** for acute situations; add **Sulphur** if chronic.

- **BELLADONNA-** when the nose is stuffed up.
- **HEPAR SULPH CALCAREA-** (*antibiotic substitute*) painful, worse from touch, yellow to green secretions, aggravated by drafts.
- **HYDRASTIS-** thick yellow ropey secretions, coated tongue, constipation.
- **KALI BICHROMICUM-** *thick, stringy sticky* discharge, green secretions or crusty nose, pain at root of nose, pain in spots.
- **KALI MURIATICUM-** thick discharge, whitish/grey color, asthma with gastric complaints.
- **KALI SULPH-** thick yellow discharge, stuffed nose, loss of smell.
- **PHOSPHORUS-** pus mixed with blood.
- **PULSATILLA-** worse getting wet, desires cold drinks, sobs or whines in pain, no thirst, fever with chilliness.
- **SANGUINARIA-** nasal obstruction, better with open air, watery discharge, headache, better from sleep, vomiting, and/or passing gas.
- **SILICEA-** tendency to catch colds, sharp pain, scanty discharge.

THE BANERJI PROTOCOL™ FOR SINUSITIS

FIRST LINE MEDICINES

- **SANGUINARIA CANADENSIS 200C-** two times per day, if acute, repeat every 3 hours until there is substantial relief, then two doses daily.

If there is acute pain, with or without fever, add **BELLADONNA 3C**, every 30 minutes.

SECOND LINE MEDICINES
- **KALI BICHROMICUM 30C-** 2-3 doses per day.
- **LYCOPODIUM 30C-** for a nose that is blocked, one dose every 1-2 hours, as needed.

THIRD LINE MEDICINES
- **CALCAREA CARBONICA 1000C in liquid-** if there is blocked nose, runny nose and/or sneezing, 1 dose per day.
- **SANGUINARIA CANADENSIS 200C-** two doses daily.
- **ARSENICUM ALBUM 6C-** for acute sneezing and runny nose, every hour until there is relief.

ACUPUNCTURE & TRADITIONAL CHINESE MEDICINE (TCM)

Treating patterns of Sinusitis may be seen as damp-heat with fluid congestion; wind-cold with fluid congestion or accumulation of toxic heat. Some forms of TCM may be chosen singly or together for the best treatment plan and holistic response.

SINUSITIS REMEDY CHART:

INFLAMATION OF THE LINING OF PARANASAL

CAUSES:
- Upper respiratory infection or any infection in the ear, nose or throat
- Allergies

SYMPTOMS:
- Headache; may have fever with chilliness
- Discharge from nose or post-nasal drip
- May include otitis (ear pain)

SANGUINARIA:
nasal obstruction, acrid discharge with streaks of blood, headache

KALI MUR:
thick discharge whitish/greyish color, asthma with gastric complaints

PULSATILLA:
sobs in pain; worse getting wet, desires cold drinks

KALI BIC:
thick gooey discharge, yellow or green

KALI SULPH:
thick yellow discharge, stuffed nose, loss of smell

HEPAR SULPH CALC:
thick yellow discharge, smells like cheese

HYDRASTIS:
Post-nasal drip, thick discharge Burning, followed by itching, snoring

Copyright © 2018 Elena Upton, PhD

SLEEP ISSUES (SEE INSOMNIA)

SORE THROAT

Your throat is a tube that carries food to your esophagus and air to your windpipe and larynx (also called the voice box). The technical name for the throat is pharynx. You can have a sore throat for many reasons. Often, colds and flu cause sore throats.

CAUSES
- Allergies
- Mononucleosis
- Smoking
- Strep throat
- Tonsillitis (an infection in the tonsils)
- Straining the voice from yelling, excess singing, etc

CONVENTIONAL TREATMENT

Treatment depends on the cause. Sucking on lozenges, drinking lots of liquids, and gargling may ease the pain. Over-the-counter pain relievers can also help. Children should not take aspirin.

NATURAL TREATMENT

Gargling with warm water and salt when a sore throat arises is one of many ways of naturally improving a sore throat. Further suggestions are:

- Making a tea of honey and lemon (with cayenne pepper also) to soothe a sore throat.
- Tea made with fresh ginger, lemon and honey to taste.
- Apple cider vinegar with honey and lemon to taste is good to gargle with throughout the day.
- Gargle with warm water and hydrogen peroxide.
- Licorice root tea.
- Chinese Herbs.
- Suck Cloves, they are anti-bacterial and anti-viral.

Balance pH to discourage growth of pathogens.

HOMEOPATHY

The following are *symptom specific* remedies:

- **BELLADONNA-** bright red sore throat, alternate with **MERC SOL OR MERC VIV**.
- **HEPAR SULPH CALCAREA-** when there is yellow mucus, sensation of a plug or splinters on swallowing.
- **LACHESIS-** left tonsil, purple throat, pain extends to ear, worse with hot drinks, cannot stand anything wrapped around throat.
- **LYCOPODIUM-** right tonsil, swollen, ulcerations, worse cold drinks, as if a wall is rising
- **MERCURIUS SOLUBILIS-** tonsils enlarged, bluish/red swelling or throat covered with white spots, hoarse voice, swollen glands on getting cold. Coughs up larghe lumps of mucus. Usually occurs at change of season.
- **PHYTOLACCA-** burning pain root of tongue, dark red or bluish sore throat, pain radiating to ears or nape of neck, sensation of lump in throat, tenacious mucus. Cannot swallow anything hot.

ACUPUNCTURE & TRADITIONAL CHINESE MEDICINE (TCM)

Treating patterns of Sore Throat may be seen as wind-heat invasion and/ or accumulation of toxic heat. Some forms of TCM may be chosen singly or together for the best treatment plan and holistic response.

TENDONITIS

Tendons are flexible bands of tissue that connect muscles to bones. They help your muscles move your bones. Tendonitis is the severe swelling of a tendon.

Tendonitis usually happens after repeated injury to an area such as the wrist or ankle. It causes pain and soreness around a joint. Some common forms of tendonitis are named after the sports that increase their risk. They include tennis elbow, golfer's elbow, pitcher's shoulder, swimmer's shoulder, and jumper's knee.

Doctors diagnose tendonitis with your medical history, a physical exam, and imaging tests.

CONVENTIONAL TREATMENT

The first step in treatment is to reduce pain and swelling. Rest, wrapping or elevating the affected area, and medicines for pain. Ice is helpful for recent, severe injuries. Other treatments include ultrasound, physical therapy, steroid injections, and surgery.

NATURAL TREATMENT

Holistic therapies can help tendonitis by naturally bringing down swelling, relieving pain and restoring normal energy flow to the area to encourage healing.

ACUPUNCTURE & TRADITIONAL CHINESE MEDICINE (TCM)

Treating patterns of Tendonitis may be seen as Liver blood and Kidney yin deficiencies. Some forms of TCM may be chosen singly or together for the best treatment plan and holistic response.

HOMEOPATHIC REMEDIES

- **ARNICA-** to help relieve pain and bring down swelling.
- **RHUS TOXICODENDRON-** for inflammation following exertion.
- **RUTA GRAVEOLENS-** in tincture form can be applied to the inflamed area.

THE BANERJI PROTOCOL™

FIRST LINE MEDICINES

- **SYMPHYTUM OFFICINALIS 200C-** two doses daily
- **CALCAREA PHOSPHORICA 3X-** two doses daily

SECOND LINE MEDICINES
- **RHUS TOXICODENDRON 30C-** two doses daily
- **CALCAREA PHOSPHORICA 3X-** two doses daily

THIRD LINE MEDICINES
- **RUTA GRAVEOLENS 200C-** two doses daily
- **HYPERICUM PERFORATUM 200C-** two doses daily

TONSILLITIS

Your tonsils and adenoids are part of your lymphatic system. Your tonsils are in the back of your throat. Your adenoids are higher up, behind your nose. Both help protect you from infection by trapping germs coming in through your mouth and nose.

Sometimes your tonsils and adenoids become infected. Tonsillitis makes your tonsils sore and swollen and causes a sore throat. Enlarged adenoids can be sore, make it hard to breathe and cause ear problems.

SYMPTOMS

- Sore throat
- Pain on swallowing
- Fever
- Body ache
- Nasal discharge

Tonsillitis is often associated with ear infections (Otitis media), sinusitis, rheumatism or pneumonia.

CONVENTIONAL TREATMENT

The first treatment in allopathic medicine for infected tonsils and adenoids is antibiotics. If you have frequent infections or trouble breathing, surgery will be advised. Surgery to remove the tonsils is a tonsillectomy. Surgery to remove adenoids is adenoidectomy.

NATURAL TREATMENT

Homeopathy can be *very successful* at treating tonsillitis. You will be able to overcome the antibiotic rollercoaster and certainly save the tonsils from being cut out. Gargling with salt and warm water, or **Calendula** frequently can help to relieve pain. The following are symptom specific and the remedy must be changed as the symptoms change.

- **APIS-** redness and swelling of the throat; stinging and burning pains; tongue and uvula swollen (looks like a water blister); thirstless; desires cool room and cold drinks.
- **ARSENICUM ALBUM-** burning throat; thirsty for repeated sips of cold water; restless and anxious; worse at midnight.
- **BELLADONNA-** right sided; throat dry and bright red; burning, unable to swallow; high fever; intense red face and possibly ears; throbbing pain that extends to ears; very thirsty, craves lemonade; can have enlargement of glands.

- **BAPTISIA-** purplish red tonsils; swelling and painless, comes on rapidly; can swallow fluids only; complete exhaustion; feels as if there are two of him.
- **CROTALUS-** left sided; may have blood poisoning; bleeding from orifices; gangrenous throat; much swelling of glands; cannot swallow liquids; throat slightly constricted; mumbles.
- **HEPAR SULPH CALC-** ulcers in throat; sensation of fish bones or splinters; pain extends to ear when yawning, swallowing or turning head; prefers warm drinks; feels cold; fever with perspiration, wants to be covered; objects to open doors or windows.
- **KALI BICHROMICUM-** deep, scooped out ulcers on tonsils; saliva is sticky and stringy.
- **LACHESIS-** left sided or left to right; sensation of fullness in neck; difficult breathing; difficulty going to sleep or swallowing; worse from warm drinks; purple throat; pain, worse swallowing saliva.
- **LAC CANINUM-** alternating right to left; throat red, glazed and shiny with silver-grey spots; pain better from swallowing cold or hot drinks.
- **LYCOPODIUM-** right side or right to left; better from warm drinks; pain extends into ears; no problem sleeping.
- **MERCURIUS SOL or VIV-** dark-red throat; fullness and stiffness of neck; dry, swallowing difficult; coated tongue with teeth marks, breath odor, sub-maxillary glands enlarged; great weakness and trembling; warm drinks aggravate.
- **PHYTOLACCA-** swollen glands; thick mucus; worse at night; bones ache; body feels bruised and sore; bed feels hard; better from cold liquids; warm drinks aggravate; pain and stiffness in cervical region.
- **EUPATORIUM PERFOLIATUM-** can be used as a mother tincture with **HEPAR SULPH CALC, MERCURIUS + BELLADONNA.**

After an acute attack subsides, **HEPAR SULPH CALC 200C,** taken twice daily is continued for at least 3 months to complete the cure and ensure no re-occurrence.

ACUPUNCTURE & TRADITIONAL CHINESE MEDICINE (TCM)

Treating patterns of Tonsillitis may be seen as wind-heat invasion; toxic heat; phlegm stagnation. Some forms of TCM may be chosen singly or together for the best treatment plan and holistic response.

TONSILLITIS REMEDY CHART:

CAUSES:
Tonsillitis is inflamation (swelling) of the tonsils. Infection may also be seen in other parts of the throat.

SYMPTOMS:
- Ear Pain
- Fever & Chills
- Headache
- Sore throat that lasts longer than 24 hours
- Tenderness of jaw and throat
- Difficulty swallowing, eating, breathing

The following remedies are specific to right sided/left sided pain and pain made better by heat/warmth (being wrapped up warmly, a heated room or warm food and drink); or cold (desire for cold drinks and food, wanting to be uncovered, needs air).
The correct remedy can work quickly to lessen the severity of an agonizing sore thorat.

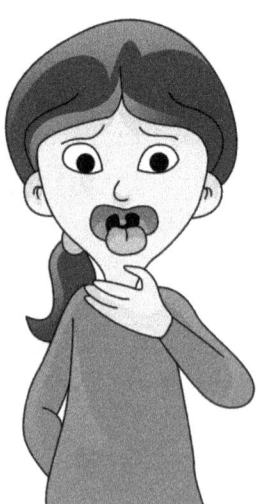

LEFT SIDED PAIN:
Rhus Tox
Lachesis
Sabadilla
Lac Caninum
Merc Iodatus Ruber

RIGHT SIDED PAIN:
Apis
Belladonna
Phytolacca
Lycopodium
Mercurious Sol or Viv

RELIEF FROM HOT/WARM
Hepar Sulph Calc
Belladonna
Lycopodium
Rhus Tox
Sabadilla
Silicea

RELIEF FROM COLD:
Apis
Lachesis
Phytolacca
Lac Caninum

Copyright © 2018 Elena Upton, PhD

TOOTHACHE (TOOTH DECAY, CAVITY)

You call it a cavity. Your dentist calls it tooth decay or dental caries. They are all names for a hole in your tooth. The cause of tooth decay is plaque, a sticky substance in your mouth made up mostly of germs. Tooth decay starts in the outer layer, called the enamel. Without a filling, the decay can get deep into the tooth and its nerves and cause a toothache or abscess.

To help prevent cavities:

- Brush your teeth after meals with non-toxic toothpaste or baking soda.
- Clean between your teeth every day with floss or another type of between-the-teeth cleaner.
- Be careful who you kiss.
- Snack smart – limit sugary snacks.
- See your dentist or oral health professional regularly.

NATURAL TREATMENT

Tooth decay can be avoided early on in life by taking the correct preventative steps. Homeopathic remedies and herbal preparations can keep your mouth clean and lower the germ load. (See GINGIVITIS for more on keeping gums clean and safe from infection.)

HOMEOPATHY

There are numerous Homeopathic remedies that can resolve dental issues. A 'Constitutional' remedy dispensed by a Homeopath to support the immune system is one method of treatment. The following suggestions are symptom specific.

- **Sides of teeth-** Mezereum, Staphasagria, Thuja.
- **At the roots-** Fluoricum Acidum, Mercurius, Mezereum, Silicea, Syphilinum.
- **Rapid decay-** Arsenicum, Barita Carbonicum, Calcarea Carbo-nicum, Calcaria Phosphorum, Fluoricum Acidum, Sepia.
- **Premature decay in children-** Calcaria Carbonicum, Calcaria Fluoricum, Calcarea Phosphoricum, Fluoricum Acidum, Kreosotum, Staphasagria.
- **Decay at edge of gums-** Calcarea Carbonicum, Syphalinum, Thuja.
- **Loss of enamel-** Calcarea Fluoricum.
- **Toothache, gum abscess, swollen jaw or difficult dentition-** Hecla Lava
- **Dental Abscess-** Hepar Sulph Calcarea (*anti-biotic substitute*).

ACUPUNCTURE & TRADITIONAL CHINESE MEDICINE (TCM)

Treating patterns of Toothache may be seen as wind heat invasion; Kidney yin deficiency and Stomach heat. Some forms of TCM may be chosen singly or together for the best treatment plan and holistic response.

URTICARIA (SEE HIVES)

VARICOSE VEINS

Varicose veins and spider veins are swollen, twisted veins that you can see just under the skin. They usually occur in the legs, but also can form in other parts of the body. Hemorrhoids are actually a type of varicose vein.

Your veins have one-way valves that help keep blood flowing toward your heart. If the valves are weak or damaged, blood can back up and pool in your veins. This causes the veins to swell, which can lead to varicose veins.

Varicose veins are very common. You are more at risk if you are older, a female, obese, don't exercise or have a family history. They can also be more common in pregnancy. They are not just a cosmetic problem, varicose veins can be an early symptom of serious vascular disease. Skin ulcers near the ankle are usually a tell-tale sign.

Doctors often diagnose varicose veins from a physical exam. Sometimes you may need additional tests.

CAUSES

- Heredity
- History of blood clots
- Hormone Replacement Therapy (HRT)
- Hormonal changes, pregnancy, menopause
- Birth Control Pills
- Obesity
- Prolonged standing
- Poor circulation

SYMPTOMS

- Achy or heavy legs
- Burning
- Throbbing
- Cramping
- Swelling
- Itching

CONVENTIONAL TREATMENT

Exercising, losing weight, support stockings; elevating your legs when resting and not crossing them when sitting can help keep varicose veins from getting worse. Wearing loose clothing and avoiding long periods of standing can also help. If varicose veins are painful or you don't like the way they look, your doctor may recommend procedures to remove them.

Another conventional treatment is Sclerotherapy. It is a procedure where a concentrated solution of saline (salt) solution, or a specifically made detergent is injected directly into the vein. This causes the vein to disappear gradually over a few weeks.

There are also a number of newer methods to relieve varicose veins, including Endovenous laser treatment. It is a method of light being pulsed into the vein, which causes it to collapse.

Radio-frequency occlusion is a small catheter inserted into the vein that delivers a radio frequency to the vein wall. This creates heat and causes the vein to collapse.

NATURAL THERAPIES

The best method of combating varicose veins is by prevention, especially if there are other members in the family who have, or have had this issue. By keeping your weight optimum, having a good diet, exercising and supplementing with remedies that encourage proper circulation they can be prevented. If the problem already exists, there are a number of natural options.

- **Apple Cider Vinegar** can improve circulation by drinking daily.
- **Witch Hazel** applied topically can be a powerful astringent and help to shrink spider veins.
- Veins can be **massaged with oils** such as clove, lemon, jojoba, avocado, mustard, and/or almond oil.
- **Herbs can increase circulation** such as, nettle, cayenne pepper, ginger and turmeric.

ACUPUNCTURE & TRADITIONAL CHINESE MEDICINE (TCM)

Treating patterns of varicose veins may be seen as blood stagnation and Spleen qi deficiency. Some forms of TCM may be chosen singly or together for the best treatment plan and holistic response.

GEMMOTHERAPY

- **HORSE CHESTNUT-** 3-15 drops daily; It has an amazing action against edema; helps to restore vein tone and increases capillary permeability.

As a protocol combine the following:
- **SERVICE TREE-** 10 drops before breakfast.
- **SWEET CHESTNUT-** 10 drops before lunch.
- **LEMON TREE-** 10 drops before dinner

HOMEOPATHY

Within Homeopathy veins are viewed as secondary organs, whereas the Liver, Ovaries, Uterus, Spleen and Intestines are considered primary organs. To relieve a secondary issue primary organs must be treated to ameliorate the secondary organ symptoms.

Enlargement of organs may be obstructing circulation. As an example, a swollen liver can cause varicose veins in the right leg. An enlarged spleen may be the cause in the left leg. Ovaries that are enlarged can be responsible for varicose veins in either leg and also the slowness of the large intestine. This is another example of how natural medicine looks to treat the whole person, not just the site of the symptom.

According to the Drs. Banerji, who have Homeopathically treated thousands of patients in their fifth-generation medical clinic in Kolkata, India; **Hamamelis Virginica 200C + Arnica Montana 3C,** taken together, are very effective and specific for absorbing blood clots, thrombosed arteries and veins.

WEIGHT LOSS

Weight loss has become a huge issue in the US. Americans have the highest rate of obesity than any other country in the world. The saddest aspect is that it has reached epidemic proportions among children. It is no news flash that the number one reason is the American diet. Our food supply is contaminated with:

- Chemical fertilizers and fungicides
- Genetically modified organisms (GMOs)
- Chemical additives not required to be listed on labels
- MSG and other artificial flavor enhancers
- Bad fats (saturated and hydrogenated)
- *PRESERVATIVES!*

Living in California I have access to some of the best fresh organic foods grown in the country. Unfortunately, this is not the case in many other areas. In some regions of the country very little fresh food is brought in because it is too expensive to ship and also in some areas, believe it or not, it is not purchased because of the dependence on packaged foods.

For weight loss to be successful and lasting, there needs to be a diet rich in fresh, nutritious food and regular exercise. There are two more extenuating factors, attitude and pH balance. *(Refer to the section previously in this chapter explaining the importance of maintaining proper pH)*.

DIGESTION

Unless you maintain proper digestion weight gain will always be an ongoing battle. Also, any underlying pathogens, such as Candida, parasites and latent bacteria must be cleared to have long-term success. Successful weight loss can be achieved by combining the rebalancing of body chemistry for proper digestion and assimilation.

The most important issue is to not be too hard on yourself. Take baby steps to improving your lifestyle and the changes will be long lasting.

DIET

There are numerous diet books, theories and protocols. Choose one that is not a 'fad', does not sound too good to be true and one that you actually like. If you are not happy with what you are eating it will be impossible to stick to.

ACUPUNCTURE & CHINESE MEDICINE

Seeing an Acupuncturist can put you on the road to being balanced and help to energetically support your process. When the body is fine-tuned in this way you will feel encouraged to stay on task and reach your goals.

GEMMOTHERAPY

Digestion is not the only key to successful weight loss. The entire body needs to function properly. If you do not have sufficient kidney and bladder drainage, or if your liver does not filter the blood efficiently, or if the bowels are impacted, there is NO diet that will help you to regain your healthy weight. The following is a list of Gemmos that can help to restore function to the emunctories (organs) necessary to keep you in optimum health.

- **Bladder-** COWBERRY
- **GI Tract-** Intestines- COWBERRY, EUROPEAN ALDER, FIG and ROSEMARY
- **Kidneys-** WHITE BIRCH, JUNIPER, SILVER BIRCH
- **Liver-** JUNIPER, ROSEMARY, HAZEL, RYE
- **Lung-** HAZEL, WAYFARING TREE
- **Lymphatic-** SWEET CHESTNUT
- **Nerves-** LINEN TREE, FIG
- **Pancreas-** WALNUT
- **Stomach-** FIG, EUROPEAN ALDER

HOMEOPATHY

A professional Homeopath trained in classical Homeopathy would dispense a "Constitutional" remedy. The remedy would represent your mental, emotional and physical attributes and help you to feel grounded and balanced to assist in your weight loss journey.

SUPPLEMENTS

I am not a huge fan of supplements, especially since most choose supplements by something they heard, or what someone told them, rather than through the advice of a professional. The money you would waste on these supplements could be better spent on a visit with a qualified practitioner. There are a few supplements that can be beneficial to all however. They are as follows:

- **OMEGA 3 Fish Oil-** (Pharmaceutical grade) helps with hormonal balance.
- **COMPLEX B VITAMINS-** (derived from a raw food source) helps with stress management.
- **COLLOIDAL MINERALS-** (more important than a multi-vitamin) minerals play an important role in all bodily functions.

- **GARCINIA CAMBOGIA** (Malabar tamarind) is a fruit grown in Southeast Asia and India and thought to control appetite. It inhibits the enzyme Citric acid lysase which in some studies was shown to help weight control.

If you need to be concerned with balancing your *blood sugar level* consider:

- **FENUGREEK**
- **CHROMIUM**
- **CINNAMON**
- **VANADIUM**

WEIGHT LOSS AND MALNUTRITION

There are times people lose weight unintentionally, even though there have been no changes in their lifestyle or diet. Many medical conditions such as diabetes, celiac disease and various gastrointestinal conditions can result in malabsorption and subsequent weight loss.

If this is the case it is important to see your doctor and be testing to confirm or rule out any such health concerns. Once other more serious health issues are ruled out the following are the **Banerji Protocol**™ for unassociated weight loss.

FIRST LINE MEDICINES

- **ABROTANUM 6C-** two doses per day.

SECOND LINE MEDICINES

- **IODIUM 200C-** in liquid, two times daily.
- **CALCAREA PHOSPHORICA 3X-** two times daily.

THIRD LINE MEDICINES

- **CHINA OFFICINALIS 200C-** one dose every other day
- **CHELIDONIUM-** (mother tincture) drops, two doses daily

ACUPUNCTURE & TRADITIONAL CHINESE MEDICINE (TCM)

Treating patterns of weight loss as malnutrition may be seen as Spleen qi deficiency and yin/yang/qi/blood deficiencies. Some forms of TCM may be chosen singly or together for the best treatment plan and holistic response.

CHAPTER VII
WHAT'S IN YOUR HOME PHARMACY?

Throughout this book a number of remedies, herbs, supplements, creams and other product suggestions have been made. I have no financial interest in any of the brands or therapies suggested. They are listed because over the years, through much trial and error, they are the products and therapies that have worked consistently.

Below is a list of the most important products to have on hand if you want to be prepared for emergencies, small and large. Most of them are sold in health food stores, natural pharmacies and online. Even some of the practitioner only products can now be found on the world-wide-web.

BUILDING A HOME PHARMACY

Anyone interested in natural healing must have a Homeopathic kit at home, in your car, your camper, your office; anywhere you would have a first-aid kit. I suggest buying a kit with 30C potency. It is the most commonly used potency for most acute situations.

You can also flip through the book to find your particular health issues and those of your family and make a list. Be sure the remedies you need are included in the kit you buy. Homeopathy is safe for babies, the elderly and everyone in between. Even for your pets.

The best resource for Homeopathic kits is online. The following are a few of my favorite places to shop. (NOT listed in order of preference)

Dana Ullman's site is a gold mine of information if you are interested in learning more about Homeopathy. Not only are there numerous books, training CDs and lectures, but also hundreds of pages filled with information on the use of remedies for just about any situation. Dana Ullman is one of the most prolific Homeopathic authors in America. Supporting his site is supporting the message of Homeopathy.

Found here is an assortment of remedy kits. A must-have for successful treatment when you need a remedy immediately.

https://homeopathic.com/product-category/medicines/homeopathic-medicine-kits-with-great-discounts/

Some of my favorite kits are manufactured by Hahnemann Labs. You can find them here:

https://hahnemannlabs.com/cgi-bin/start.cgi/hahnemannlabs.com/home-first-aid-kit.html

Another gold mine for Homeopathic information, kits and rare remedies is OHM Pharmacy.

http://ohmpharma.com/

A popular site offering a selection of kits is ABC Homeopathy:

https://abchomeopathy.com/kits.php

Here you will find a number of choices by one of the standard manufacturers.

http://www.1-800homeopathy.com/homeopathic-kits/homeopathic-remedy-kits.html

If you like to shop Amazon, they carry 2 great brands, Helios and Washington Homeopathic.

https://www.amazon.com/s/ref=nb_sb_noss_1?url=search-alias%3Dhpc&field-keywords=helios+homeopathic+kits

There are more sites that sell remedy kits, have fun looking for the one that suits your needs. The kits are filled with basic remedies that I repeatedly mention throughout the book. There are a number of remedies I write about that you will never find in a health food store, a kit, or even a pharmacy. They will need to be sourced online. Here are three resources to find anything you might want in just about any potency.

- Hahnemann Labs: http:/ www.hahnemannlabs.com/
- OHM Pharma: http:/ ohmpharma.com/
- Helios: https:/ www.helios.co.uk/

Helios is located in England, but shipping to the US is simple and faster than you might think.

Basic single remedies can always be purchased at health food stores and natural pharmacies. They usually carry 6X, 12X and/or 30C potencies. A few carry 200C. All work well, but as I mentioned previously, 30C is my go-to potency. For acute situations it is advantageous to stock 200C. You will be pleasantly surprised at the price. Homeopathy is very inexpensive. Pricing is usually $6.00-$8.00 for each remedy. When buying kits, they are considerably less.

Always have on hand creams for broken skin (an antiseptic) and for bruised, injured skin.

Calendula cream is a must for cuts, scrapes, skin rashes, etc. It can take the place of allopathic antibacterial creams. It is made in cream or gel form. I prefer cream over gel, since some gels contain alcohol and can irritate skin. There are numerous brands to choose from.

A great 'sports' cream for closed injuries like bruises is **Topricin**®. It is a combination of *Arnica and Hypericum* in a higher potency than other creams.

Other popular brands:

Traumed® or **Traumeel®** by HEEL.

MARCOSPORT BLUE COOLING GEL or MARCOSPORT GREEN MASSAGE CREAM; both can be sourced online.

ASAP365® **Silver Gel** is a must for skin issues from poison ivy & oak, to eczema, psoriasis, bug bites, stings, burns, and more. It can also be used as an antiseptic ointment under bandages.

Colloidal Silver spray is excellent to have on hand for all types of skin injuries, especially burns. You can spray in your mouth for a sore throat or dental issue.

Colloidal silver is great for colds and flu. It can be transferred to a nasal spray bottle for sinus issues if you can't find a silver nasal spray.

Can you tell I love colloidal silver! Two excellent brands are **Silver Biotics®** by American Biotech Labs® and **Sovereign Silver.** They each have different manufacturing methods. The first adds an extra molecule of hydrogen so that silver residue does not linger in the body. The second is a nano-silver, meaning the particles are smaller and accomplishes a similar result.

American Biotech Labs has also developed a tooth gel called **SilverSol®**. It is great for cleaning the buggies in the mouth that cause gingivitis. I brush with another brand of toothpaste first, then use the SilverSol® ToothGel and do not rinse. It is a wonderful disinfectant.

LUFFEEL® nasal spray is my number one go-to for most types of nasal conditions, including chronic sinus infections. It is imported from Germany and can be accessed online.

REBOOST™ is the American off-shoot of Luffeel. The formula is somewhat different, but the combination of five homeopathic remedies specific to sinus issues, from cold/flu to allergies, can be very effective.

Xlear® nasal spray is good for any nasal irritation. Studies have shown it to be anti-bacterial and can help to balance bacteria in the case of nasal and ear infection. Good to have on hand and also for travel. It can be especially helpful if there is a history of chronic strep infection.

Clove oil is anti-bacterial, anti-viral and anti-fungal. It also works amazingly well for joint pain, injury, arthritis, etc. This essential oil is a multi-use product that is a must to have in your medicine cabinet or first-aid kit..

Peppermint oil is efficient as a digestive aid, for respiratory problems, nausea, headache (put a drop at the back of your neck, or on temples), fever, pain relief and even bowel spasms. It is one of the world's oldest medicines.

OSCILLOCOCCINUM- one of the most effective remedies for stopping the flu in its tracts; can be found in most pharmacies and health food stores. You will want to pick up a pack so when achy flu symptoms start to creep in you can take immediately. Easy to dispense to children also.

UMCKA- a homeopathic combination remedy that shortens the duration, speeds recovery and reduces the severity of the common cold, nasal, throat and bronchial irritations. This syrup is for colds than flu and wonderful for children also.

For **Cold Sores** there is a product called **Oleavicin™**. It treats herpes sores, even genital. It is made from Olive leaf extract, which is anti-viral, a natural anti-biotic and a powerful antioxidant. The olive leaf extract is combined with St John's Wort, Bee Propolis, Allantoin and Aloe Barbadensis. It is known to stop outbreaks quickly and reduces frequency.

VITAMIN C- I can't stress enough the importance of Vitamin C. The issue for many with Vitamin C is that they find it difficult to tolerate the recommended dose necessary for the highest benefit. Look for, **Sufficient-C® Lemon Peach Immune-Ade drink mix.** They have managed to pack into each dose 4,000 mg of non-GMO Vitamin C along with generous doses of L-Lysine, Bromelain and a 94% pure Green Tea Extract; all in a natural stevia sweetened formula that is non-GMO, gluten and sugar-free.

ZINC- In the 2007 edition of *Integrative Medicine*, University of Wisconsin professor David Rakel, MD, says that 25 mg of zinc sulfate with 250 mg of Vitamin C taken orally daily can prevent cold sore outbreaks altogether in some people and reduce the duration of symptoms to one day in others. Topical preparations that contain 0.01% to 0.025% zinc sulfate produce similar effects.

Zinc supplements typically cost less than prescription antiviral drugs and offer the additional benefit of being non-toxic.

For red, swollen gums, or periodontal disease, a remedy manufactured by DesBio®, is **Gum Therapy.** I have recommended this combination homeopathic to many clients over the years and they are always amazed at the improvement in their gum health (and so is their dentist).

GEMMOTHERAPY

Gemmotherapy tinctures are mentioned frequently throughout this book. There are a few options for purchase. Concentrated and diluted versions alike are effective. It is only the number of drops per dose that differs.

Imported from Belgium, **Gemmo Base** brand may look more expensive at first glance, but they are concentrated and a dose is fewer drops than diluted brands. Enter the name of the Gemmo you are looking for in the search bar.

> http://www.gemmospharmacy.com/

Amazon is one of a number of distributors of the **Boiron** brand of Gemmos. They are a diluted version.

> https://www.amazon.com/s/ref=nb_sb_noss_1?url=search-alias%3Daps&field-keywords=boiron+gemmotherapy

Unda is another reliable brand of Gemmotherapy sold through Amazon and other sites.

> https://www.amazon.com/s/ref=nb_sb_noss?url=search-alias%3Daps&field-keywords=unda+gemmotherapy&rh=i%3Aaps%2Ck%3Aunda+gemmotherapy

Lauen Hubele has written a book on Gemmotherapy and imports tinctures for sale.

http://vitalextract-com.3dcartstores.com/

Dr. Garber's Natural Solutions line of formulas contain plant stem cells, as well as glandulars and elements. They are condition specific.

https://drgarbers.com/

PHENOLIC THERAPY

If you are interested in learning about desensitization of allergens go to:

http://desbio.com/

They can direct you to a practitioner who specializes in this type of therapy and offer further information on the purchase of their products.

TRACE MINERAL THERAPY (OLIGOTHERAPY)

https://www.amazon.com/s/ref=nb_sb_noss?url=search-alias%3Dhpc&field-keywords=oligotherapy

DON'T FORGET THE BASICS

Sterile gauze, cotton bandages, steri-strips, round nose plyers (to remove splinters and foreign objects), sterile syringe (10ml) for pressure cleaning wounds, latex gloves, scissors and a flashlight.

Be sure to have on hand the simple age-old remedies:

- Baking Soda
- Hydrogen Peroxide
- Ethyl Alcohol
- Witch Hazel

Baking Soda is a very underutilized and necessary component to a complete home pharmacy. It is mentioned throughout this book for specific health issues and should be remembered for much more than absorbing odors in your refrigerator and baking. Keep a fresh box on hand to treat bug bites by making a poultice, addressing acid indigestion, cleaning your teeth, and a soothing bath to ease aches and pains, to name a few.

Hydrogen Peroxide can be used for everything from mouthwash, to cleaning bacteria from surfaces, to fungus on your toes, to whitening your laundry.

Ethyl Alcohol is an excellent disinfectant and helps to heal burns.

Witch Hazel is a wonderful astringent for your skin. It can assist with hemorrhoids, a sore throat, disinfecting a cut, sunburn and even varicose veins.

A homeopathic kit plus a few other items mentioned above covers most emergencies. A kit will last a long time. If you store your kit carefully out of the sun and heat they will survive the expiration date. The dates are an FDA requirement, but there are homeopathic tinctures over 100 years old still in use.

Remember to grab the most important first-aid remedies when you travel so you are prepared. You can purchase travel kits specifically for this purpose. Books are also an important addition to your home pharmacy. Whether they be printed books or eBooks, you will be much more prepared if you continue to add to your library. You may want to purchase a pediatric book of remedies, or one that specializes in female issues, or whatever is important to your concerns, or that of your family. Use this book as a stepping-stone into a life free of medical disasters by continuing to expand your knowledge.

Being prepared means stepping into your power and knowing how to tend to your needs and the needs of your family when called upon.

LEARN MORE ABOUT HOMEOPATHY

There are numerous books, blogs, seminars and on-line classes that offer the opportunity to gain greater knowledge about the use of homeopathy. The following are a few suggestions:

Dana Ullman offers a number of methods for further education. They include a library of free articles on his website to audio tapes you can purchase to learn at your own pace. They are listed here:

> https://homeopathic.com/category/how-to-learn-homeopathy/

The National center for Homeopathy has an extensive on-line free library as well as other opportunities here:

> http://www.homeopathycenter.org/homeopathic-education

Joette Calabrese has a website and blog that offers an extensive library of free articles and blog posts. She also has downloadable courses on particular topics of interest.

> https://joettecalabrese.com/

Washington Homeopathic has a number of free resources to further the education of homeopathy.

> https://homeopathyworks.com/categories/the-learning-center.html

Boiron, the largest manufacturer of homeopathic remedies in the US offers some on-line training here:

> https://www.boironusa.com/education-training/online-training/

NOTES

CHAPTER I
HOW DID WE GET HERE?

H. Coulter, 1981, Homeopathic Science and Modern Medicine: The physics of healing with microdoses; North Atlantic Books, Richmond, CA

H. Coulter, 1975, Divided Legacy, The Patterns Emerge Hippocrates to Paracelsus, Volume I, Center for Empirical Medicine, Washington, D.C.

H. Coulter, 1982, Divided Legacy, The Conflict Between Homeopathy and the American Medical Association, Volume III; North Atlantic Books, Berkeley, CA

I I. Coulter, 1994, Divided Legacy, Twentieth-Century Medicine: The Bacteriological Era, Volume IV; North Atlantic Books, Berkeley, CA

https://www.homeopathic.com/Articles/Introduction to Homeopathy/A Condensed History of Homeopathy.html

http://www.healthy.net/Health/Article/ The Unique Preparation of Homeopathic Medicines/664

Institute for Health Metrics and Evaluation http://www.healthmetricsandevaluation.org/gbd/visualizations/country

FLEXNER REPORT

http://www.hindawi.com/journals/ecam/2012/647896/

Flexner, 1908, 'The American College, New York: The Century Company, pp. 215-216

http://lcweb2.loc.gov/service/mss/eadxmlmss/eadpdfmss/2003/ms00 3042.pdf

CHAPTER II
EXPLORING NATURAL MEDICINE

ACUPUNCTURE & TRADITIONAL CHINESE MEDICINE

http://www.acos.org

http://www.nccaom.org/effectiveness-of-acupuncture-and-oriental- medicine-studies

Personal Interview with Ryan Cashman, MA, LAc, DNBAO, CSCS

CHIROPRACTIC

https://www.acatoday.org/level3 css.cfm?T1ID=13&T2ID=61&T3ID=149 Murray Goldstein, ed1975, 11-17, 25, 43 (Vol IV)

HOMEOPATHY

Homeopathic Science and Modern Medicine: The physics of healing with microdoses; North Atlantic Books, Richmond, CA

H. Coulter, 1994, Divided Legacy, Twentieth-Century Medicine: The Bacteriological Era, Volume IV; North Atlantic Books, Berkeley, CA

http://hpathy.com/ http://www.homeopathic.com/

NATUROPATHIC MEDICINE

http://www.bastyr.edu/academics/areas-study/study-naturopathic- medicine/about-naturopathic-medicine

Waters, E. The Herbal Medicines of the mid-19th Century Botanical Societies.

Pharm.Hist (London) 2000 June; 30(2): 34-36 http://ncanp.com/about-ncanp/history-of-naturopathic-medicine

Flannery, Michael A. John Uri Lloyd. The Great American Eclectic. Southern Illinois University Press. Carbondale. 1998. P.xiii

http://doctorschar.com/archives/eclectic-school-of-medicine/

John Milton Scudder, 1887, The Eclectic Physician. Twenty First Edition, Fifth Revision. Cincinnati. John K. Scudder. . P.28-32

Scudder, John Milton, 1874, Specific Medication and Specific Medicine. Fifth Edition. Wilstach, Baldwin and Co. Cincinnati.

Berman, Alex. The Eclectic Concentrations and American Pharmacy (1847- 1861); Pharmacy in History. Vol.XXII, No.3, 1980. P.91-103

Boyle, Wade, 1988, Herb Doctors: Pioneers in 19th Century American Botanical Medicine and A history of the Eclectic Medical Institute of Cincinnati; Buckeye Naturopathic Press.

OSTEOPATHIC MEDICINE

http://www.aacom.org/about/osteomed/pages/history.aspx

Still A.T. 1897; Autobiography, Pulbished by the Author. Kirksville, Mo., p 19, 20

https://www.westernu.edu/osteopathy/osteopathy-departments/omm-nmm- pages/osteopathy-omm history/

http://www.osteodoc.com/sutherland.htm (Sutherland) http://www.osteopathic.org/insideaoa/about/affiliates/Pages/default.aspx

Personal Interview with Arsen Nalbandyan, D.O.; July 2016

CHAPTER III
ADVANCES UNDER THE RADAR

CELL SALTS

Jan Scholten, in Homeopathy And Minerals,

Schuessler, W. H. 1984; Biochemic Handbook: Guide to Using Dr. Scheussler's Tissue Salts; UK

Carey, G.W. 2005; The Biochemic System of Medicine; B. Jain Publishers Ltd., New Delhi, Inia

LIittlefield, C; 1910, Man, Minerals and Masters, Kessinger Publishing, LLC

Littlefield, C W; 1919, Beginning and Way of Life, Metropolitan Press, Seattle, WA

GEMMOTHERAPY

http://www.phytembryotherapie.com/EN/Bourgeon.php

Tetau, M (1998), Gemmotherapy, A Clinical Guide; Canada, Editions du Detail Inc.

SEROYAL, UNDA, GEMMOTHERAPY, Practitioner Guide; Canada

Rozencwajg, J, (2016) Dynamic Gemmotherapy. Beyond Gemmotherapy, New Zealand; Natura Medica Ltd.

ORGANOTHERAPY

http://www.nature-reveals.com/media/mconnect uploadfiles/r/o/rozen cwajg-organ-otherapy drainage and detoxification-reading excerpt and content pages.pdf

http://www.dratiq.com/academy/organo.html

PHENOLIC THERAPY

www.des-bio.com

Gardner, R.W., 1994, Chemical Intolerance: Physiological Causes and Effects and Treatment Modalities, CRC Press, Boca Raton, Florida, 1994.

Remington, D.W., Harper, D. D. April 1989. "Allergy Treatment with Phenolic Compounds," A copyrighted patient bulletin issued by Dr. Remington, 1675 North Freedom Blvd. Provo, UT.

TRACE MINERAL THERAPY (OLIGOTHERAPY)

Marco Pharma International- Physicians Reference Manual

Dr. Jeffrey Marrongelle, DC, CCN, The Somaplex Connection: Interface of Biological & Energetic Therapies, lecture presented by Marco Pharma International, LLC; Jan 16, 2007

CHAPTER IV
HOW WE GET SICK AND HOW TO FIX IT

Dr. H.J. Carl; engineer, mathematician, biochemist, scientist and researcher

CHAPTER V
FIRST-AID A-Z CONVENTIONAL WISDOM & NATURAL RELIEF

CONVENTIONAL DESCRIPTIONS OF CONDITIONS

http://www.nlm.nih.gov/medlineplus/ency/article/001439.htm

HOMEOPATHY REFERENCES

Phatak, Dr. S. R. (1999) Materia Medica of Homeopathic Medicines, Second Edition; B. Jain Publishers (PVT.) Ltd., New Delhi

Phatak, Dr S. R.. (2005) A Concise Repertory of Homeopathic Medicines, Fourth Edition; B. Jain Publishers (P) Ltd., India

Murphy, R, (1995), Lotus Materia Medica, Pagosa Springs, CO: Lotus Star Academy

Murphy, R (2005), Homeopathic Clinical Repertory, Blacksburg, VI: Lotus Health Institute

Vermeulen, F. (2012) Synoptic Reference I; Belgium, Europe; Emryss

Shepard, D (1977), Homeopathy For The First Aider, Devon, England; Health Science Press

Horvilleur, A (1986), The Family Guide to Homeopathy, Health and Homeopathy Publishing Inc., Virginia

Vermuelen, F, (1994), Concordant Materia Medica, Netherlands: Merlijn

Nauman, E (2000); Homeopathy 911; Kensington Publishing Corp., New

York, NY

Ratera, Dr. M (2016); FIRST AID with HOMEOPATHY, Narayana Verlag, Kandern, Germany

Shroyens, Dr. Frederik (1997) Edition 7, Synthesis, Repertorium Homeopathicum Syntheticum; B. Jain Publishers, Ltd., New Delhi, India

ALLERGIES

NAET

https://en.wikipedia.org/wiki/Nambudripad%27s Allergy EliminationTechniques

Clove Oil

http://www.aobjournal.com/article/S0003-9969%2811%2900051-3/abstract

Insulin Shock

Cryer PE. Hypoglycemia. In: Melmed S, Polonsky KS, Larsen PR, Kronenberg HM, eds. Kronenberg: Williams Textbook of Endocrinology. 12th ed. Philadelphia, Pa: Saunders Elsevier; 2011: Chap 34.

CHAPTER VI
COMMON CONDITIONS A-Z; CONVENTIONAL WISDOM & NATURAL RELIEF

CONVENTIONAL DESCRIPTIONS OF CONDITIONS

http://www.nlm.nih.gov/medlineplus/

HOMEOPATHY REFERENCES

Phatak, Dr. S. R. (1999) Materia Medica of Homeopathic Medicines, Second Edition; B. Jain Publishers (PVT.) Ltd., New Delhi

Phatak, Dr S. R.. (2005) A Concise Repertory of Homeopathic Medicines, Fourth Edition; B. Jain Publishers (P) Ltd., India

Murphy, R, (1995), Lotus Materia Medica, Pagosa Springs, CO: Lotus Star Academy

Murphy, R (2005), Homeopathic Clinical Repertory, Blacksburg, VI: Lotus Health Institute

Vermuelen, F, (1994), Concordant Materia Medica, Netherlands: Merlijin

Shroyens, Dr. Frederik (1997) Edition 7, Synthesis, Repertorium Homeopathicum Syntheticum; B. Jain Publishers, Ltd., New Delhi, India

Horvilleur, A (1986); The Family Guide to Homeopathy, Health and Homeopathy Publishing Inc. Virginia

Pitt, Richard (2015) Comparative Materia Medica, Integrating Old & New Remedies; San Francisco, CA; Lalibela Publishing

Banerji, P, (2013) The Banerji Protocols; W Bengal, India, PBH Research Foundation

Degroote, F. (1992) Physical Examination and Observations in Homeopathy; Homeoden Bookservice; Gent, Belgium

Shepard, D (1995), More Magic of The Minimum Dose, Hillman Printers (Frome) Ltd., Great Britain

Geraghty, B, (1997), Homeopathy for Midwives; Churchhill Livingstone, London, England

Rozencwajg, J (2010), Organotherapy Drainage & Detoxification; Holland, Netherlands, Emryss Publishers

Vermeulen, F1996; Synoptic Materia Medica II; Merlijn Publishers; Haarlem, The Netherlands

Dr Carey Reams (pH)

http://www.phoenixinstituteonline.com/2012/06/the-reams-equation-of-perfect-health/

http://www.newtreatments.org/reams

Weston Price (Nutrition)

http://www.westonaprice.org/health-topics/weston-a-price-dds/

Weston A. Price, DDS, 1939; Nutrition and Physical Degeneration; Price- Pottenger Nutrition Foundation,

ACID-REFLUX

The complete article describing the theory of the use of Vitamin B3 in resolving digestive issues can be found at:

http://orthomolecular.org/library/jom/2001/articles/2001-v16n04-p225.shtml

CANKER SORES

Canker sores http://www.drweil.com/drw/u/ART02954/Canker-Sores.html Cholesterol

http://www.ncbi.nlm.nih.gov/pubmed/21296318%20

COLDS

http://articles.mercola.com/sites/articles/archive/2009/12/03/how-to- prevent-the-flu-easy-as-1-2-3.aspx

COLIC

http://www.radiantlifecatalog.com/product/life-start-infant-bifidum/ baby-child-care

http://hpathy.com/clinical-cases/crying-infant-colicky-baby/

Buteyko Method

http://www.buteyko.com/method/index method.html

DEMENTIA

http://philosophers-stone.co.uk/wordpress/2013/02/dementia-can-be-reversed-naturally/

http://www.acupuncturetoday.com/mpacms/at/article.php?id=28184

DMSO

http://www.dmso.org/articles/information/muir.htm

HYPERTENSION

Carditone-https://www.ayush.com/store/cardiovascular-and-metabolic-support/carditone-60-cardiovascular-support-60-caplets

Seanol- Fisheries Science, 72(6): 1292-1299

MENOPAUSE

Ikenze, I, (1998), Menopause & Homeopathy, Berkley, CA; North Atlantic Books P-54-68

PARASITES

Omar Amin, M.D., (2005); OPTIMAL DIGESTIVE HEALTH, A Complete Guide;, Edited by T. W. Nichols, MD & N. Faass, MSW, MPH, Healing Arts Press, Rochester, Vermont, P. 133

http://www.betterhealthguy.com/images/stories/PDF/parasites.pdf

http://www.parasitetesting.com/about.cfm

http://www.kpho.com/story/16666981/cdc

INDEX

A

abdomen, 159, 174–75, 192, 210, 252–53

abscesses, 74, 110–13, 235–36, 285

    chronic, 178

aches

    joint, 108

    muscular, 254

acid environment, 170, 191, 263, 267

acid foods, 118, 193

acid indigestion, 116–17, 297

acidosis, 158, 170, 190, 202, 208, 221, 262

    chronic metabolic, 183

    chronic systemic metabolic, 118

    reversing, 267

acid-reflux, 114, 116–18, 192, 202, 305

ACID-REFLUX & GERD, 202

acid test, 192

acne, 17, 30–32, 41, 121–25, 172, 231

    cystic, 122

    juvenile, 125

    pustular, 121–22, 172

acne rosacea, 125

acute bronchitis, 137–38, 152, 163

Acute illness, 15

adenoids, 282

ADHD, 231

adrenals, 34, 238

    rejuvenate, 248

air pollution, 45, 137

alkaline, 115, 117–18, 192, 262

alkaline state, 121, 125, 142, 197

ALKALIZE & HYDRATE, 264

allergic reactions, 35, 54–55, 127–29, 198, 212–13, 250

    severe, 104

ALLERGIC RHINITIS & HOMEOPATHY, 130

allergies, 35–36, 41–42, 126–27, 129–30, 132, 163–64, 170, 174, 180, 197–98, 204, 212, 259, 263, 274, 278

    dairy, 129

    seasonal, 129, 231

    wheat, 208

allergy desensitization, 22

Allergy Elimination Techniques, 303

allergy shots, 35, 126–27, 133, 197

Allergy Treatment, 302

altitude sickness, 56

aluminum cooking pans, 249

aluminum cookware, 204

AMENORRHEA, 245

Amin, Dr. Omar, 257–58, 260–61, 306

Anaphylactic Shock, 54

anemia, 18, 30–31, 41–42, 112, 191, 204, 209, 246

    iron deficiency, 265

Anemia-Ferrum Phos, 242

anger, 34, 91, 93, 168, 193, 245

    excessive, 156

animal bites, 57–58

    poisonous, 53

ankles, 106, 182, 184, 270, 280, 286

anti-aging, 219, 248

anti-anxiety, 168

antibacterial remedies, 234

anti-biotic substitute, 152, 285

anti-depressants, 135, 237, 265

antidotes, xix, 60

antifungal, 58, 61, 64, 71, 139, 177, 295

antihistamines, 96, 163, 170, 265

Anti-nausea medicines, 265

antioxidants, 45, 153, 178, 255

anxiety, 31, 34, 56, 74, 80, 83, 90–92, 102, 104, 109, 174–75, 199, 227–28, 231, 238–39, 241–42

aplastic anemia, 246

apple cider vinegar (ACV), 47, 100, 122, 127, 135, 138, 142, 145, 151, 170–71, 180, 183, 190, 192, 278, 287

Arsen Nalbandyan, 301

arteries, 61, 149, 205, 214, 218

arthritis, 41, 188, 206, 253, 263–64, 295

    rheumatoid, 231, 265

artificial sweeteners, 231

asthma, 24, 41–42, 53, 92, 129, 132–33, 152, 163, 198, 231, 270, 275

athlete's foot, 134, 143, 190, 267

Autoimmune diseases, 185

autoimmune reactions, 231

Ayurvedic Medicine, 9–10

B

babies, 26, 52, 72, 83, 90, 94, 139, 145, 156–60, 176–77, 180, 212, 234–35, 293

backache, 108, 246, 252, 254

Baker's cysts, 108

baking soda solution, 180, 183, 190

Banerji Protocols, 16, 110, 112, 116, 125, 147, 161, 171, 189, 201, 203, 208, 236, 240, 275, 280

bed wetting, 135, 245

Bee Pollen, 133

Bee Propolis, 296

belching, 32, 56, 91, 160, 191–93, 203, 221, 252

    constant, 116

Beverly Joubert, xviii

Birth Control Pills, 244, 286

bites, 53, 55, 57–59, 96, 108–9, 112

    bug, 18, 295, 297

    insect, 53, 104, 129, 257

    snake, 60

bladder control, 135

bladder drainage, 290

Blastocystis hominis, 257

bleeding disorders, 99

bleeding gums, 196

bleeding nose, 164

blisters, 31, 53, 63, 65, 87, 90

bloating, 35, 91, 116, 129, 174, 191, 204, 231, 233, 239, 244

blood clots, 286

blood deficiency, 162

blood poisoning, 283

blood pressure, 79, 104, 127, 214

blood stagnation, 125, 162, 189, 214, 223, 253, 287

blood sugar, 79–80, 94–95, 171, 216, 251

Blood thinners, 33, 99

blood vessels, 79, 99, 110, 125, 199, 214

bone density, low, 84

bones, 10, 29, 31, 64, 66, 76, 79, 84, 86, 103, 106, 112, 118, 205, 274, 280

    spinal, 135

bones ache, 283

Botulism, 82

bowel movements, 161, 174, 208

    incomplete, 193

bowels, 116, 136, 206, 290

brain, 19, 23, 29, 46, 69–70, 78–80, 85, 111, 204, 206, 223–25, 232, 239, 242, 249–50, 265

brain fog, 204, 259, 264

breast, infected, 234

breast abscess, 112, 236

breastfeeding, 158, 234–35

Breast infections, 234–35

breathlessness, 164

breath odor, 283

bronchitis, 41, 132, 137–38, 152

bruising, 52, 55, 64, 71, 74, 78, 84, 86, 101–2, 106, 188, 254

burns, 53, 58, 63, 65–66, 87, 104, 107, 134, 171, 180, 210, 255, 268, 295

Buteyko Method, 93, 305

C

Calabrese, Joette, 298

calcium, 30, 114, 117, 182, 205, 219

cancer, 184–85, 205, 228, 253

candida, 140, 142–43, 170, 174, 190–92, 216, 241, 289

canker sores, 145–46, 305

Canola, 141

Carbon Monoxide Poisoning, 68

CARPAL TUNNEL SYNDROME (CTS), 23–24, 147

Cashman, Ryan, 300

Castor oil packs, 47

cavities, 149, 210, 285

cayenne pepper, 48, 278, 287

Celiac, 119

Cell Salts, 30–31, 71, 123, 142, 175, 219, 301, 319

Cell Salt Therapy, 29

CELL SALT/TISSUE SALT CHART, 31

chelation, 205–6

chemical burns, 66

Chemical Intolerance, 36, 302

chest, sore, 152

chest aches, 164

chest constriction, 132

chest discomfort, 151

chest pain, 68, 91, 115, 202

    chronic severe, 128

Chest pain and changes in breathing, 96

chest tightness, 137
child, fussy, 74
children
    sensitive, 136
    whiny, 136
children teething, 145
child rubs ears, 133
Chinese Medicine, 3, 5, 9, 19–21, 124, 129, 138, 189, 232, 248, 251
Chiropractic Medicine, 8–9, 11, 23
chlorella, 206
cholesterol, 34, 149–50, 207
Cilantro, 46
circulation, 19, 33, 46–47, 76, 125, 152, 161, 188, 238, 271, 286–87
Classical Homeopathy, 12, 15, 290
claustrophobia, 91
Clostridium bacteria, 82
clove oil, 113, 134, 143, 163, 227, 267, 295, 303
cluster headaches, 199
cold/allergy, 130
cold compresses, 100, 240
Cold/Flu, 153
coldness, 77, 168, 272
colds, 30–31, 99, 151–54, 165, 186, 220, 275, 278, 295–96, 305
    chronic, 133
    frequent, 18, 117
colds and flu, 151, 220, 295
colic, 156–60, 305
colitis, 41–42, 115, 211
Colitis Insomnia, 128
Colloidal Silver, 51, 58, 61, 64–65, 71, 111, 236, 267, 295

colon, 45–46, 161, 174, 260, 266
colon cleanse, 46
COMMON CONDITIONS A-Z, 303
concentration, 41, 113, 220
concussion, 69, 85, 88
Condylomata, 133
congested ears, 31
congestion, 30–31, 274
    pulmonary, 152
    respiratory, 139
    venous, 217
congestive headache, 107
conjunctivitis, 78
constipation, 127, 135, 156, 160–62, 175, 200, 204, 208, 235, 239, 241, 245, 275
constipation/diarrhea, 115
Constipation- Lycopodium, 119
Constipation Menstrual Disorders, 128
convulsions, 59, 85, 185
COPD (chronic obstructive pulmonary disease), 92, 163
cortisol, 94, 150, 248
    elevated, 217
cough, 13, 17–18, 31, 132–33, 137, 139, 151–53, 163–65, 177, 186, 241, 272, 274, 279
    heavy, 186
coughing, 70, 79, 126, 137, 163–64, 200, 241
Coughing and post-nasal drip, 197
Coulter, 299–300
CPR, 54, 57, 59, 61, 66–69, 72, 76, 80, 88, 105
cracked ribs, 85
cracked skin, 171

cramping, 57, 116, 159, 175, 204, 239, 286
    pelvic, 244

cramps, 31, 174, 231, 247, 257, 259, 273
    abdominal, 54, 82, 127

Crohn's Disease, 174, 231, 257–58

croupy cough, 132

crying baby, 157

Cullen, William, 13

Cuts, 71, 104

CYP1B1 enzyme, 254–55

cystitis, 41, 53
    interstitial, 255

cysts, 110–11, 117

D

Dairy Intolerance, 119

DAIRY SENSITIVITY, 176, 194

Dana Ullman's site, 293

Dandelion, 46, 183

Dandruff, 31

Daniel David Palmer, 24

dark-field microscopy, 109

decongestants, 99, 274

dehydration, 72, 80, 82, 104, 107, 161, 174–75, 185, 226

DEMENTIA, 305

DENTAL ABSCESS, 112

Dental and jaw infections, 176

dental caries, 149, 285

dental issues, 74, 176, 285, 295

dental trauma, 74, 108

dentist, biological, 176, 196, 261

depression, 34, 41–42, 48, 91, 109, 130, 149, 167–69, 199–200, 204, 231, 245–47, 249, 254, 265

dermatitis, 170–72, 180–81, 259

DesBio, 37, 296

desensitization, 197, 250, 297, 319

desensitize, 36, 198, 213

detoxification, xx, 33, 45–48, 117, 141, 170, 264, 319
    lung, 47–48

detoxify, 34, 48, 206–7, 218

Devi Nambudripad, 129

diabetes, 79–80, 94–95, 149, 189, 206, 216–17, 265, 292

diaphragm, 115, 210

diarrhea, 82–83, 98, 104, 127, 132, 152–53, 156, 174–75, 193, 203–4, 208–9, 221, 231, 233, 239, 241
    severe, 174

Diarrhea/constipation, 259

digestion, 46–47, 56, 114–15, 118–19, 125, 127, 144, 158, 192, 202, 233, 238, 250, 259, 264, 289–90

DIGESTION REMEDY REFERENCE CHART, 119

digestive issues, 83, 119, 130, 132, 192–93, 204, 218, 223, 238–39

disappointed love, 168

discharges, 13, 266
    acrid, 197
    cottage-cheese type, 140
    foul smelling, 177
    green, 152, 178, 246
    stringy sticky, 275

disinfectant, 53, 58, 61, 64, 71, 109, 123, 295

dislocated joints, 76
distress, emotional, 80, 245
Diverticulitis, 120
dizziness, 56–57, 68–69, 72, 79–80, 83, 88, 91, 98, 102, 185, 204, 216, 238
DMSO, 255, 305
dopamine, 36, 48, 169, 250, 265
drainage, 33, 45, 132, 170, 184, 206, 319
    lung, 47
    lymph, 46–47
drainage remedies, herbal, 46
drowsiness, 59, 138
dry cough, 138, 152, 210, 259
dry mouth, 72, 91, 130, 193
dry skin brushing, 46–47
Dynamic Gemmotherapy, 301
Dyslexia, 128
DYSMENORRHEA, 246
dyspepsia, 83, 154, 193, 221

E

earache, 13, 132, 152–53, 177–78
ear infections, 133, 152, 176–78, 186, 253, 282, 295
eating disorders, 247
    emotional, 239
eczema, 30, 41–42, 122, 127, 172, 180–81, 231, 268, 295
edema, 182–84, 204, 242–43, 287
elbows, 52, 158, 270
    left, 70, 81, 105, 238
    tennis, 280
Electrical burns, 66
electrolytes, 73

energy, xxi, 8–9, 11–12, 14–16, 20, 27, 205, 216, 240, 250
Energy Medicine, 11
Entamoeba bhistolytica, 257
enteritis, 211
Enurisis, 135, 185
enzymes, 33, 41–42, 48, 116, 118, 194, 214
epinephrine, 48, 54, 127
EpiPen, 54
esophagus, 140, 191, 193, 202, 210, 278
estrogen, 123, 237, 242
exhaustion, 53, 98, 107, 174, 200, 252, 283
    adrenal, 42
eyes, 66, 78, 85, 126, 130, 133, 152, 184, 197–99, 224
    irritated, 125
    red, 240
    watery, 126, 130, 197
eyes burn, 132, 153

F

facial neuralgias, 168
fainting, 54, 56, 72–73, 79–80
Fallon, Sally, 159
fatigue, xvii, 30, 42, 108, 151, 175, 204, 226, 231, 244–46, 259
    chronic, 117, 133, 231
fear, 53, 56, 74–75, 91, 136, 145, 152, 156, 167–68, 185, 193, 224, 234–35, 239, 254
    anticipatory, 227
FEMALE REMEDY REFERENCE CHART, 242

fever, 13, 17–18, 30–31, 74–75, 82, 92, 137–38, 151–52, 174, 177, 185–86, 235, 247, 254, 274–75, 282–83

    high, 72, 185, 234–35, 282

Fibromyalgia, 231

First Aid A-Z, 51–52

flatulence, 32, 159, 192–93

Flexner Report, 5–7, 299

fluid congestion, 129, 198, 276

food allergies, 120, 127, 129, 145, 161, 192, 208, 232–33, 266

food intolerances, 174, 203, 232, 266

food poisoning, 53, 82–83, 95, 174–75, 216, 221, 257, 266

    unresolved, 221

foods

    acidic, 114, 117

    alkaline, 118

fractures, 53, 64, 66, 84–86, 188, 254

free radicals, 44–45, 65, 121, 183, 206

frontal headaches, 42, 132

frontal sinus headache, 130

frostbite, 53, 63, 87

fungal infections, 33, 121, 134, 142–43, 170, 174, 190–91, 207, 232, 241, 263, 267, 274

G

Gaba, 169

gall stones, 117

Gardner, Robert W., 36, 128

Gastritis, 117

gastroenteritis, 53, 211

gastrointestinal tract, 171, 180, 194

gel, colloidal silver, 63, 134

Gemmos, 148, 181, 206, 232, 248, 290, 296

    antifungal, 143

    anti-viral, 146

Gemmotherapy, 33, 168, 172, 180, 184, 206, 209, 218, 224, 232, 241, 248, 287, 290, 296–97, 301

GEMMOTHERAPY-Canker sores, 146

GEMMOTHERAPY-DRY ECZEMA, 181

Genetically modified organisms (GMOs), 116, 249, 289

GERD, 116, 163, 191–92, 194, 202, 210, 221

German Biological Medicine, 122, 319

Giardia lamblia, 221, 257–59

Gingivitis & Tooth Decay, 74, 196, 285

Gintis, Bonnie, 26

glands, 31, 46, 64, 121, 219, 282–83

gluten intolerance, 35, 203

Goldstein, Murray, 300

grief, 81, 93, 167–68, 175, 215, 224, 240, 245, 247, 254

growths, 112, 204, 228, 278

gums, 196, 285

gut, 121, 144, 158, 180, 190–91, 196, 207, 221, 231–33, 249, 260, 266

H

hacking cough, 132, 165, 198

    dry, 133, 185

Hahnemann, Dr. Samuel, 13

Hahnemann Labs, 294

hair analysis, 205

hair loss, 240

hay fever asthma, 132

hay fever symptoms, 198

HAZEL PARCELL'S FORMULA, 264

HBP, 214, 265

headache, 15, 56, 59, 68–70, 94, 96, 98, 107–8, 132, 151–52, 199–201, 204, 234–35, 239–40, 244–46, 274–75

    bursting, 235

    children's, 200

    migraine, 199

head injuries, 53, 69, 85, 88

head sweats, 177, 235

heart, 46, 79–80, 91, 104, 114, 210, 214, 250, 286

heart attack, 92, 104, 202, 210

heartburn, 17, 114–16, 191–94, 202–4, 210, 221, 239, 252

heat exhaustion, 88, 185

heat rash, 90, 239

heat stroke, 88

heaviness, 186, 203, 221, 246

heavy metals, 140, 204–7

hemorrhoids, 162, 208, 239, 286, 297

hiatal hernia, 114–15, 192, 202, 210–11

high blood pressure, 79, 99, 139, 149, 194, 214

histamine response, 271

hives, 41, 53–54, 117, 127, 129, 153, 212–13, 286

HMOA73, 7

hoarseness, 56, 164, 228, 274

Homeopathy, xvii, xix, 3–6, 8, 10–17, 21–22, 62–65, 70–71, 73–74, 83, 100–102, 105–7, 233, 293–94, 298–301, 303–4

home pharmacy, 16, 51, 53, 154, 178, 293, 297–98

hormonal balance, 169, 290

hormonal changes, 121, 145, 199, 258, 286

hormones, 33, 35, 94, 121, 123, 125, 192, 199, 216, 237, 242, 249, 251

    bio-identical, 237

hot flashes, 18, 237–38, 241, 248

H-Pylori, 192, 221

HRT (Hormone replacement therapy), 237, 286

hydration, 48

hydrogen peroxide, 51, 57–58, 61, 64, 71, 101, 151, 278, 297

hypertension, 214–15, 305

hyperventilation, 91–92

hypoglycemia, 94–95, 216–17, 303

hypothyroidism, 41, 191, 248

I

IBS (Irritable Bowel Syndrome), 174, 182, 231, 257–58

Ikenze, Dr. Ifeoma, 306

immune system, 22, 45, 110–11, 127–28, 139–40, 142–44, 151, 153–54, 177–78, 185, 218–20, 258, 261, 275, 285

Incontinence, 241

indigestion, 15, 32, 115–16, 120, 194, 201, 221, 224

    chronic, 192

infection, 58, 64–65, 74, 83–84, 91–92, 101, 108–12, 136–37, 142–43, 151–52, 176, 178, 190–92, 234, 257–58, 267

    bacterial, 41, 108, 114, 137, 266, 274

    candida, 170

    chronic sinus, 295

    chronic strep, 295

    frequent, 282

    intestinal, 144

nail, 190
   parasitic, 258–60
   reoccurring sinus, 274
   systemic Candida, 274
   upper respiratory, 41, 100, 154
inflammation, 33, 44, 47–48, 78, 110–11, 121, 125, 137, 207, 271, 280
   chronic, 231–32
influenza, 186, 254
insomnia, 41, 56, 168, 223–24, 226, 231, 239, 241–42, 259, 278
   chronic, 239
Insulin Shock, 94, 216, 303
internal abscesses, 113
iodine, 41, 238
irritability, 18, 31, 116–17, 159, 192, 216, 221, 226, 239–40, 244–45, 249
itch, jock, 172, 267
itching, 54, 63, 87, 90, 126–27, 130, 132, 140, 164, 170–71, 180, 245, 247, 265, 267–68, 270
itchy nipples, 235
itchy nose, 130
itchy skin condition, 269

J
jaw infections, 176
Jet Lag, 226
joints, 23, 76, 112, 270
Joubert, Beverly, xviii

K
Kegel exercise, 241
Keto-acidosis, 92
kidney cleanse, 46, 182, 184

kidney deficiencies, 165, 218, 250
kidneys, 45–48, 85, 94, 111, 143, 150, 182–83, 206, 214, 217, 241, 262, 272, 290
kidney stones, 117, 182
kinesiology, 21
knee, 52, 80, 159, 271

L
Lacerations, 71
laryngitis, 41, 132, 152, 164, 228–29
LDL cholesterol, 95, 217
L-dopa, 169, 250
Leakey, Richard, xviii
leaky gut syndrome, 231, 233
leg cramps, 30, 117, 239
lemon, 47, 120, 122, 125, 151, 153, 196, 228, 278, 287
ligaments, 53, 106, 148, 188
LIittlefield, Dr., 301
lips, pursed, 54, 92, 130, 235
liver, 34, 45–47, 111, 122, 143, 150, 170, 206–7, 216–17, 226, 248, 258, 288, 290
liver detoxification, 47, 122, 170
Lyme disease, 108, 258
Lyme disease and intestinal disease, 196
Lymph blockage, 259
lymph nodes, 182

M
malabsorption, 191, 259, 292
malnutrition, 292
Marco Pharma International, 302
mastitis, 234
memory loss, 13, 41, 206, 249–50, 259

Meniere's Disease, 98

menopause, 125, 132, 188, 237–38, 240–42, 244, 249, 286, 306

menopause symptoms, 169, 237

MENORRHAGIA, 246

Menstrual issues, 244, 265

meridians, 11, 19

metabolism, 41–42, 171, 238

Milton, John, 300

minerals, 11, 20, 29–30, 33, 41, 73, 88, 114, 118, 123, 145, 153, 178, 182, 206, 301

Morgellon's syndrome, 260

morning sickness, 251–52

motion sickness, 53, 98

mouth sores, 145

mucus, 112, 132, 137–38, 163–64, 175–76, 252, 259, 274, 279

N

NAET (Nambudripad's Allergy Elimination Technique), 129, 303

nail fungus, 142, 190

nasal discharge, 130, 132, 152–53, 197, 282

nasal obstructions, 274

Nattokinase, 214

nausea, 56–57, 59, 68–69, 82–83, 85, 98, 116, 152, 174–75, 192–93, 201, 203, 233, 235, 246–47, 251–52

    constant, 252

nausea and vomiting, 53, 59, 82, 98, 104, 251

neck, 79, 100, 108, 111, 121, 199, 205, 235, 238, 240, 279, 283, 295

    stiff, 108, 199

nervousness, 92, 117, 228, 241

nervous system, 23, 55, 82, 104, 169, 217, 224–25, 253

neurotransmitters, 36, 169, 249–50

Nixon, Richard M., 7

nose

    broken, 99

    clogged, 126, 197, 276

    crusty, 275

    dripping, 132

nosebleeds, 99–100, 152, 186

numbness, 31, 59, 69, 76, 84–85, 87, 91, 94, 147, 204, 271

nutrition, 28, 115, 124, 129, 133, 138, 140, 147, 200, 249, 304–5

O

obesity, 3, 286, 289

OHM Pharmacy, 294

oils

    castor, 47, 123, 196

    coconut, 141, 143, 150, 196

Oligotherapy, 41–42, 297, 302

Osteopathy, 5, 22, 26–27, 77, 188, 198, 200, 266, 272

osteoporosis, 42, 84, 237

otitis media, 24, 176, 253, 282

oxidative stress, 44, 65, 121, 183

P

pain, 23–24, 57–59, 63–66, 74, 85–87, 101–2, 140, 145–48, 159, 199, 234–35, 244–47, 253–55, 271–73, 278–80, 282–83

    abdominal, 59

acute, 208, 236, 240, 275

burning, 145, 180, 235, 252, 282

chronic, 204, 253, 263

cramping, 175, 235

darting, 132, 152

gnawing, 70, 252

joint, 23, 35, 117–18, 149, 188, 212–13, 231, 259, 295

rheumatoid, 112

severe, 92, 112, 177, 199, 208, 221

spasmodic, 31, 159, 245

pain and swelling, 59, 70, 76, 102, 148, 188, 280

Painful periods, 246

Palmer, David, 23

palpitations, 56, 91, 203, 233

panic attack, 91–92

parasites, xvii, 57, 82, 109, 111, 135, 139, 174, 185, 191–92, 204, 257–61, 289, 306

Parasitology Center, 261

Parcells, Hazel, 264

Parkinson's disease, 265

peanuts, 127, 141

pelvis, 26, 241, 245

period, 21, 83, 145, 219, 223, 237

periods

extended, 75, 123, 205, 208, 219, 241

heavy, 246–47

perspiration, 252, 268, 283

pesticides, 116, 207

Phenolic Charts, 169

phenolic therapy, 21, 28, 35–37, 123, 128–29, 169, 198, 213, 224, 250, 297, 302, 319

PHYSOSTIGMA-flashes of light, 78

PMS (PRE-MENSTRUAL SYNDROME), 231, 234, 244–45, 265

pneumonia, 92, 282

poison ivy/oak, 170, 172, 295

poisonous neurotoxin, 58

pollens, 126, 128, 133, 170, 197, 212

post-nasal drip, 35, 126, 197, 274

Post-partum depression, 243

potency choice, 16

pregnancy, 92, 121, 175, 182, 202, 208, 244, 251, 254, 265, 286

pregnenolone, 237

pre-hyper-tension, 149

preservatives, 119, 121, 289

Price, Weston A., 140, 304–5

psoriasis, 41–42, 122, 172, 206, 213, 231, 295

Ptomaine poisoning, 82

pulmonary embolism, 92

R

rashes, 18, 108, 125, 140, 170, 212, 269

diaper, 170, 172

Reams, Dr. Carey, 262, 304

Rectal itching, 259

remedy kits, 293–94

respiration, 132, 153

Respiratory failure, 54

restlessness, 85, 90, 93, 104, 130, 132, 152, 174, 185, 213, 224

intense, 113

retina, 78

Revici, Emanuel, 118

rheumatism, 42, 193, 282

ribs, broken, 102
Ringworm, 134, 142, 190, 267–68
root canals, 111, 176
rosacea, 125, 231
Rozencwajg, Dr. Joseph, 301, 304
runny nose, 35, 130, 132, 151, 197, 218, 276

S

sadness, 31, 167–68, 247
Salinsky, Phil, 114
saliva
    excess, 146
    increased, 112
Salmonella, 82
Salsolinol, 36
salt, 29, 48, 88, 117, 119, 137, 182–83, 196, 228, 239, 252, 278, 282, 287
    pink Himalayan, 48, 117, 182
Salvestrol, 254–55
sauerkraut, 118–19, 233
scabies, 269
scalp, 193, 199, 268
scalp ringworm, 267
scarring, 65, 123
Scheussler's Tissue Salts, 301
Scholten, Jan, 301
Schuessler, Wilhelm, 29
sciatica, 19, 23, 128, 271–73
scrapes, xvii, 52, 55, 71, 96, 104, 294
scratches, 71, 180
scratching, 134, 213, 268–70
Scudder, John K., 300
seasonal allergies mimic, 151

secretions, 115, 164, 213, 232, 275
seizures, 69, 79, 85, 95
SELENIUM, 42, 123, 207, 220
Selinsky, Phil, 210–11
sepsis, 55, 60, 92, 105, 109
Septic shock, 104
septum, deviated, 99
serotonin, 168–69, 250
sexual abuse, 168
shock, 16, 53, 55, 57, 59, 64–68, 76, 81, 86, 89, 93, 96, 101–2, 104–5, 135, 167–68
    cause anaphylactic, 104
shoulder blades, 188, 252
shoulders, 121, 159, 188, 199, 235
    frozen, 188–89
sinus congestion, 240
sinus drainage, 177, 274
sinuses, 274–75
sinus headaches, 199
sinus infection, 176, 275
sinusitis, 17, 41, 99, 139, 274–76, 282
    chronic, 274
skin, 45–48, 54–55, 63–66, 87, 90, 96, 105, 107–9, 111, 121–23, 126–27, 170–72, 180–81, 212, 260–61, 268–70
    baby's, 90
    cracking, 58, 101, 145, 235, 267, 270, 294
    damaged, 139, 294
    dry, 72, 88, 117, 198
    inflamed, 65, 171, 294
    spotted, 45
skin abscesses, 111
skin conditions, 30–31, 122, 257

skin rashes, 57, 180, 231, 259, 269, 294

sleep, xix, 53, 98, 136, 164, 199, 223–24, 238–40, 252, 265, 275, 283

smell, 130, 132, 153, 206, 240, 252, 275

smoking, 125, 163, 192, 210, 221, 228, 278

sneezing, 126, 130, 132, 152, 197–98, 272, 276

sore throat, 13, 31, 151–53, 177–78, 186, 197–98, 274, 278–79, 282, 295, 297

spasms

    bowel, 295

    intestinal, 159

spider veins, 286

spinal cord, 70, 84

spirochetes, 109, 196

Spleen, 223, 250, 288

splinters, 101, 279, 283, 297

sports injuries, 69, 84–85

sprains, 23–24, 53, 106, 188, 254–55

Staphylococcus, 82, 234

stings, 55, 60, 65, 87, 96, 104, 107, 172, 295

stomach acids, 154, 191, 193, 220, 228, 263

stools, 156, 161–62, 174–75, 208, 233, 257

straining vocal cords, 228

strains, 23–24, 27, 53, 106, 188, 240, 254

stress, 30, 91–92, 117, 121, 135, 145, 147, 167–68, 191, 199, 212, 214–15, 221, 245, 257, 266

stress management, 290

sugar, 48, 95, 117, 136, 140–42, 193, 208, 216, 233, 239

sunburn, 107, 129, 182, 297

sunstroke, 53, 88–89

suppress symptoms, xxi, 11, 14, 52, 110, 164, 170, 199, 202

sweating, 57, 88, 94, 96, 104, 178, 185, 204, 206

swelling, 54–55, 57–59, 70–71, 74, 76, 78, 84, 86–87, 102, 106–7, 109–10, 112, 182, 184, 234, 282–83

    relieve, 170

    severe, 280

Swelling of legs, 226

Swelling of tongue and throat, 59

swollen, 76, 90, 130, 132, 180, 198, 208, 213, 234–35, 274, 279, 282, 286

    breasts, 235

    uvula, 282

swollen glands, 235, 279

swollen gums, 296

swollen jaw, 285

swollen lips, 212

swollen liver, 288

swollen tongue, 72

T

tapeworm, 132, 257–58

Tapping, xix

teeth, 74, 108, 111–12, 140, 145, 174, 196, 285, 297

teething, 31, 74–75, 177, 219

tendons, 26, 53, 103, 106, 147–48, 188, 204, 280

testosterone, 123, 149, 237

tetanus shot, 109

tetanus vaccine, 112

thirstless, 13, 252, 282

Thompson, Bill, 191

throat, 54, 56, 59, 126–27, 130, 137, 152, 154, 163–64, 191, 193, 197–98, 228–29, 274, 278–79, 282–83

    dry, 229

    purple, 279, 283

Throat Disorders, 163

thrush, 140, 142

thyroid issue, 41–42, 206, 237–38, 248

thyroid levels, 238, 250

tick bite, 108–9

tickling cough, dry, 130, 152

tinnitus, 98, 242

tissues, damaged, 110, 123, 260

tissue salts, cell salts, 29–30

toes, 86–87, 267, 271, 297

tonsillitis, 278, 282–83

tooth extraction, 112

tourniquet, 59, 61

Toxic shock, 247

toxins, 29, 41, 48, 66, 82, 122, 126, 153, 161, 178, 205–6, 231, 260–62

Toxoplasma gondii, 257

Trace Mineral Therapy, 41–42, 215, 220, 240, 297, 302, 319

trauma, emotional, 135, 227, 258

Trichinella spiralis, 257

Trichuris trichiura, 257

tummy, distended, 159

tumors, 14, 84, 112, 216

U

ulcers, 145, 180, 191, 215, 221, 232, 270, 283

Ullman, Dana, 293, 298

urinary tract, 72, 79, 104, 135–36, 205–6, 241, 247

urticaria, 130, 212, 286

uterus, 235, 244, 254, 288

V

vaginal, atrophy, 242

Vaginal dryness, 237, 243

Vaginitis, 140

Valerian, 169

Valley fever, 258

Varicose veins and spider veins, 286

veins, 27, 61, 286–88

    inflamed, 208

Vermeulen, Frans, 303–4

viruses, 82, 99, 111, 137, 139, 158, 174, 185, 258

vision, 78–79, 199

    blurry, 80, 94

    tunnel, 240

vocal cords, 228

vomiting, 53, 56–57, 59, 68, 70, 82–83, 98, 104–5, 108, 152, 156, 175, 186, 192, 247, 251–52

    intense, 104

W

Wagstaff, Dr. Craig, 21–22, 37

Washington Homeopathic, 294, 298

water, distilled, 117, 120, 122, 141, 206–7

weakness, 31, 59, 68–69, 73, 82, 85, 91, 94, 96, 105, 147, 151, 241, 245, 247, 254

    muscular, 186

Weepy/Depressed, 242

weight loss, 289–90, 292

weight problems, 184

Weil, Andrew, 231

wheezing, 54, 132, 137

white discharge, 31, 235, 247

whooping cough, 132–33, 152

Witch Hazel, 121, 287, 297

World Health Organization (WHO), 6, 80, 109

worms, 56, 134–35, 258, 261, 267

worthlessness, 167

wound healer, great, 112

wounds, 30–31, 53, 55, 57, 61, 71, 76, 101, 111–13, 184, 254, 297

X

Xlear, 295

Y

Yeast, 140–41, 190

ABOUT THE AUTHOR

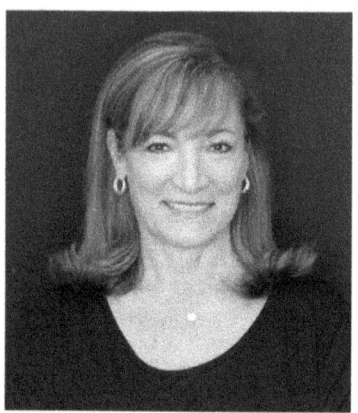

ELENA UPTON, Ph.D. is a classically trained Homeopath, avid researcher, writer and product development specialist with nearly thirty-years' experience in the natural health field. Having followed a graduate program in Homeopathy at a time when natural medicine was in its resurgence in America, she studied with some of the finest Homeopaths of our time.

During and after developing a successful clinic, The Holistic Resource Center in Southern California, Upton continued her education with numerous medical experts from around the world. As a result, her practice extends to include many modern uses of Homeopathy, as well as other holistic modalities.

Upton is the mother of two sons and five grandchildren.

CONTINUING YOUR JOURNEY TO VIBRANT HEALTH...

For a more in-depth understanding of the information contained in this book reference, **THE ALTERNATIVE, CONTINUED; Secrets to Success;** your companion guide to **THE ALTERNATIVE, Your Family's Guide to Wellness**.

Contained in this compelling volume is a more in-depth explanation of the five holistic modalities discussed in Chapter II, as well as an expanded list of energetic modalities not mentioned in Volume I.

Eight chapters outline:

- Top Homeopathic remedies and their uses
- Top Chinese Herbs and their uses
- Flower Essences (little-known combinations)
- Cell Salts and their uses
- Gemmotherapy tinctures and their uses
- Trace Mineral Therapy and their uses
- Phenolic Therapy for desensitization

and... the use of *German Biological Medicine* for detoxification and drainage.

Also included are numerous *Cases* so you can gain a better understanding of how to choose remedies and protocols, as well as how to put them together. As an added bonus, there are multiple practitioner interviews further explaining many of the therapies.

The last chapter is an expanded version of resources for finding the tools you need to render you "ready to go" when health needs arise.

The combination of these two volumes is a life-long resource of information important to a library you will reference time and again for many years to come.

www.ingramcontent.com/pod-product-compliance
Lightning Source LLC
Chambersburg PA
CBHW080355030426
42334CB00024B/2879